Foot and Ankle Trauma Injuries

Walter Daghino • Alessandro Massè
Daniele Marcolli

Foot and Ankle Trauma Injuries

Atlas of Surgical Procedures

Springer

Walter Daghino
CTO Hospital
University of Turin CTO Hospital
Turin
Italy

Alessandro Massè
CTO Hospital
University of Turin CTO Hospital
Turin
Italy

Daniele Marcolli
Orthopedic division
Azienda Ospedaliera Ospedale Civile di L
Milano
Italy

ISBN 978-3-030-09901-5 ISBN 978-3-319-69617-1 (eBook)
https://doi.org/10.1007/978-3-319-69617-1

Softcover re-print of the Hardcover 1st edition 2018

Printed on acid-free paper

This Springer imprint is published by the registered company Springer International Publishing AG part of Springer Nature
The registered company address is: Gewerbestrasse 11, 6330 Cham, Switzerland

Foreword 1

Orthopaedics, like all surgical specialties, has definitely evolved versus sub-specialization.

Foot and ankle surgery is one of these established sub-specialties. The impressive increase in knowledge and techniques justifies this evolution. Comprehensive textbooks offer the generic knowledge for every surgeon, while monographs offer the superspecialists the details they need. Thanks to information technology (IT), the access to scientific data is no longer a problem. On the contrary, we are confronted to an information overload. We need a sound selection of information based on clinical experience. A given clinical problem has usually many different possible solutions. To illustrate all of them with all details needed for practical implementation is impossible in a conventional publication and would only produce uncertainty. A group of surgeons, in one or more institutions, can and has to choose and define a "house doctrine" taking into account the local circumstances. This is the basis of what can become an ideal monograph, like the present one about foot and ankle trauma. The vast amount of available data is "filtered" and based on clinical experience of the group. This does not mean to present only "the single and only solution" to a given problem but a limited number of alternatives for which the group of authors have solid experience. To know that there are different solutions to a given problem and that science evolves continuously, i.e. that there is no definitive certitude, is a fundamental attitude to be transmitted to younger surgeons. This open-mindedness is crucial to allow progress and avoid "blindly following fashion".

This monograph covers the relevant topics of foot and ankle trauma. The described solutions, validated by experience, are well illustrated. Therefore, the authors satisfy the wish of today's users for application in daily practice. The decisional algorithms proposed are very useful in this respect. All chapters include detailed and useful paragraphs about classification, indication, timing and access.

The iconography consists of a sound balance between instructive drawings and clinical photos. It is meritorious to have also included nonskeletal trauma like Achilles tendon ruptures.

Lugano, Switzerland, AO Foundation Honorary Trustee — Pietro Regazzoni

Foreword 2

My friendship with Walter started about 20 years ago, at the time he was a young neo-specialist, and I had a few more years, both busy with the daily activity of a Hospital Orthopedic Division. Already at that time, I was struck by his manner to face the clinical problems: precision, rigour and extremely schematic, clear and defined paths, in a word: "method". During the time, we had the opportunity to share the interest in the pathologies of the foot and the ankle; after his reassignment to the CTO Hospital of Turin, Walter continued to deepen the topic and in particular the aspects related to traumatic lesions.

Over the years, Walter gained considerable practical experience on the subject, becoming a real point of reference; this amount of work has allowed the creation of a well-designed theoretical and practical annual course that allows participants to have a complete overview on the problems related to the traumatology of foot and ankle. I was therefore very pleased to discover this book, *Foot and Ankle Trauma Injuries: Atlas of Surgical Procedures*, that is the graphic translation of the course.

It is a truly interesting and original volume, in which all the traumatic injuries from the ankle to the forefoot are described, with a very appealing graphic presentation. For each topic, the general aspects are discussed (traumatic mechanisms, classifications, pathological anatomy, etc.), but the presentation is mainly focused on the surgical treatment that has the greatest space. The reader is accompanied step by step in the planning and execution of the surgical procedure, from the patient's positioning, to the surgical access, to osteosynthesis; each passage is presented in a meticulous way, with many tips and tricks useful for optimizing the result. A very strong asset of this book is related to the illustrations, carried out in collaboration with the anatomical drawing course of the "Accademia Albertina di Belle Arti" of Turin; the drawings result at once schematic and full of details that make the already clear exposition even more explicit. The operating theatre images are particularly beautiful: in these, the artists have masterfully rendered the three-dimensionality and depth of the illustrations describing the surgical fields. Reading the texts and looking at the illustrations, the exposure is so clear and detailed that one gets the feeling that even the most complex surgeries (and very often they are "really" complex procedures) are indeed easy and within everyone's reach.

Therefore, most sincere congratulations to my friend Walter for the well-done work, which goes to fill a gap in medical publishing on the subject; we all know how much effort and time taken away from rest and family is required to accomplish a work of this kind.

Good reading and good consultation!

Alba (CN), President of Italian Society of Foot and Ankle (SICP) — Luigi Milano

Preface

Professor Giacomo Pisani, one of the founding fathers of foot surgery in Italy and around the world, usually presented his courses, always appreciated and attended by many surgeons, with a simple and effective formula; it has proposed them as "… his home kitchen …"; this formula left the participants free to express a more or less complete acceptance to the presented techniques, introducing the concept of taste, clearly personal and subjective.

But all participants knew well that given the great fame that the "Prof." had gained over the years following his scientific value and the consolidated results of his surgical activity, those he presented as advices were indeed precious information that would necessarily become paramount guides in their daily clinical activity.

When I first time took into consideration this work, immediately and automatically I remembered those words, and I realized that it was possible only by proposing the result with the same humility, considering this book like our home recipes.

This is the goal of this volume: systematize and organize over 15 years of activity in a superspecialist field such as foot and ankle traumatology in a particularly favourable environment such as the Orthopedic Traumatology Center of Turin, so to easily transmit the results. In this centre, the continuous peer review and consideration of scientific literature, the coexistence with high professionalisms also in disciplines related to orthopaedics and the availability of the best technology and the most modern instrumental equipment for surgeons have possibly made very specific experiences to mature, extensively tested on the field over time, which have been collected in these pages.

We don't think that these "recipes" are the only way to behave, but we hope that they can be a useful assistance to the surgeon who must treat difficult cases in the challenging field of orthopaedic surgery.

In the "2.0 era", it is not possible to approach the traditional book without a clear target to pursue: our aim was to give support to surgeons who approach these injuries through pictures that can help them in order to understand and simplify the problems. The previous statement clarifies the choice of creating not a text but an atlas, with many didactic pictures that, through the effort made with the artists, will deliver to the surgeon a clear message. For this reason, all surgical illustrations use colours to underline what the surgeon should see and transparencies to indicate the anatomical structures that the surgeon should not see, but he must know that they run near the surgical field, for the best execution of the procedure.

Before I conclude this introduction, it is appropriate to make some acknowledgements. First of all, I would like to thank Prof. Alessandro Massè, co-author of this work. I am grateful to him not only because he recognized and shared my efforts but mainly because he also taught me the importance of essentiality and sharpness in the surgical gesture, of the rigour in the scientific method and of the clarity during transmission of information and knowledge. I would like to thank Dr. Daniele Marcolli, a young coworker in the English version of this book, who accurately solved all translation problems from the Italian version.

I then would like to thank Prof. Paolo Belgioioso, a fundamental referent for the images of this volume, who has coordinated the work of illustration in a perfect manner, with full integration between different skills. I also thank the collaborators of Professor Belgioioso: Fabrizio Lavezzi,

Kim SooGyeong and Debora Quaglino, and I congratulate them for the ability to adapt the graphic sign to the difficult requests of illustration.

Again, I would like to thank Prof. Pietro Regazzoni, one of the most important trauma surgeons in the world, who honoured me by writing a foreword of this book. I yet thank another friend, Dr. Luigi Milano, now president of Italian Society of Foot and Ankle (SICP), who has realized the Preface, from which I learned the passion for foot surgery and which represented a point of reference over time for my technical growth, with his always valuable advices and lessons. I also thank all the great Italian surgeons who converge in this prestigious Specialistic Society: they always have been my models and now they honour me with their friendship; I thank them also for their continuous stimulus to the comparison and discussion that they transmit not only at official scientific meetings of the society, which represent the state of the art of this surgery in Italy, but on every occasion of meeting, also if informal.

Finally, I thank all the collaborators of this book and all the colleagues with whom I have worked with over the years: they have participated and contributed to the daily management of this specific and specialized surgical activity, and it is right and due to share with them the results achieved.

The last thought necessarily goes to my dear ones who always gave me strength to get through every trouble: I apologize for the time I took from them for the realization of this work.

Turin, Italy Walter Daghino

Acknowledgement

We acknowledge those who have assisted us in the preparation of this work.

Contents

1 Tibial Pilon Fractures

Contents

1.1 Tibial Pilon Fractures

A tibial pilon fracture is a bony lesion that involves the distal meta-epiphyseal tibia associated with an important cartilage involvement [1].

These injuries represent about 1% of the lower limb fractures [2, 3] and are typically associated with an important soft tissue involvement. The entity and the management of the latter are the main prognostic factors [4].

1.1.1 Classification

According to the AO classification [5], these fractures correspond to the 43A category if they are extra-articular, 43B if there is a partial articular involvement and 43C if there is an involvement of both medial and lateral column, with complete disruption of the joint portion from the tibial diaphysis (Fig. 1.1). The latter are the more properly defined tibial plafond fractures, and it is useful to further divide them in subgroups regarding their comminution: C1 if there are only big fragments and there is no comminution, C2 if there is only comminution of the extra-articular metaphyseal part and C3 if there is comminution of both articular and extra-articular components.

Such subdivision is not only descriptive, but it is related to the traumatic mechanism that generates the fracture, usually a low kinetic energy event with mainly torsional stress in the less comminuted fractures and high energy event with mainly compressive stress in the more comminuted cases [2, 6, 7].

Since during the fracture evaluation it is possible to encounter borderline cases regarding the fragmentation and the correct definition of the comminution, practically the fracture is assigned to the C2 and C3 categories, with high complexity features, only if there are one or more fragments halfway the main ones, and it is not possible to obtain a complete contact between the latter even after the fracture reduction [2, 5–8].

W. Daghino et al., *Foot and Ankle Trauma Injuries*, https://doi.org/10.1007/978-3-319-69617-1_1

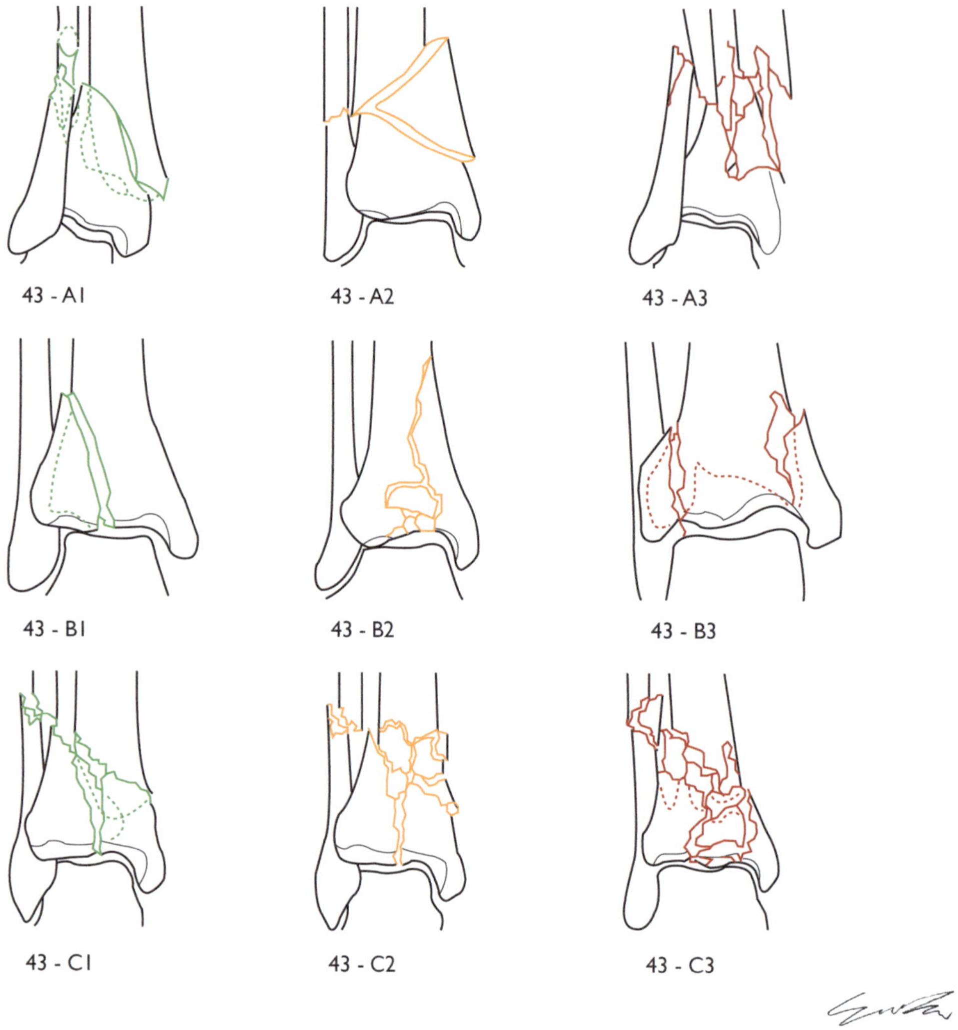

Fig. 1.1 AO classification of the distal tibia epiphysis fractures; subgroup A indicates the extra-articular fractures, B subgroup the partially articular fractures and subgroup C the fractures of the tibial pilon, in which the joint involvement is complete with an entire separation between the diaphysis and the joint part

1.1.2 Treatment and Indications

Being articular fractures, the ideal treatment should be the anatomical reduction and stable internal fixation, to reduce the arthritic joint degeneration through a precise reconstruction of the joint surface and to allow early joint mobilization, aiming to preserve the range of motion, thanks to the protective function of the mobilization on the cartilage [9–12]; the constant soft tissue involvement greatly complicates the previous treatment and needs to be carefully managed to avoid complications that can be very severe [2, 13–15].

If there is bony exposition and soft tissue loss of substance, it is convenient to proceed if possible before 24 h from the injury with an external fixator positioning and through the debridement of the soft tissues [16–18].

It is advisable during this procedure to irrigate the wound with saline solution to facilitate the removal of foreign bodies and to reduce the bacterial concentration [17]; this procedure should be performed avoiding high-pressure irrigation, for which there is no evidence of efficacy, while recent publications show a higher rate of complications [19–21].

The closure of the wound during the acute phase is associated with a high risk of complications, and it is advisable to consider the use of interrupted stitches or to delay the wound closure, through second intention healing, that becomes imperative in the more severe wounds, in which the use of a skin graft can be necessary.

The use of vacuum-assisted closure (VAC®) has a key role to obtain the best results when plastic surgery is needed and more broadly to obtain the best healing for the soft tissues [22].

The antibiotic therapy with first-generation cephalosporin, begun within 3 h from trauma, is proven to reduce significantly the infection rate of open wounds [18].

Even closed injuries require a treatment specifically orientated in the management of the extra-osseous anatomy: around the ankle there is a poor representation of soft tissues, and there are no muscles that protect the deep planes; for this reason there is a dangerous and precarious biology that highly exposes to complications an open reduction and internal fixation procedure [4].

To avoid such risk, the more effective strategy appears to be a staged treatment [3, 4, 10, 13, 23–28], through an external fixation of the fracture performed immediately and then in a second time proceeding to a definitive open osteosynthesis when the soft tissues are in good conditions [29].

Because the time window in which the soft tissue stabilization is achieved and the open reduction and synthesis are possible is brief, it seems to be advisable to establish a trauma management protocol that considers all the variables and helps the surgeon to choose the more appropriate moment to take the decisions regarding the indications.

An example of this protocol, concerning complete articular fractures (AO 43C), is depicted in Fig. 1.2: we advise in these injuries to obtain in emergency a temporary fixation through an external fixator, even if the soft tissues seem to be unharmed, to avoid complications of the latter [30].

After a waiting and clinical supervision period, reported in literature as a minimum of 4 days and maximum of more or less 14 days from trauma [13, 24, 26, 29, 31, 32], the choice of definitive treatment must be subordinated to soft tissue condition and pattern of the bone injury: if the skin appears to be healed or not affected by any complications and if the surgeon on the base of the preoperative planning believes that a stable osteosynthesis is achievable, the indicated surgery will be an open reduction and internal fixation; if, otherwise, the soft tissues are suffering even after 2 weeks of external fixation treatment with the fracture in distraction, or if the fracture comminution will lead to an unstable fixation that will not permit an early mobilization of the limb, it will be preferable to achieve a definitive fixation with an external fixator, less dangerous for the soft tissues, eventually associated with a minimal osteosynthesis of the main fracture fragments [22, 23, 33].

The same considerations are valid for the partial articular and the extra-articular fractures (43B and 43A), normally more simple to synthetize but equally exposed to soft tissue problems.

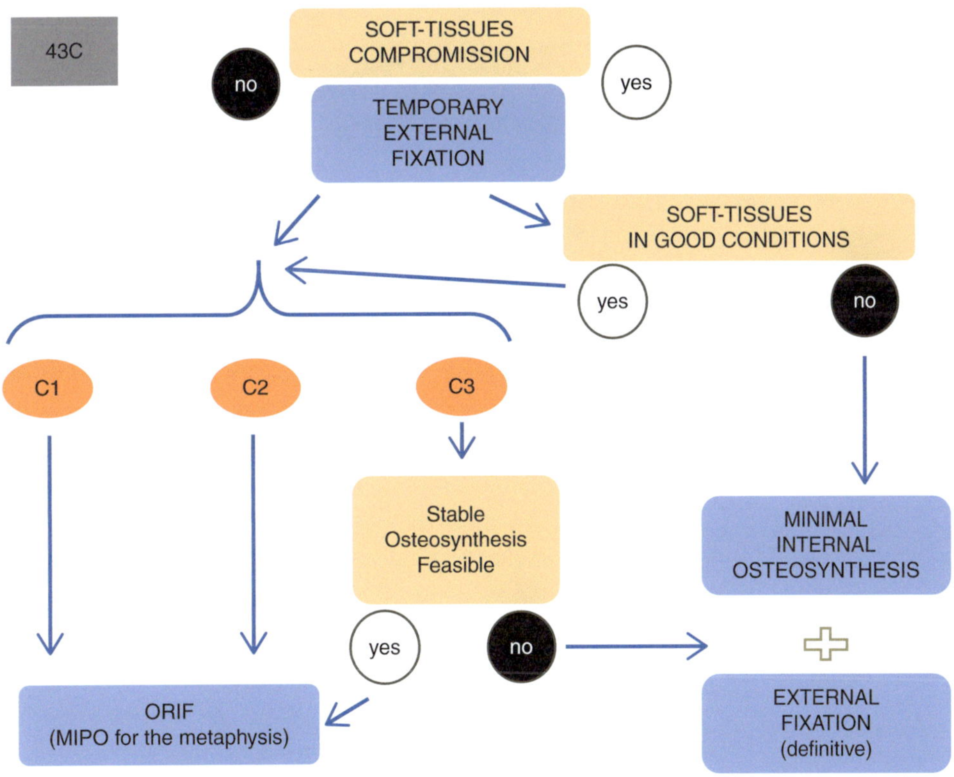

Fig. 1.2 Example of decisional procedure that takes care of the complete joint fractures of the tibial pilon (43C considering the AO classification)

1.1.3 Temporary Stabilization

1.1.3.1 Goals

The objective is to neutralize the stress on the soft tissues derived from the loss of continuity induced by the fracture and the consequent hematoma induced by the bone bleeding.

This is achieved through the bridge distraction obtained with an external fixator, roughly realigning the bony segments by the traction of the capsular and ligamentous components.

The aim is to gain a sufficient stability that reduces fracture bleeding and allows the non-bearing position manageable by the patient, creating the best conditions for the unswelling of the soft tissues, necessary to facilitate the next surgical steps.

The external fixator positioning necessary to achieve these objectives must not jeopardize the future surgical options.

If trans-skeletal tractions are avoided, the patient's nursing is easier, with a more simple mobilization for the hygiene, and if the skin conditions are not seriously compromised, it is possible to discharge temporarily the patient before the final surgery.

Furthermore the possibility to perform a CT scan with the bony fragments distracted and realigned is essential, because it permits a better interpretation of the fracture characteristics and "personality", allowing a more simple and reliable final surgical planning.

1.1.3.2 Surgical Technique

All the configurations of the external fixator must have the screws positioned without interfering with any vascular, nervous, tendon and muscular structures and distant from the planned skin incision to avoid contamination of the surgical access [2].

Considering such external fixation as a "portable traction", namely, a pure temporary stabilizer, to leave in site only for a few days before the definitive osteosynthesis, it is possible to reduce at minimum the fixation elements and exoskeleton and consequently minimize the surgical aggression, allowing the use in a normal emergency room, with a simple sedation and without the use of X-rays [34].

The patient is positioned supine with the injured limb elevated from the healthy side with a cushion (Fig. 1.3); this will allow an easy access to the operator that will stay on the opposite side of the fracture. The limb is left free to move in the sterile surgical field, including the knee to enable assessment of limb rotation.

The necessary instrumentation includes, besides a motorized drill, specific drill bits and screwdrivers, this basic dotation: three Shanz screw self-drilling and self-tapping with a 5–6 mm diameter stem, one of them with a thread part diameter reduced to 4 mm, three carbon fiber rods used for the

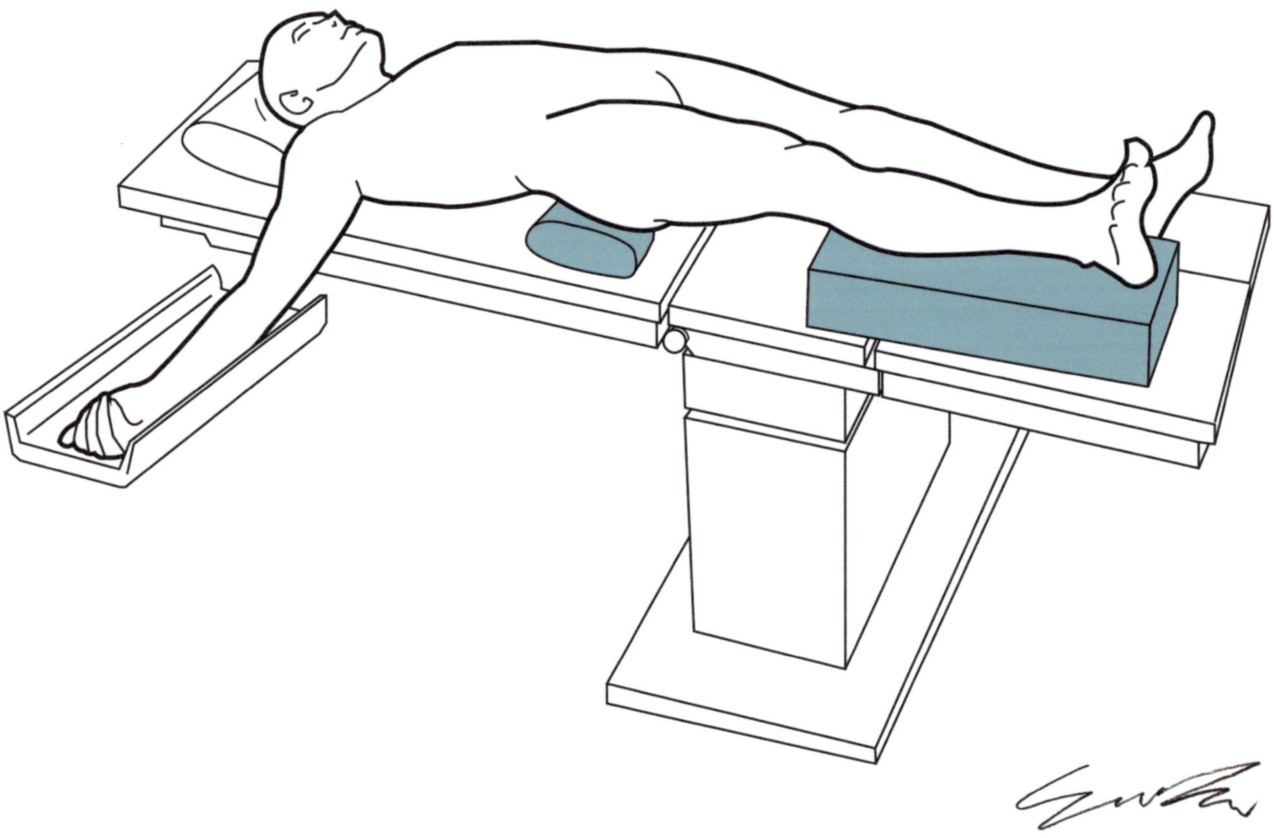

Fig. 1.3 Ankle spanning external fixator for emergency treatment of tibial pilon fracture: patient positioning

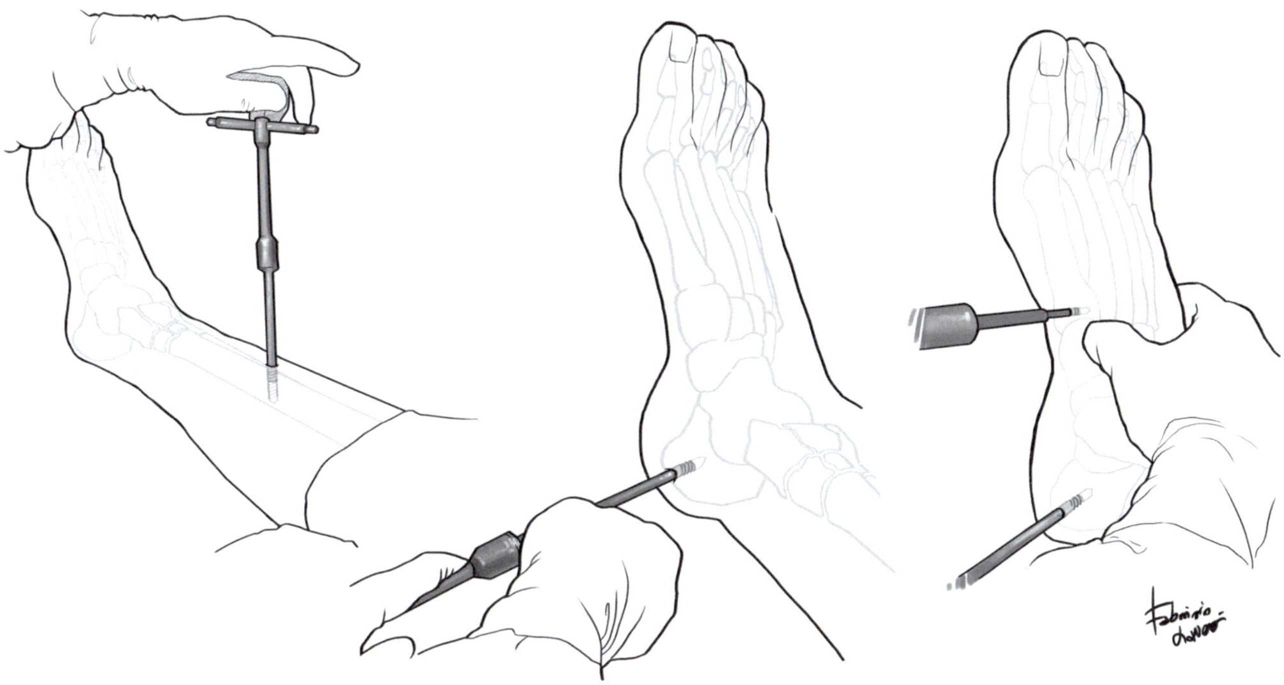

Fig. 1.4 Ankle spanning external fixator for emergency treatment of tibial pilon fracture: self-drilling and self-tapping screw positioning in the tibia with the use of a motorized screwdriver for the first part and then manually tightened without the need of intraoperative fluoroscopy; with the same technique, the calcaneal and first metatarsal screws are positioned

composition of the frame, fast connecting rod-to-pins clamps and rod-to-rod clamps in number of three for each type.

With the patient in anaesthesia, the pins are positioned; initially using the motorized drill to pass the first cortex, when the self-drilling and self-tapping screws are sufficiently tightened in the bone, they are finally fixed manually; in this way it is possible to feel the moment in which the screw passes through the second cortex, a moment in which it is possible to feel a peak in the tightening force; from now on the pin needs to be turned for 4–5 half turns of the screw, gaining in this way the right deepness of the pin. With this technique and a sensibility that is gained after a few cases, the surgeon is able to correctly insert the screws without the use of any X-rays to check the correct positioning.

The tibial screw is inserted as shown previously in the anterior crest, with a vertical anterior-posterior way, to avoid to cross the area of an eventual sliding plate positioned on the medial or lateral tibial surface during the definitive fracture stabilization and most distantly possible from the ankle. The second screw is inserted in the posterior tuberosity of the calcaneus, with a medio-lateral direction, in a horizontal plane, perpendicular to the tibial screw, and the third screw, which has a reduced thread pitch of 4 mm, is inserted with the same direction in the base of the first metatarsal bone (Fig. 1.4).

If the surgery is performed with a sedation anaesthesia, it is possible to start to awaken the patient, because the more aggressive part of the treatment is finished and the only part that remains is to build the frame of the external fixator.

To do so, three rod-to-screw clamps are positioned, one for each screw, and the two screws positioned on the foot are connected through a short rod that represents the base of the frame triangle (Fig. 1.5a); after, with three rod-to-rod clamps, the base of the triangle is united to the apex of the triangle, represented by the tibial screw, locking the clamp of the base and leaving free to slide the clamps at the apex of the figure (Fig. 1.5b).

Keeping as a fixed point the tibial pin, the fractured bone segment is realigned through distraction acting on the base of the fixator; once enough traction and a correct fracture realignment are achieved, the stabilization is completed locking all the clamps and finishing the surgical treatment (Fig. 1.6a, b).

1.1.4 Definitive Treatment

1.1.4.1 External Fixation

Goals

The aim of an external fixation is to restore the metaphyseal alignment and simultaneously the best reduction of the epiphysis, achievable through the distraction applied to the fractured segments acting on the soft tissues connected that are put under tension from the traction induced by the fixator (ligamentotaxis) [35, 36].

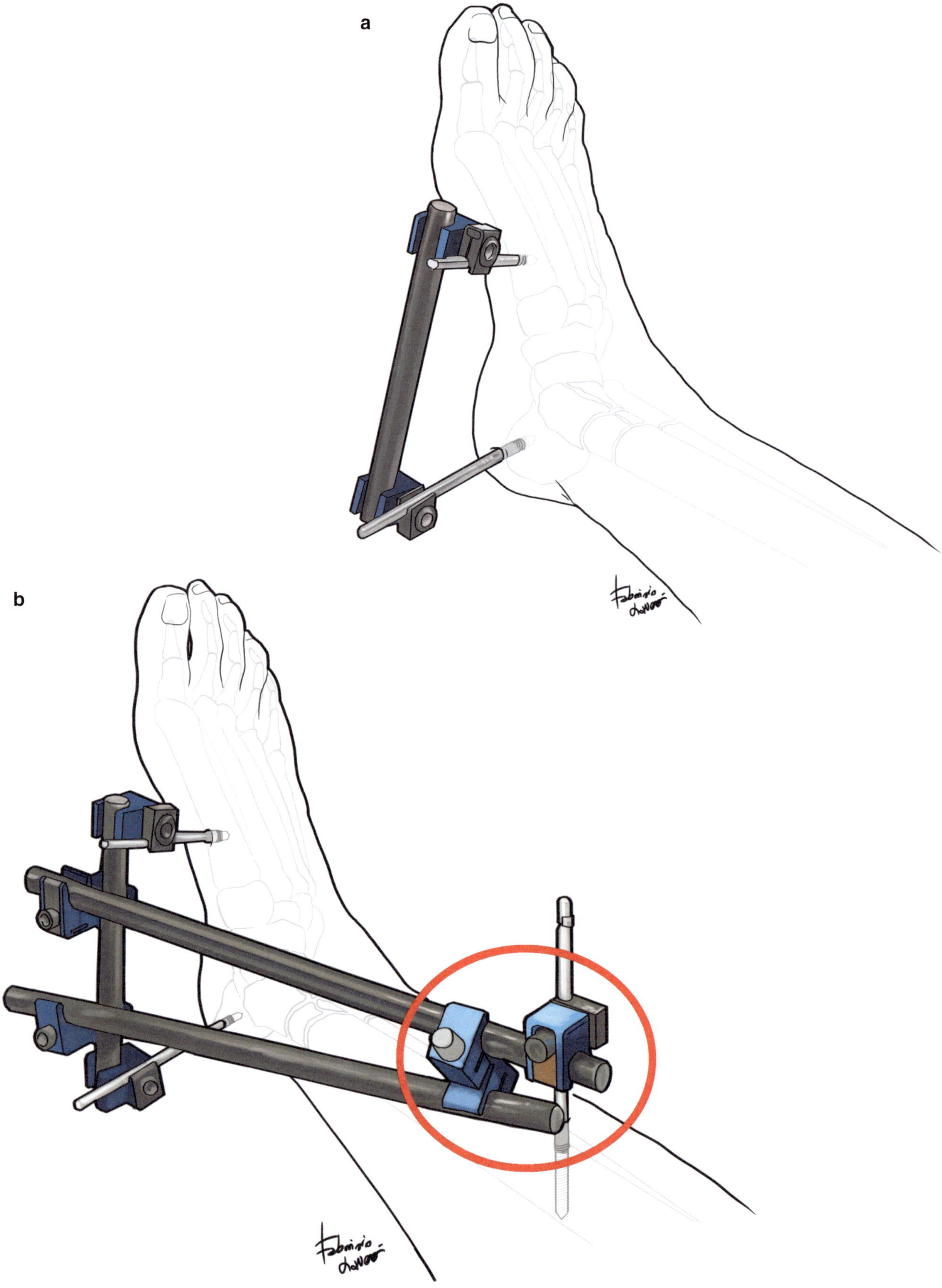

Fig. 1.5 Ankle spanning external fixator for emergency treatment of tibial pilon fracture: a short rod is connected by "rod-to-screw" clamps to the two screws previously inserted in the foot, to create the base of the triangle (**a**); with a third "rod-to-screw" clamp and three "rod-to-rod" clamps, the triangular frame is completed (**b**), leaving the proximal clamps temporarily free to move, shown in the red circle

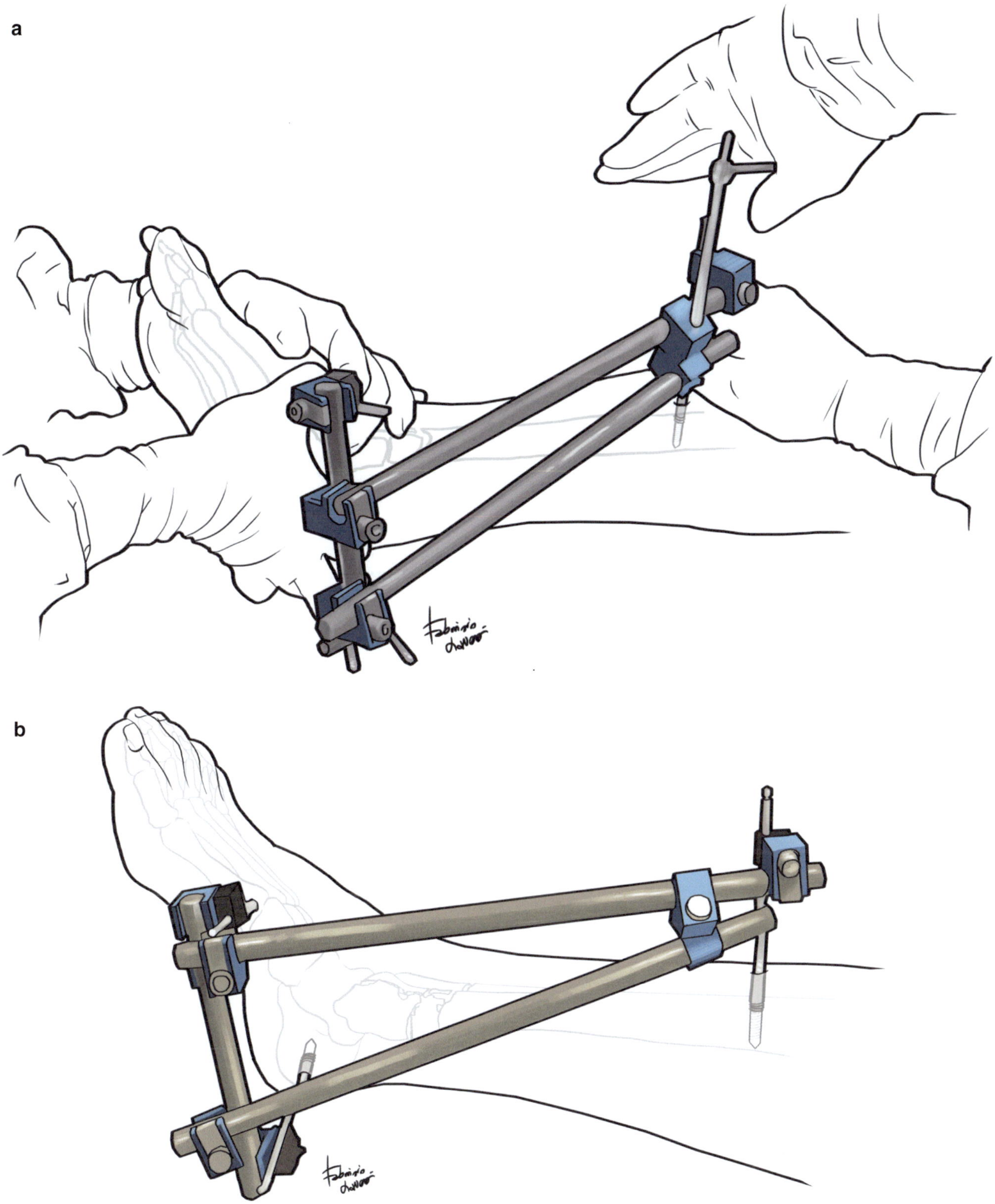

Fig. 1.6 Ankle spanning external fixator for emergency treatment of tibial pilon fracture: acting on the proximal screw as a fixed point, the fracture is reduced through a traction applied on the base of the triangle (**a**); once a good clinical reduction is achieved, the proximal clamps are fixed, completing the building of the external fixator (**b**)

When the traction induced by the tension of the soft tissues is not enough to achieve a good joint morphology, a mini-invasive reduction of the epiphyseal fragments can be associated as far as possible through limited cutaneous incisions and eventually through a consequent osteosynthesis with metallic wires or cannulated screws, always with the objective to restore at the best the joint line, avoiding further risk of complications on the soft tissues [22].

Surgical Technique

The patient is positioned on a radiolucent table, supine with the injured limb free to move in the surgical field and including the knee to enable assessment of limb rotation; a cushion is put under the gluteus to limit extra-rotation of the affected lower limb, while the contralateral limb can be flexed and elevated on a support to facilitate access to the surgeon, which will stay on the medial side, as well as to favour the lateral X-ray projections (Fig. 1.7).

The hardware used to fix the healthy bone at the extremity of the fracture is represented by screws or wires, passing through the safe anatomical routes avoiding the noble vascular, nervous and tendinous structures and maintaining the ankle flexed in a functional position during the inserting manoeuvres; the frame arhitecture can lead or not to a joint immobilization. The spatial configuration of the fixator can consist in a simple axial architecture, using connecting clamps between the screws and the frame, or hybrid type, with wires and circular rings at the periarticular level and clamps in the diaphyseal zone; more frequently because more adaptable, the circular configuration,

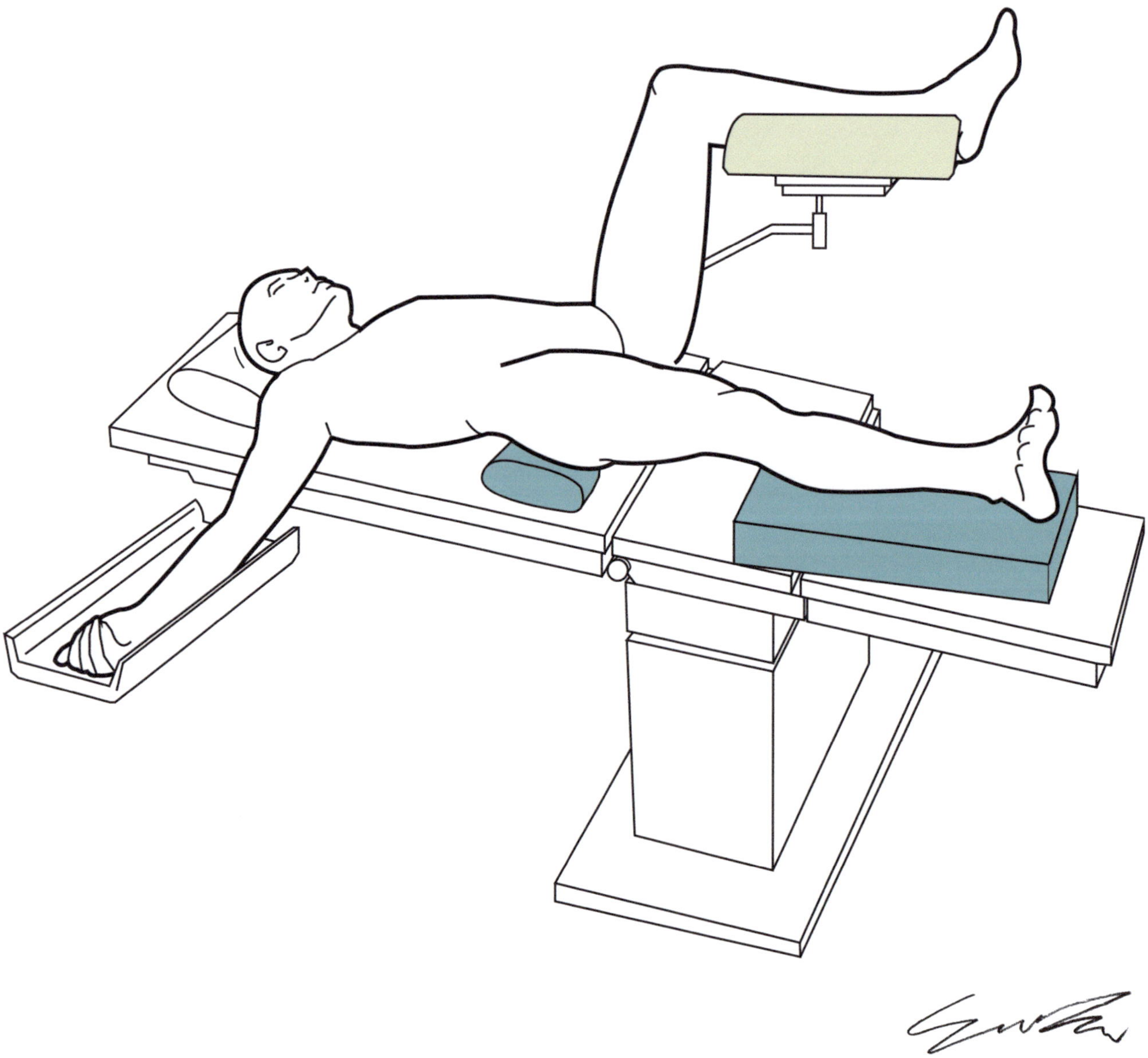

Fig. 1.7 Circular external fixator surgical technique as a definitive treatment of pilon tibial fractures: patient positioning

using both periarticular and diaphyseal rings, results the best way to perform the stabilization with the external fixation.

In this case the first ring positioned is the more proximal, on the tibial diaphysis, acting as a fixed point, and the second ring positioned is the more distal (usually an half ring or a 5/8 circle ring) on the foot, bridging the ankle joint, fixed with Kirschner wires or screws at the calcaneus and eventually at the first and fifth metatarsal bone, to avoid equinism of the foot.

This second element is used as a tie rod for the joint distraction through ligamentotaxis.

The two parts of the extremities of the frame are considered the main ones; the other rings, between the latter, are two or three: one of this is always positioned on the distal tibia, very near to the joint space and fixed with wires; at least one of the wires of this ring must also transfix the peroneal bone (avoiding in this way it's internal fixation, that for certain authors appears to be detrimental) [36]. The other one or two rings are positioned metaphyseally, and they allow through K-wire traction, in consequence of their elasticity, to apply translational forces that realign the diaphyseal elements on the frontal and lateral plane, before proceeding with the stabilization of the latter and completing the final preparation of the external fixator (Fig. 1.8).

The joint block through ligamentotaxis is maintained for 6 weeks and then removed in the outpatient clinic, allowing from that moment to start joint mobilization without weight bearing; full weight bearing is allowed after 12 weeks, to protect the joint element; the tibial part of the fixator is removed after a few months, only when the X-ray performed in the four projections shows the complete fracture union.

1.1.4.2 ORIF

Goals

If and when it is possible to perform an open reduction and internal fixation, more specifically in absence or after full recovery of soft tissue involvement, the main objective is the anatomical reconstruction of the fractured joint line, the realignment of the diaphyseal fractured bone and the stable fixation that allows early joint mobilization, conditions necessary to reduce the chondral injuries and arthritic joint degeneration and to avoid abnormal solicitations on the joint in consequence of a malunion [9–12].

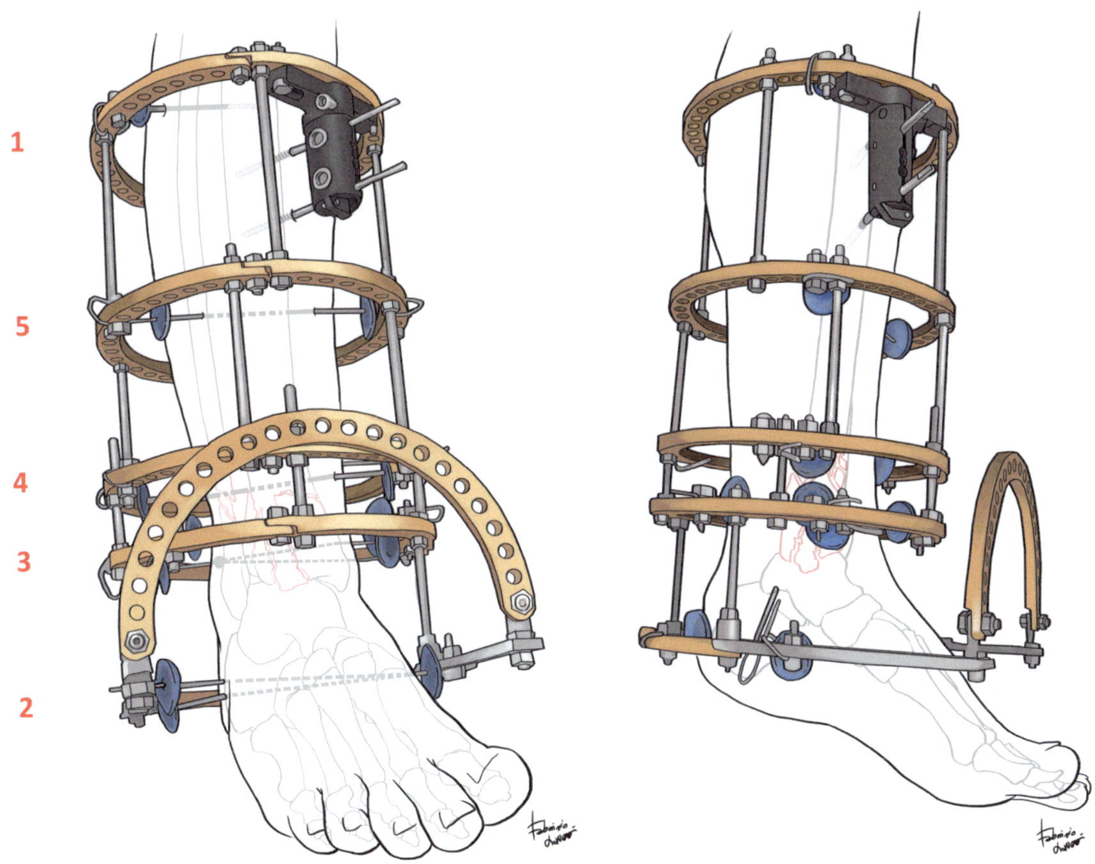

Fig. 1.8 Circular external fixator surgical technique as a definitive treatment of pilon tibial fractures: circular external fixator completed, visible on a lateral and frontal view. On the side the connecting sequence of the circular frames to the bone grips that are, respectively, screws for the diaphyseal part and Kirschner wires for the meta-epiphyseal part is reported

It is mandatory to always perform this surgery with the full protection and respect of the soft tissues, avoiding every kind of traction or abnormal stress on the latter.

Surgical Technique

The patient positioning is the same used for the circular fixator procedure, with a tourniquet applied on the thigh (Fig. 1.9).

The surgical instrumentation must have silicone laces to protect the superficial peroneal nerve if an anterolateral access is chosen; an AO large distractor; Kirschner wires for temporary fixation; AO LCP 3.5 blade system, with medial and lateral plates; mouldable reconstruction plates if an anterior access is chosen; and poly-L-lactic (PLLA) rods and screws for the synthesis of little osteochondral fragments and synthetic bone graft if needed and when iliac crest grafting is not an option.

The difficulty of these fractures is that treatment does not leave any space for unpreparedness: the surgery must always begin from the preoperative planning, performed on the basis of the CT scan achieved with the fracture distracted by the external fixator priorly positioned; this allows the surgeon to understand correctly the "personality" of the fracture, sensing the pathologic anatomy and translation of the unreduced fragments (Fig. 1.10).

The preoperative planning must grant a strategy well acknowledged before surgery, with all the key points enlighten: the bony segment to start from, if a peroneal fracture is associated, the surgical access for the tibia, the modality of fracture reduction and the choice of osteosynthesis.

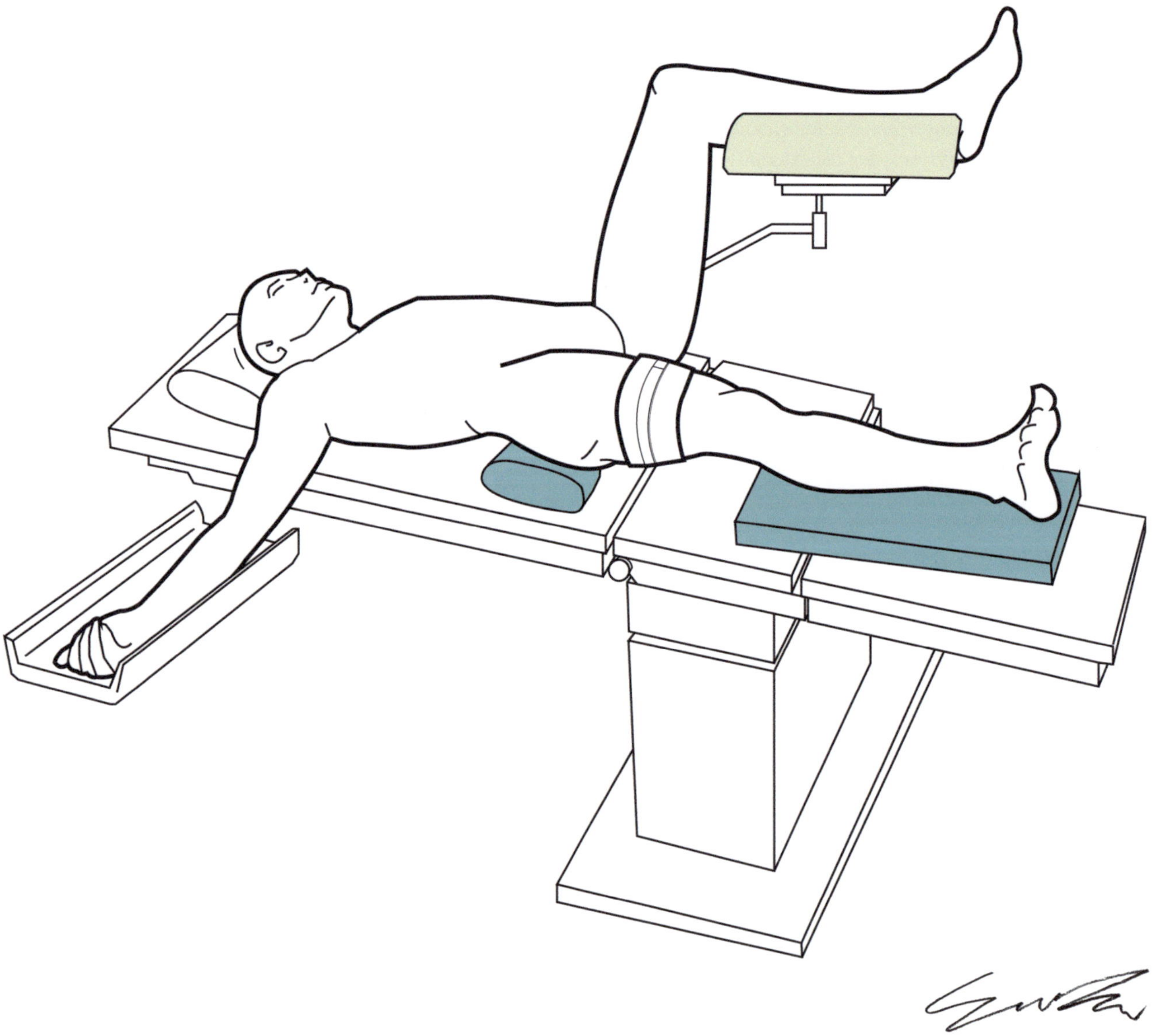

Fig. 1.9 Open synthesis of a pilon fracture: patient positioning

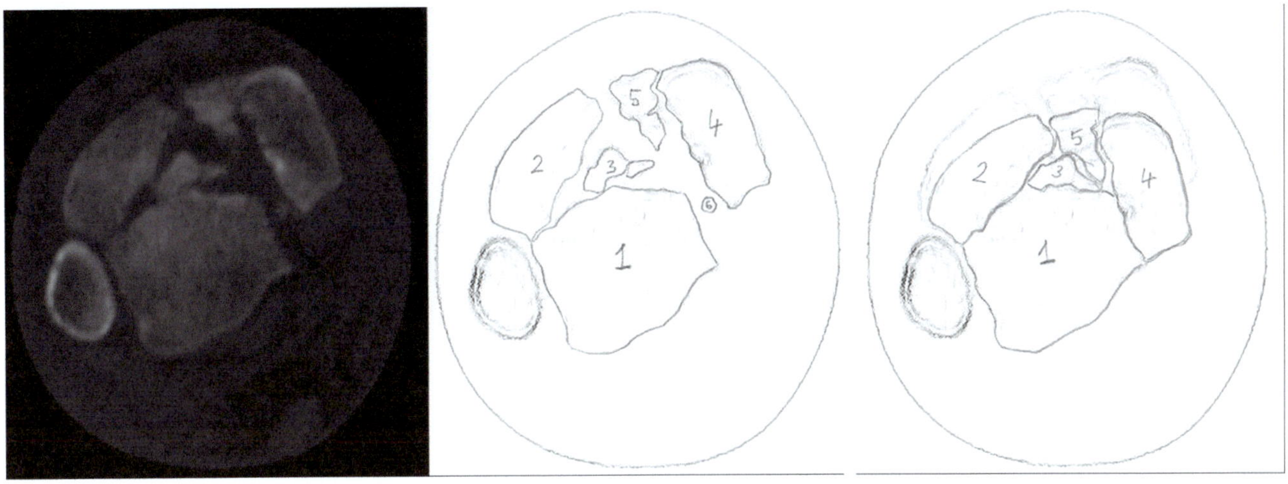

Fig. 1.10 Preoperative planning of the ORIF of a pilon fracture: the axial cut, just proximal to the joint line, is broken up into simple graphic elements. The latter are evaluated to understand the pathological anatomy of the injury and the necessary reduction manoeuvres

Priority of Surgical Aggression

When a peroneal fracture of the mid-distal third part is present, it is usual to start from the latter, because the restoration of the fibular length, due to the tough ligamentous bond of the syndesmosis, determines the reestablishment in the anatomical position of the anterolateral part of the tibia that is the key fragment and the fixed point on which the pilon fracture reduction is achieved [2].

An exception of this rule is when it is not possible to achieve an anatomical reduction of the fibula as a result of its excessive fragmentation: even if proceeding to the reduction of the peroneal bone, the main tibial fragment could result unreduced, leading to the anatomical restoration of the pilon fracture impossible; in these cases the reduction of the tibial epiphysis for first results less dangerous, leaving for second the peroneal reduction and synthesis with a bridging plate, aiming only to the restoration of its length and rotation [37, 38].

In consideration of the surgical access, modality of reduction and osteosynthesis of the fibula, nothing results different from the technique used for the malleolar fragments, described in Chap. 2.

Surgical Access to the Tibia

The aggression to the tibia can be performed through an anterior, posterior, medial or anterolateral access, in the more severe cases even with a combination of the latter to achieve the best reduction of the joint in all the planes [2].

The direct anterior access is the same usually performed for total ankle replacements procedures; it grants a good exposition of the anterior tibial pilon, but with an important capsular detachment, with a high risk of osteochondral fragment devitalization. Furthermore, the anterior incision could result too near to the fibular access, with possible suffering of the skin flap in between, above all if the width results inferior 5 cm; for these reasons, such surgical access actually results very limited in its indications [2].

The posterior aggression is realized mainly through a posterolateral route, being medially limited by the posterior tibial neurovascular bundle; it is used exceptionally and always in addition to other surgical accesses, to reduce large posterior fragments of the joint that are in other ways not dominable, performing a posterior access to the fibula and using the same incision to access to the tibia [37].

The antero-medial and anterolateral accesses are more frequently used; the choice of which of the two must be used is taken during the preoperative planning, to grant the plate positioning on the side where there is the highest comminution of the fracture: this allows the plate screw tip to be well fixed, tightening on the more reliable part of the bone [39] (Figs. 1.11 and 1.12); only in the more severe and comminuted cases it can be necessary to use a combination of the two surgical access to permit a medial and lateral blade positioning, to have a support of the two columns.

The anterolateral access is performed through a single incision on the fibula and tibia [40], beginning proximally in correspondence of the interosseous membrane and extending distally in the line of the fourth ray of the foot.

It results less invasive on the soft tissues, because the plate is covered by the muscles, but the surgical route is demanding, requesting to isolate and protect the superficial peroneal nerve branches that cross the incision (Fig. 1.13).

If the plate needs to be removed, a revision surgery can result complicated because the nerve covered by scar will be difficult to dissect, with a higher risk to develop a painful neuroma.

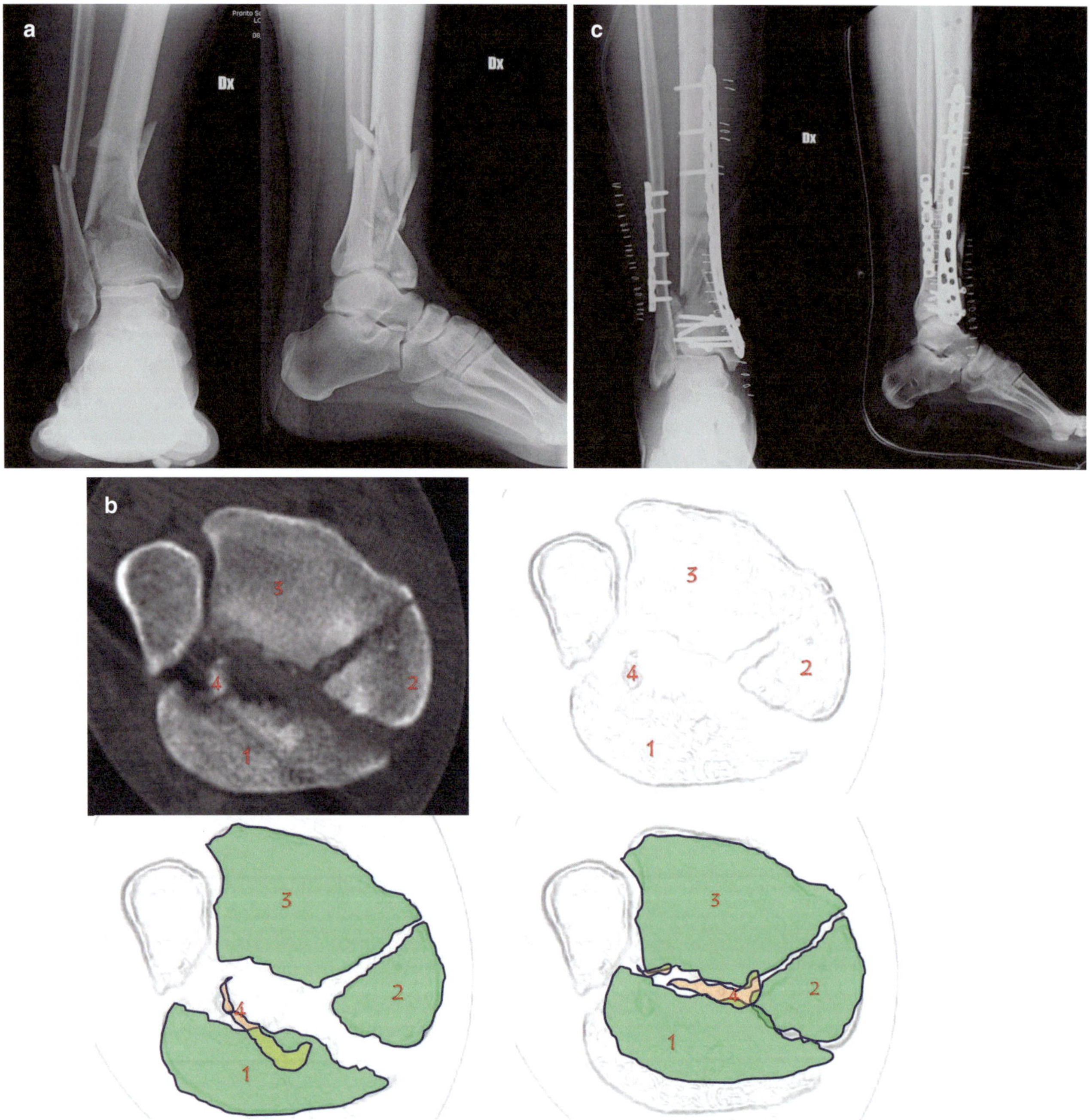

Fig. 1.11 Clinical case of a tibial pilon fracture 43C2: preoperative X-ray evaluation (**a**); preoperative planning in consideration of the CT, which shows the smaller bony portions on the medial side (**b**); postoperative check of the osteosynthesis achieved through an antero-medial access with a medial plate (**c**)

The medial access is performed through an incision in correspondence of the anterior tibial edge, slightly lateral to the latter, ending on the navicular bone (Fig. 1.14); the soft tissue dissection is done leaving the tibialis anterior and extensor tendon sheath unharmed, both of them retracted laterally (Fig. 1.15).

The capsulotomy is performed through a vertical incision, aiming the line of the antero-medial fracture, after a medial rotation of the tibial malleolar fragment, which is divided "as an open book", to grant access to the central portion of the tibial pilon.

Reduction

Once the exposure is performed, the fracture reduction strategy must have been previously studied in the preoperative planning; in the surgical field, all the fragments

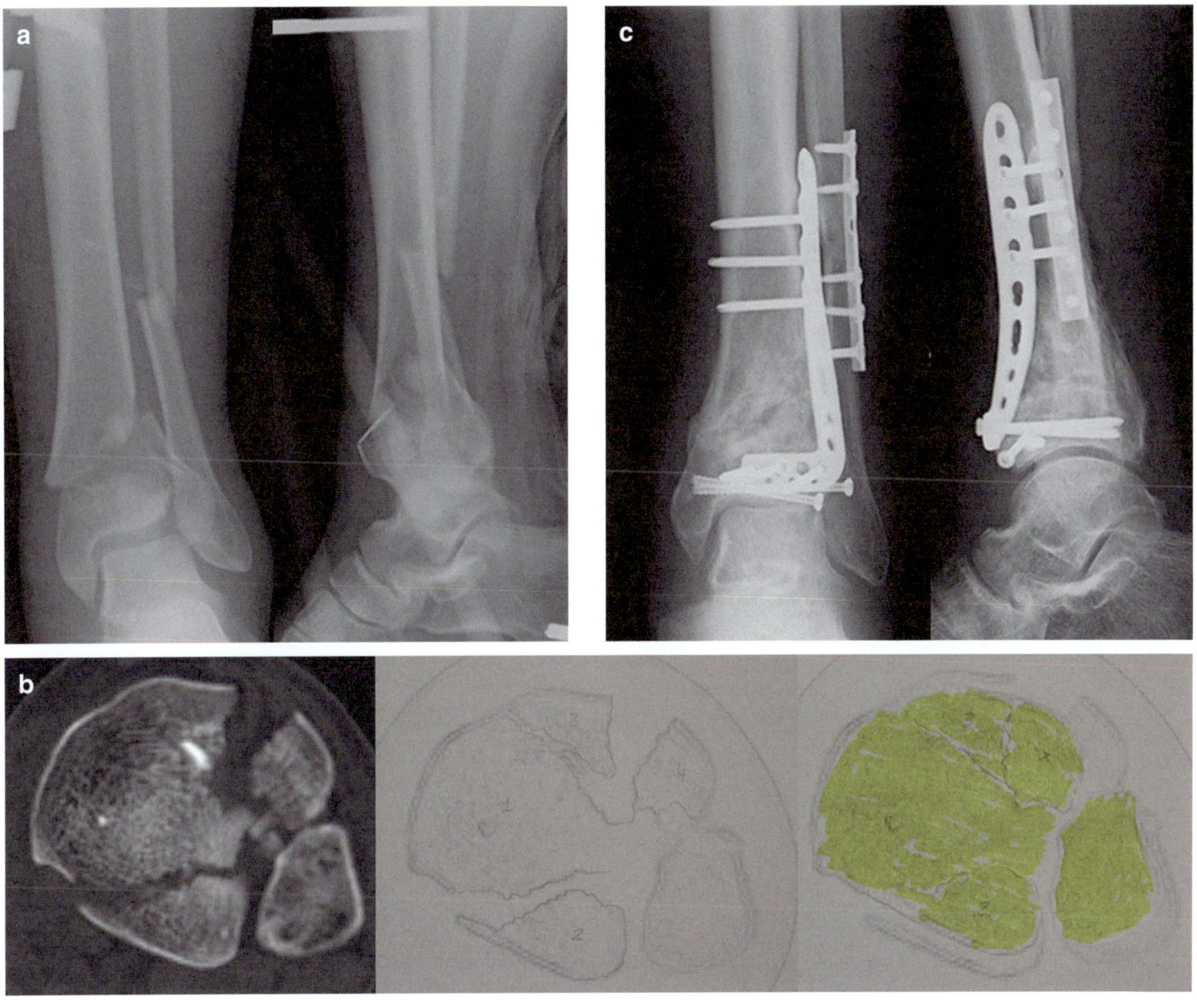

Fig. 1.12 Clinical case of a tibial pilon fracture 43C2: preoperative X-ray evaluation (**a**); preoperative planning in consideration of the CT, which shows the smaller bony portions on the lateral side (**b**); 6-month check of the ORIF, achieved through an anterolateral access with a lateral plate: fracture has healed (**c**)

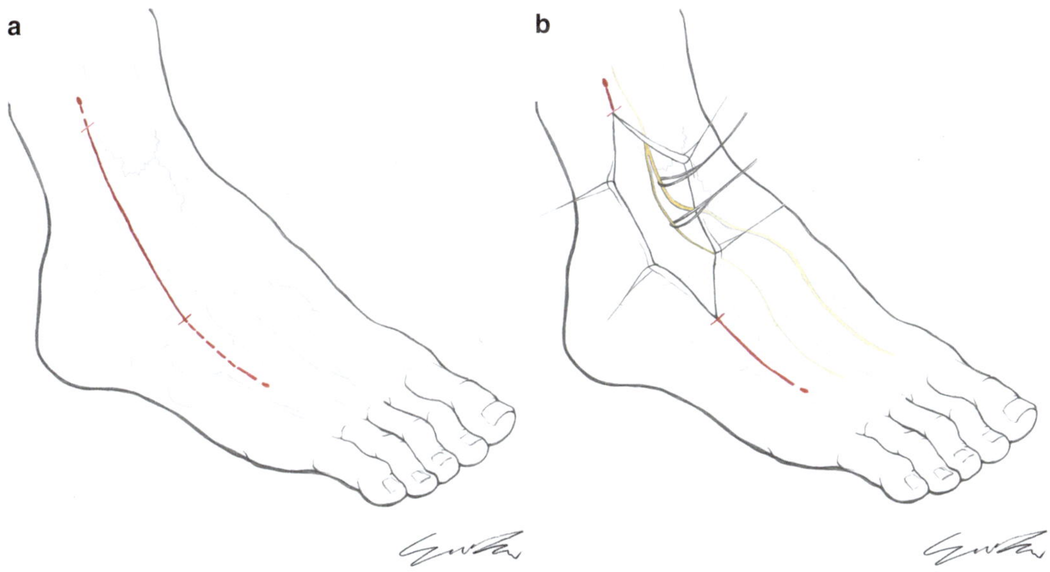

Fig. 1.13 Anterolateral access to the tibial pilon: the incision lays proximally on the interosseous line to the fourth ray distally (**a**); during the superficial dissection, it is important to isolate and protect the branches of the superficial peroneal nerve that cross the incision line (**b**)

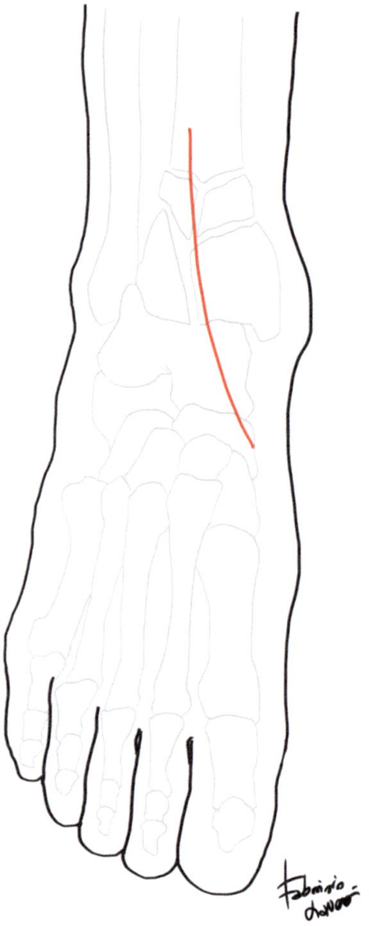

Fig. 1.14 Antero-medial access to the tibial pilon: the incision rides along the lateral side of the tibial crest to the tarsal navicular bone

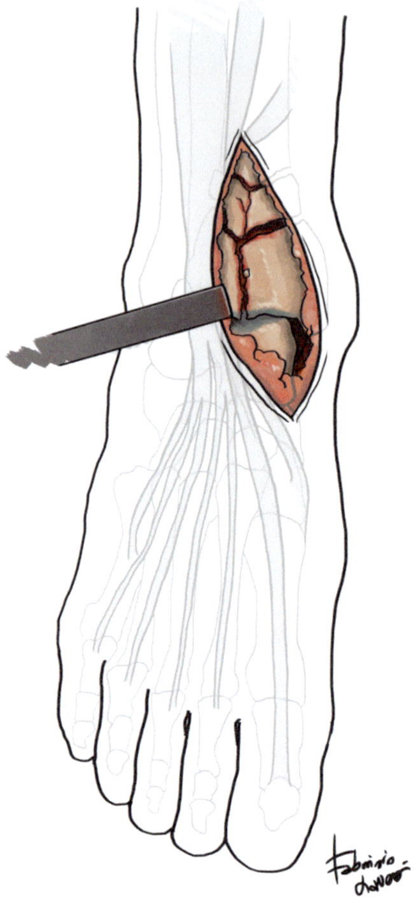

Fig. 1.15 Antero-medial access to the tibial pilon: the dissection is brought onto the bony plane with a lateral retraction of the tendons of the tibialis anterior, extensor hallucis longus and digitorum and tibialis anterior neurovascular bundle

spotted through the diagnostic imaging must be identified for first and only after must be reduced, correcting the pathologic anatomy of the lesion and fracture displacement [10, 14].

The reduction is practically performed through a window realized by the open book opening of the fragment were the capsulotomy is done and results strongly eased by the use of the AO distractor. The temporary external fixator screws can be used in association with the AO distractor, after being sterilized by an antiseptic and disinfectant solution used for the preparation of the surgical field (Fig. 1.16).

At this point all the rest of the fracture components are identified, and above all the osteochondral central fragment is recognized, normally not seen with the traditional radiology, but enlightened through the CT scan, usually found impacted proximally. This fragment represents one of the key elements to perfect the pilon reduction (Fig. 1.17).

The osteochondral fragment must be freed and repositioned at the correct height on the anterolateral and the posterior fragments, previously reduced if an anatomical reduction and synthesis of the fibula have been performed.

Then the reduction is completed through the repositioning of the fragment that was previously displaced to gain access to the fracture.

The joint portion, in this way reconstructed, is stabilized with a provisional synthesis and checked through X-ray [14]. In this phase the central articular fragment is more difficult to control, and it is always extremely challenging to keep it in correct position during the manoeuvres needed for the reduction of the other joint fragments and definitive synthesis. To achieve this, lost Kirschner wires in the bone are useful, or, to avoid leaving metallic fragments free in periarticular zones, it is possible to use absorbable PLLA pins and screws to achieve stabilization.

Osteosynthesis

Once that the joint part is reconstructed, it is stabilized with the main fracture segments with a provisional synthesis, usually with free compression screws, carefully avoiding the area where the plate will be positioned.

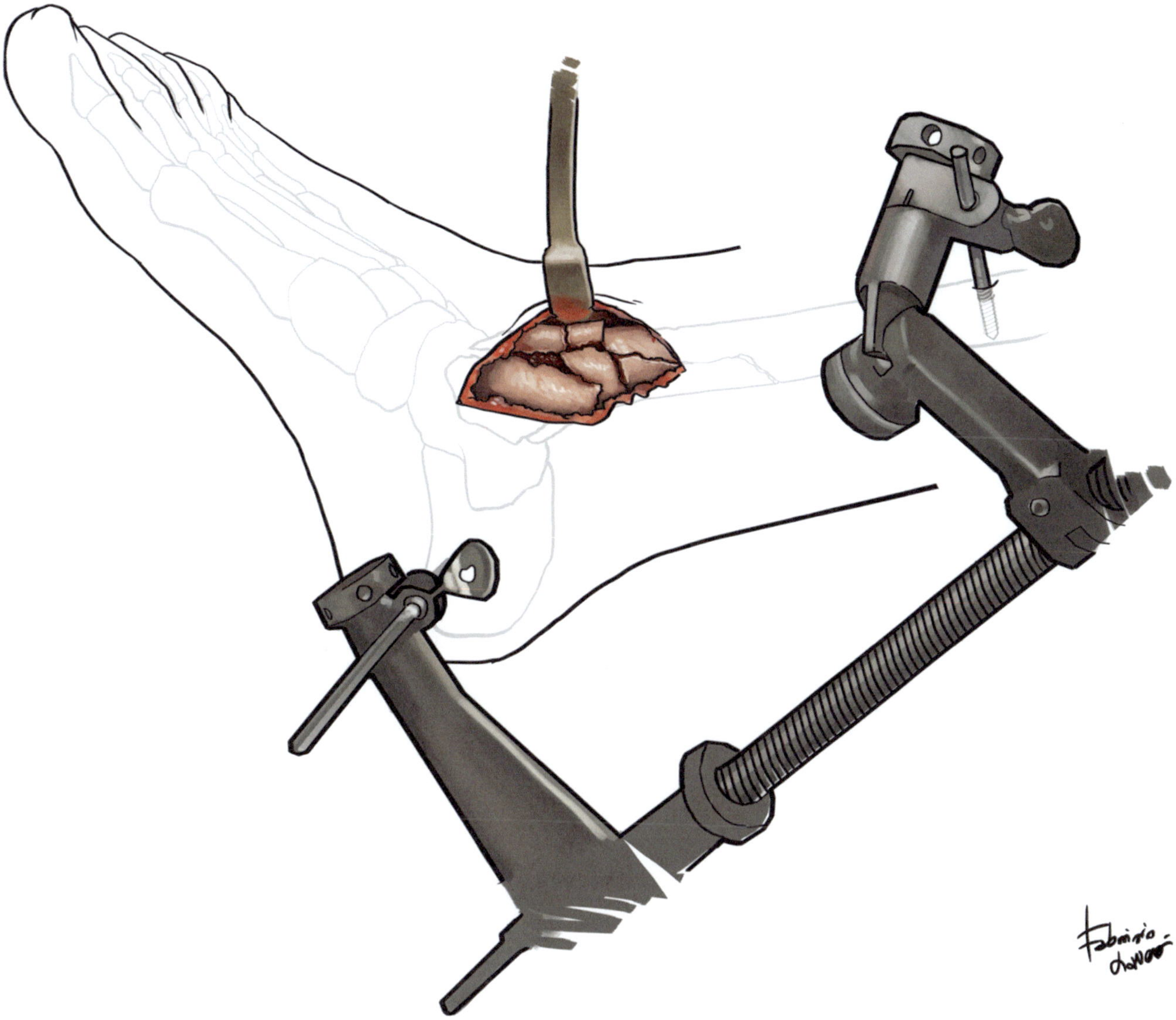

Fig. 1.16 Antero-medial access to the tibial pilon: the AO distractor can be positioned on bone grip screws as a temporary external fixator; in consideration of the distraction applied, it is possible to grant a better view of the joint surface

This type of osteosynthesis has a dual function: it permits to fix the articular part with the diaphyseal segment and, if a latest generation plate is used, it helps to reduce the metaphysis without any invasive manoeuvres on the soft tissues, fulfilling an osteosynthesis named "MIPO" (minimally invasive plate osteosynthesis).

This is essential if the metaphysis shows a multifragmentary and complex morphology: in this case, the "anatomic" plates, built to ease the positioning through a subcutaneous sliding, are introduced bridging the fracture comminution and respecting the biology of the latter but allowing to restore length and alignment of the segments. Once the plate is introduced through a subcutaneous tunnel reaching the proximal tibia (Fig. 1.18), it is possible to reduce the meta-diaphyseal segment on the plate, allowed by the anatomical conformation of the latter, even in a multifragmentary metaphyseal fracture, through conventional screws or specific instrumentation to recall the bony fragments. Once a satisfactory alignment of the axial components is achieved, controlled under fluoroscopy, the fracture is fixed with locking screws using the plate as an "internal fixator" (Fig. 1.11c) that will permit the healing of the meta-diaphyseal portion through an indirect way, with the flexibility of the segment and the formation of bone callus, respecting simultaneously the biology of the bony fragments [2] (Fig. 1.12c).

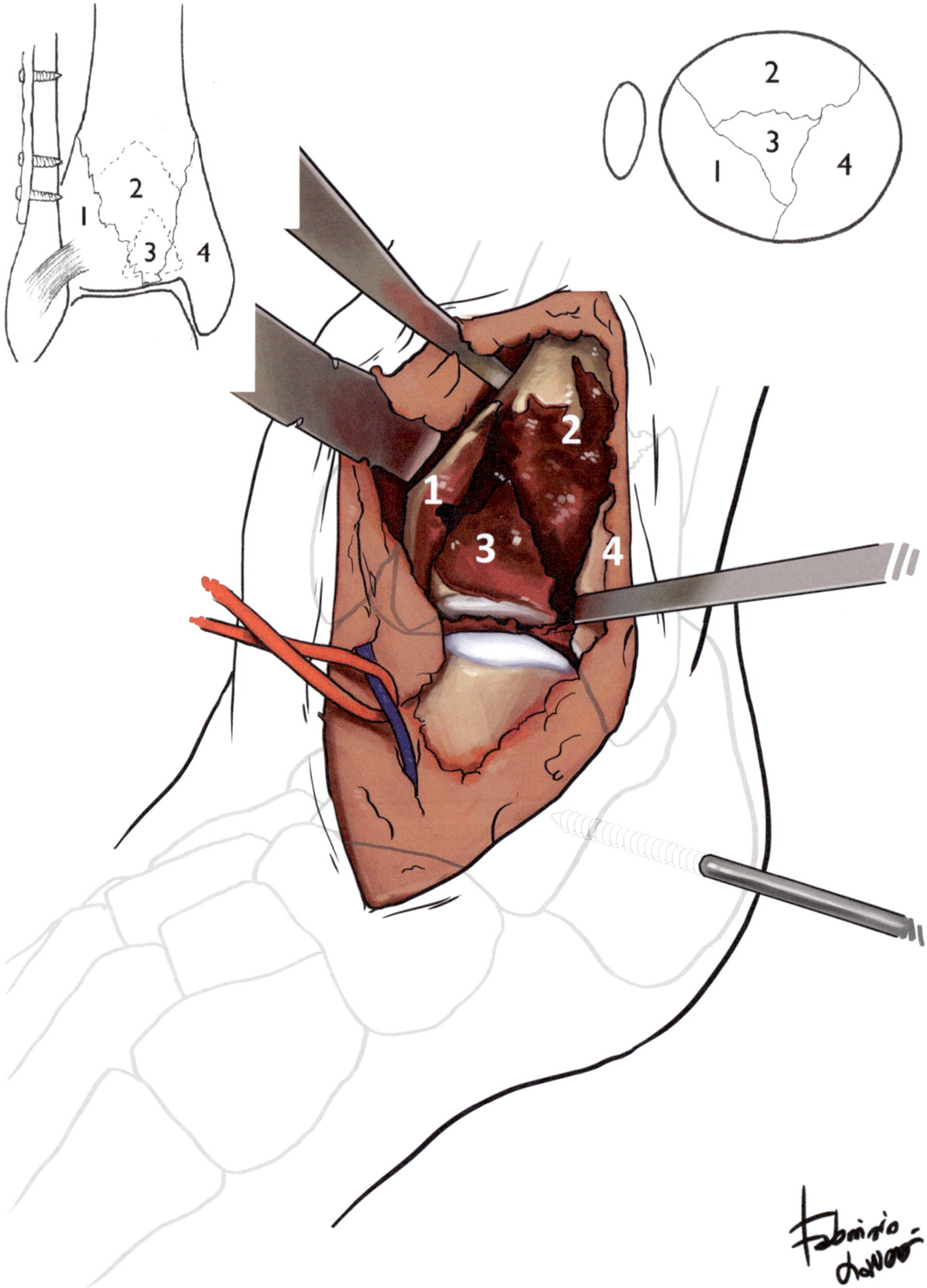

Fig. 1.17 Antero medial access to the tibial pilon: the "book wise" rotational opening of the fragment of the tibialis malleolus (n. 4) grants the access to the osteochondral impacted fragment that is migrated proximally (n. 3), that is going to be freed from the posterior and diaphyseal fragment (n. 2) and repositioned at the correct height through the reduction of the key fragment (n. 1), the whom position has been previously restored through the fibular connections and the reduction of the latter

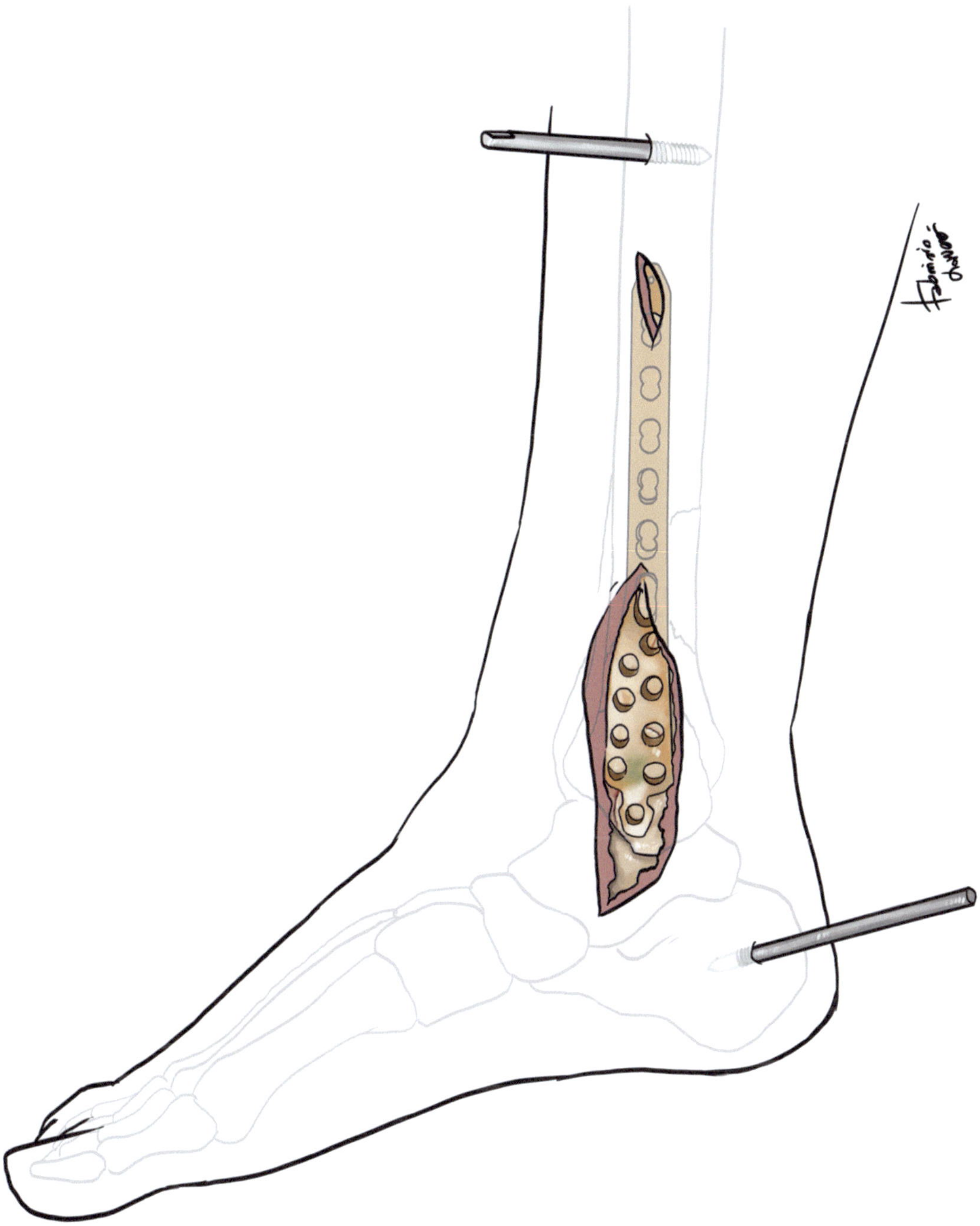

Fig. 1.18 MIPO osteosynthesis of a tibial pilon fracture: after the joint part has been reduced and stabilized with a minimal osteosynthesis, the plate is positioned through the distal wound, sliding it under the skin and proceeding to a proximal fixation through aimed mini-incisions. The anatomical form of the blade allows to reduce indirectly the comminuted metaphyseal areas

The same principle is worthy for medial column or lateral column plating (Fig. 1.19), as for an approach were both plating are required.

If the synthesis is stable, the use of bone grafting to fill the loss of substance does not have any indications, being the metaphyseal area a well-vascularized spot that usually is able to repair these defects; however the bone graft can have an important role to rise the primary stability of the osteosynthesis, especially as a support that prevents the proximal migration of the little osteochondral fragments sufficiently wide to be included in the reconstruction. When a bone graft is used, autologous or synthetic, it is necessary to keep it carefully unrelated to the joint portion to preserve functionality [14].

If the synthesis is stable, the postoperative follow-up must consider a cast immobilization as short as possible, 2 weeks at the most, to preserve the wound until the stitches are removed, followed by an intense active and passive lower limb mobilization without weight bearing to achieve the best recovery of joint range of motion.

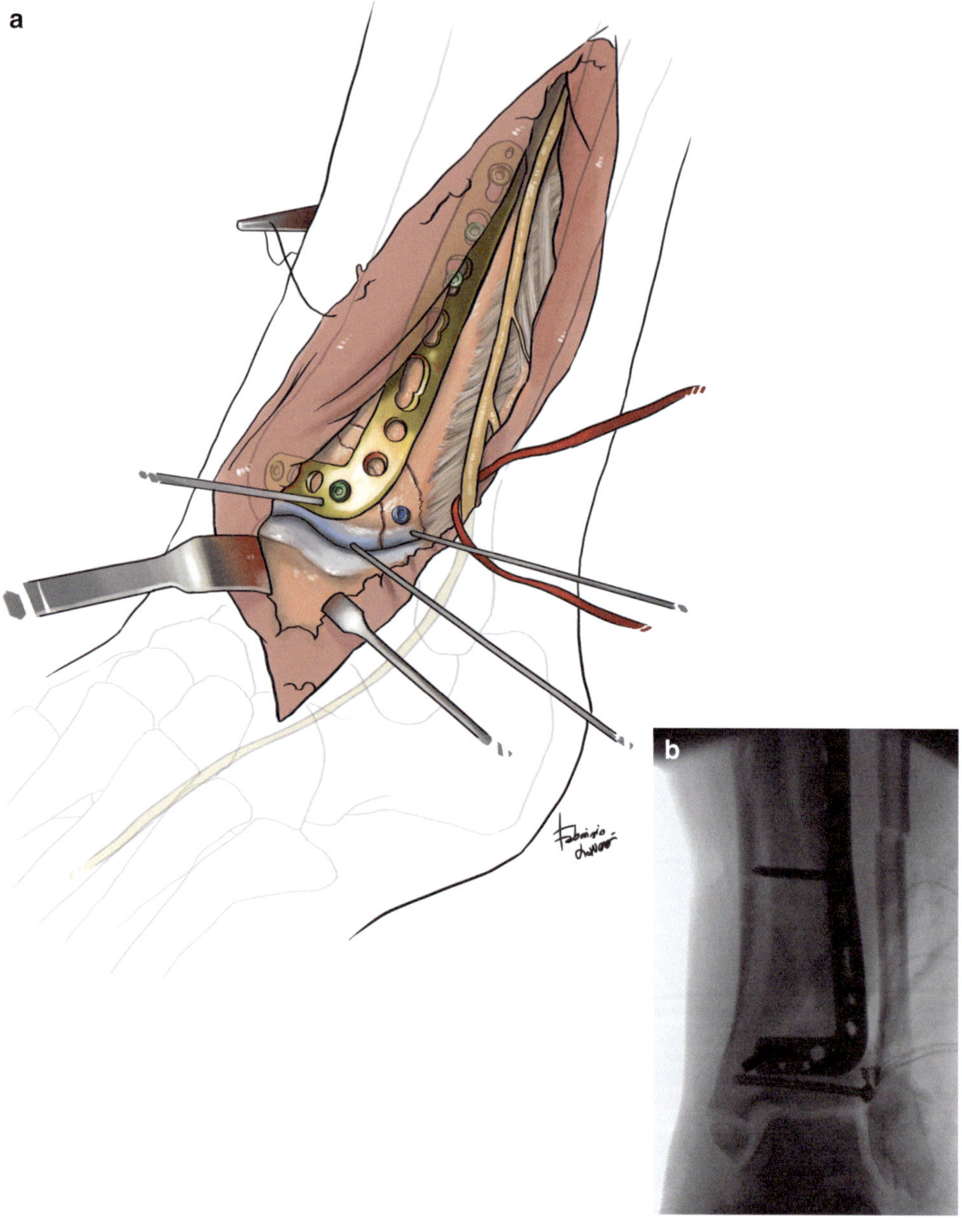

Fig. 1.19 Tibial pilon fracture osteosynthesis with an anterolateral anatomical plate: once the joint part has been reduced and stabilized with a minimal osteosynthesis, the anatomical blade, glided proximally under the skin, reflects the segmental anatomy (**a**) and allows the indirect reduction of the metaphyseal comminution (**b**)

Being an articular fracture, mutual movements of the fragments must absolutely be avoided, to not jeopardize the obtained reduction; for this reason a direct bone healing is pursued; therefore the weight bearing must be prohibited for at least 90 days from surgery [39, 41].

References

1. Destot E (1937) Traumatisme du pied et rayons X. Masson, Paris
2. Sanders RW, Walling AK (2007) Pilon fractures. In: Coughlin MJ, Mann RA, Saltzman CL (eds) Surgery of the foot and ankle, 8th edn. Mosby Elsevier, Philadelphia, pp 1941–1971
3. Koulouvaris P, Stafylas K, Mitsionis G et al (2007) Long-term results of various therapy concepts in severe pilon fractures. Arch Orthop Trauma Surg 127(5):313–320
4. Tarkin IS, Clare MP, Marcantonio A et al (2008) An update on the management of high-energy pilon fractures. Injury 39(2):142–154
5. Muller ME, Nazarian S, Koch P (1990) AO classification of fractures. Springer, Berlin
6. Kellam JF, Waddell JP (1979) Fractures of the distal tibial metaphysic with intra-articular extension- the distal tibial explosion fracture. J Trauma 19(8):593–601
7. Ruedi T, Matter P, Allgower M (1968) Intra-articular fractures of the distal tibial end. Helv Chir Acta 35(5):556–582
8. Orthopaedic Trauma Association Committee for coding and Classification (1996) Fracture and dislocation compendium. J Orthop Trauma 10(Suppl 1):v–ix, 1-154

9. Anderson DD, Chubinskaya S, Guilak F et al (2011) Post-traumatic osteoarthritis: improved understanding and opportunities for early intervention. J Orthop Res 29(6):802–809
10. Barei DP, Nork SE (2008) Fractures of the tibial plafond. Foot Ankle Clin 13(4):571–591
11. Buckwalter JA (1995) Activity vs. rest in the treatment of bone, soft tissue and joint injuries. Iowa Orthop J 15:29–42
12. Mitchell N, Shepard N (1980) Healing of articular cartilage in intrarticular fractures in rabbits. J Bone Joint Surg Am 62A(4):628–634
13. Sirkin M, Sanders R, DiPasquale T et al (2004) A staged protocol for soft tissue management in the treatment of complex pilon fractures. J Orthop Trauma 18(8):S32–S38
14. Sommer C, Baumgaertner MR (2007) Tibia, distal intraarticular (pilon). In: Ruedi TP, Buckley RE, Moran CG (eds) AO principles of fracture management, 2nd expanded edn. Thieme, New York, pp 855–869
15. Shatzer J, Tile M (1987) The rationale for operative fracture care, 1st edn. Springer, New York
16. Joshi D, Singh D, Ansari J et al (2006) Immediate open reduction and internal fixation in open ankle fractures. J Am Podiatr Med Assoc 96(2):120–124
17. Zalavras CG, Patzakis MJ, Holtom PD et al (2005) Management of open fractures. Infect Dis Clin N Am 19(4):915–929
18. Hulsker CC, Kleinveld S, Zonnenberg CB et al (2011) Evidence-based treatment of open ankle fractures. Arch Orthop Trauma Surg 131(11):1545–1553
19. Bray TJ, Endicott M, Capra SE (1989) Treatment of open ankle fractures. Immediate internal fixation versus closed immobilization and delayed fixation. Clin Orthop Relat Res 240:47–52
20. Bhandari M, Schemitsch EH, Adili A et al (1999) High and low pressure pulsatile lavage of contaminated tibial fractures: an in vitro study of bacterial adherence and bone damage. J Orthop Trauma 13(8):526–533
21. Hassinger SM, Harding G, Wongworawat MD (2005) High-pressure pulsatile lavage propagates bacteria into soft tissue. Clin Orthop Relat Res 439:27–31
22. Tarkin IS, Sop A, Pape HC (2008) High-energy foot and ankle trauma: principles for formulating an individualized care plan. Foot Ankle Clin N Am 13:705–723
23. Blauth M, Bastian L, Krettek C et al (2001) Surgical options for the treatment of severe tibial pilon fractures: a study of three techniques. J Orthop Trauma 15(3):153–160
24. Egol KA, Wolinsky P, Koval KJ (2000) Open reduction and internal fixation of tibial pilon fractures. Foot Ankle Clin 5(4):873–885
25. Dickson KF, Montgomery S, Field J (2001) High energy plafond fractures treated by a spanning external fixator initially and followed by a second stage open reduction internal fixation of the articular surface-preliminary report. Injury 32(Suppl 4):SD92–SD98
26. Bacon S, Smith WR, Morgan SJ et al (2008) A retrospective analysis of comminuted intra-articular fractures of the tibial plafond: open reduction and internal fixation versus external Ilizarov fixation. Injury 39(2):196–202
27. Boraiah S, Kemp TJ, Erwteman A et al (2010) Outcome following open reduction and internal fixation of open pilon fractures. J Bone Joint Surg Am 92A(2):346–352
28. Ketz J, Sanders R (2012) Staged posterior tibial plating for the treatment of Orthopaedic Trauma Association 43C2 and 43C3 tibial pilon fractures. J Orthop Trauma 26(6):341–347
29. Sirkin M, Sanders R, DiPasquale T et al (1999) A staged protocol for soft tissue management in the treatment of complex pilon fractures. J Orthop Trauma 13(2):78–84
30. Cierny G 3rd, Byrd HS, Jones RE (1983) Primary versus delayed soft tissue coverage for severe open tibial fractures. A comparison of results. Clin Orthop Relat Res 178:54–63
31. Lavini F, Dall'Oca C, Mezzari S et al (2014) Temporary bridging external fixation in distal tibial fracture. Injury 45:S58–S63
32. He X, Hu Y, Ye P et al (2013) The operative treatment of complex pilon fractures: a strategy of soft tissue control. Ind J Orthop 47(5):487–492
33. Kiene J, Herzog J, Jürgens C et al (2012) Multifragmentary tibial pilon fractures: midterm results after osteosynthesis with external fixation and multiple lag screws. Open Orthop J 6:419–423
34. Daghino W, Matteotti R, Pinzi D et al (2011) La configurazione "tripolare" del fissatore esterno temporaneo nel trattamento in due stadi delle fratture di pilone tibiale. Aggiornamenti CIO 17(2):37–41
35. Rammelt S, Endres T, Grass R et al (2004) The role of external fixation in acute ankle trauma. Foot Ankle Clin 9(3):455–474
36. El-Shazly M, Dalby-Ball J, Burton M et al (2001) The use of trans-articular and extra-articular external fixation for management of distal tibial intra-articular fractures. Injury 32(Suppl 4):SD99–S106
37. Di Giorgio L, Touloupakis G, Theodorakis E et al (2013) A two-choice strategy through a medial tibial approach for the treatment of pilon fractures with posterior or anterior fragmentation. Chin J Traumatol 16(5):272–276
38. Mehta S, Gardner MJ, Barei DP et al (2011) Reduction strategies through the anterolateral exposure for fixation of type B and C pilon fractures. J Orthop Trauma 25(2):116–122
39. Keita I, Perren SM (2007) Biology and biomechanics in bone healing. In: Ruedi TP, Buckley RE, Moran CG (eds) AO principles of fracture management, 2nd expanded edn. Thieme, New York, pp 9–31
40. Grose A, Gardner MJ, Hettrich C et al (2007) Open reduction and internal fixation of tibial pilon fractures using a lateral approach. J Orthop Trauma 21(8):530–537
41. Ito K, Perren S (2009) Biologia e biomeccanica della guarigione dell'osso. In: Ruedi T, Buckley RE, Moran C (eds) Principi AO per il trattamento delle fratture. CIC Edizioni Internazionali, Roma, pp 9–30

2 Malleolar Fractures

Contents

2.1 Malleolar Fractures

The malleolar fracture definition includes all the injuries that incorporate the distal portion of the tibia and fibula, without any interest of the mid-joint portion. They are relatively frequent injuries, including 9% of all the fractures, and they develop after low kinetic energy traumas, with a high torsional component.

They can interest only one malleolus, more frequently the fibula (60%) than the tibia (6%) or the posterior malleolus, or they can be associated as bimalleolar or trimalleolar fractures [1].

2.1.1 Classification

Considering the AO classification of this anatomical segment, numbered as 44, the fractures are divided into three categories on the basis of the relationship between the fibula and the tibiofibular syndesmosis; the infra-syndesmotic fractures correspond to the 44-A, the trans-syndesmotic fractures correspond to the 44-B and the supra-syndesmotic fractures correspond to the 44-C: such alphabetic progression is related to a progressive instability of the tibio-talar mortise [2, 3].

They are mixed injuries, in which the fracture accompanies a ligamentous lesion [2]. Every group of the AO classification is subdivided into three subgroups in relation with other bony injuries and ligamentous damage [4] (Fig. 2.1).

2.1.2 Indications and Surgical Timing

The malleolar fracture must be considered like articular fractures; therefore, in case of a displacement, the more appropriate indication is to obtain an anatomical reduction and stable internal fixation [3]. If there is a fracture with a joint dislocation, the primary and immediate objective is to reduce such dislocation, because this limits the bleeding and follows soft tissue suffering induced by the swelling [5].

W. Daghino et al., *Foot and Ankle Trauma Injuries*, https://doi.org/10.1007/978-3-319-69617-1_2

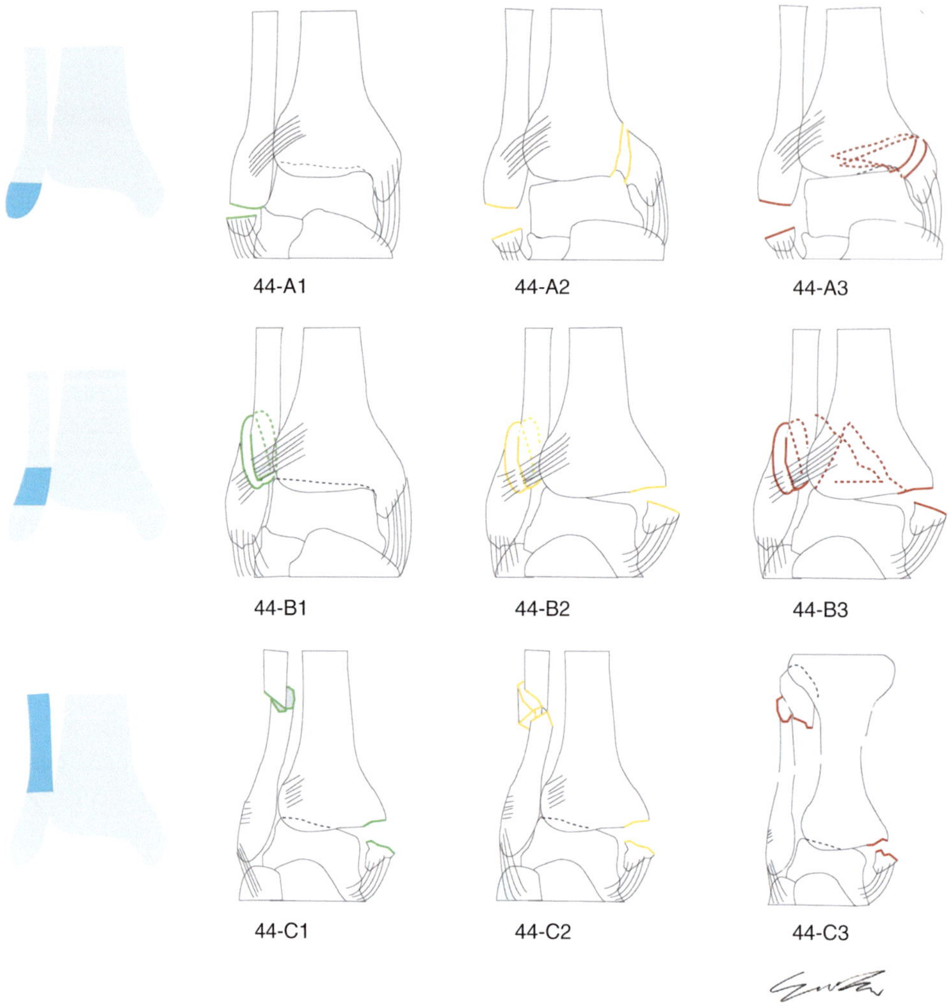

Fig. 2.1 AO classification of the malleolar fractures; for subgroups A and B, the increasing numbering shows, respectively, the involvement of one, two or three malleoli; for the subgroup C, the fracture is simple in type 1, comminuted in type 2 and proximal in type 3

When the joint reduction is achieved, it is advisable to proceed immediately to the stabilization of the injury: to achieve this we think that the best option is a closed cast, more than an open cast, because it grants a more effective conservation of the reduction and immobilization of the fracture. In all the malleolar fractures, without considering the joint dislocation, the positioning of a plaster cast immediately after the trauma and the elevation on the affected limb reduce considerably the development of complications such as hematoma and blisters and grant the best conditions for a possible surgery.

If the limb is already affected by serious oedema and soft tissue suffering, like in fractures with bone exposition, the acute treatment is the same as the pilon tibial fractures, through a temporary external fixation, and the final definitive osteosynthesis will be performed once the soft tissue involvement is reduced and in particular where the skin incision must be done [6–8].

The indication to an open anatomical reduction and internal fixation is posed when there is a 2 mm or higher fragment dislocation on plain X-rays, with lower tolerance if the patient is a young athlete with high functional demands; besides this, the surgical correction must be done if there are malrotations or shortening of the fibular malleolus and if there is a subluxation of the talus, with diastasis or instability of the ankle syndesmosis [3]. If there is a fracture of the posterior malleolus, an osteosynthesis is performed when the cartilage portion of the fragment is considerable with respect to the entire articular surface and if there is a dislocation of the fragment higher than 2 mm on the lateral X-ray view [2].

2.1.3 Goals

The aim of the malleolar fracture treatment is to achieve an anatomical reduction and a synthesis with low impact on the soft tissues that are particularly delicate and thin in this area; such osteosynthesis must be adequately stable to allow an early joint mobilization, to prevent the chondral joint degeneration and to lessen the risk of an arthritic evolution [9–11].

If there is a metaphyseal comminution of the fibula that prevents an anatomical reduction of the fracture, the aim is to restore the length and axis of the segments involved that need to be indirectly evaluated through the use of intraoperative fluoroscopy.

2.1.4 Surgical Technique

2.1.4.1 Positioning

A radiolucent table is used; the tourniquet is positioned at the thigh; in most cases the patient is positioned supine, with the lower limb involved free to move inside the surgical field, and the latter needs to be extended a few centimetres proximal to the fracture; a cushion is positioned under the gluteus of the side of the limb that undergoes surgery to abolish its rotation, and the opposite lower limb is elevated, flexed and positioned on a support (Fig. 1.9), to ease the access to the medial malleolus and the execution of the lateral X-ray projections with the image intensifier. A 45° inclination on the unharmed side or a frankly lateral decubitus is needed only if it is necessary to perform a posterior malleolus external surgical access; such positioning requires to move the patient during surgery, after the fibular and/or posterior malleolar stabilization is performed, if a reduction and osteosynthesis also of the medial malleolus fracture are needed. The positioning is terminated once anteroposterior and lateral projections are obtained through fluoroscopy, to be sure that the correct imaging is achieved, before the surgical field is prepared. Such images, kept on the memory of the computer, are useful to be compared with the ones obtained after the reduction during surgery.

2.1.4.2 Instrumentation

The best instrumentation needed for this type of surgery is composed of a basic set, reduction clamps big enough for the dimension of the segment treated; a set of screws and plates with the additional choice of locking fixation devices for the fibula; partially threaded screws, better if cannulated, for the posterior and medial malleoli; and tension bands with 1–1.8 mm diameter wires for the highly comminuted cases.

As regard the fibular hardware, we believe that one third tubular plates, with 3.5 mm screws (Synthes®) are very functional; it is possible to use version of these plates with locking screws, which is enough to manage the main problems related to this segment: this is an excellent compromise between efficient synthesis and low impact on the soft tissues. Only if there are seriously comminuted fractures or a very proximal extension of the fracture is it necessary to use plates that are thicker and less mouldable, like the reconstruction ones, or to use preformed plates, so-called anatomical.

The latter allow a combination of different diameter screws such as 2.4, 2.7 and 3.5 mm, having more holes with different directions in the distal part that grant the fixation of the more apical segments even if very little; furthermore, they are built to adapt on the normal bony anatomy; this allows the possibility to use a minimally invasive technique (MIPO). Although these are undeniable advantages, the thickness of these plates is a limitation in consequence of their bulkiness on the soft tissues, so the shared indications are the more comminuted cases, with the impossibility of an anatomical reduction, situations in which there is an important osteoporosis and in conditions where the apical segment is too little to allow the positioning of at least two screws of 3.5 mm diameter.

2.1.4.3 Surgical Approach

Usually the surgical treatment starts from the fibula, which is reached through a frankly lateral incision; it is a simple and direct access, without any specific dangers; the only attention that must be kept when performing the skin incision, which must not be too anterior, is to avoid the risk of damaging the superficial peroneal nerve that runs longitudinal just over the fibula (Fig. 2.2): it is an exclusively sensitive nerve that infrequently can be involved and damaged by the fracture fragments; but in the normal situations, the nerve is not seen because it remains inside the upper part of the surgical wound; in these cases it is best to find it and dissect it to have it protected with a lace during all the surgery. This is because if the superficial sural nerve is injured, it can lead to very painful neuromas with an important dysaesthesia that can lead to a poor clinical result of the osteosynthesis [2, 3].

The tibial malleolus is reached through a medial incision, usually straight and central or, as an alternative, curved posterior if there is the need to avoid areas of soft tissue suffering.

Even in this case the access is direct to the bone, without any structures that need to be identified in the soft tissues; the only attention that must be paid is to protect the branch of the saphenous vein that is anterior to the upper side of the malleolus (Fig. 2.3).

The posterolateral approach, seldom required, is performed through a skin incision between the Achilles tendon and the peroneal tendons and allows to dominate either the fibula, which is reached from its posterior aspect after a deep dissection through the peroneal tendons, or the third malleolus, reached posteriorly through the peroneal tendons, avoiding during dissection the sural nerve that crosses the surgical route in the soft tissues at the level of the Achilles fat pad (Fig. 2.4).

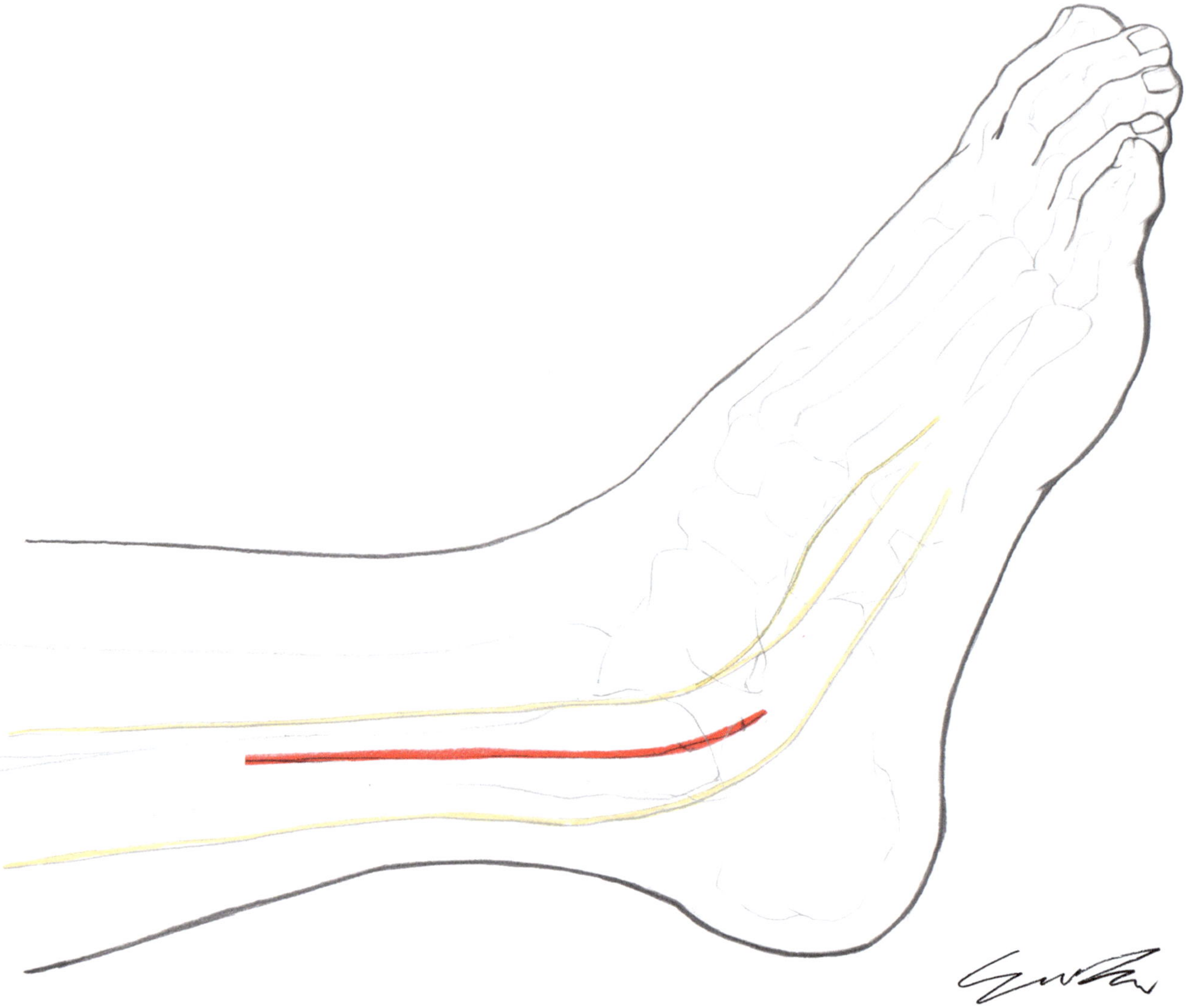

Fig. 2.2 Lateral surgical access to the fibula: the incision is longitudinal, centred over the bony component; it allows to avoid the sural nerve that passes posteriorly and more importantly to avoid the superficial peroneal nerve that runs adjacent to the anterior margin of the fibula

2.1.4.4 Reduction and Osteosynthesis

Fibula

Considering the simple pattern fractures, the transverse type represents an exception, where the reduction is easy and the compression is achieved through an asymmetrical positioning of the screws in specific plates (e.g. Synthes® dynamic compression plate), following the AO technique [2, 12]. In most of the cases, the fracture line is oblique, and a specific sequence of steps has to be followed to obtain reduction and osteosynthesis.

The reduction goal consists to restore exactly length and rotation of the fibula: this is possible by moving the distal segment, mobile, on the proximal diaphyseal segment, that is more fixed. This step is achievable through a careful surgical debridement of the bone segments, with the aim of enlightening them, without compromising the anatomy of the single fragments. This will allow seeing the successful reduction of the latter through a precise correspondence of the opposed surfaces. The key area to observe this correspondence is the posterior wall of the fibula, where the perfect match of its asperities is the necessary demonstration of a good reduction. The steps that need to be done to achieve such result are the traction to regain the correct length and the rotation to correct any torsional defect; to do so, and to perform delicate manoeuvres, pointed reduction clamps are very useful. They need to be used with extreme caution to avoid any iatrogenic additional fractures, specifically if there is an osteoporotic bone.

Once a satisfying reduction is obtained, it is very important to stabilize it through the use of a clamp that will

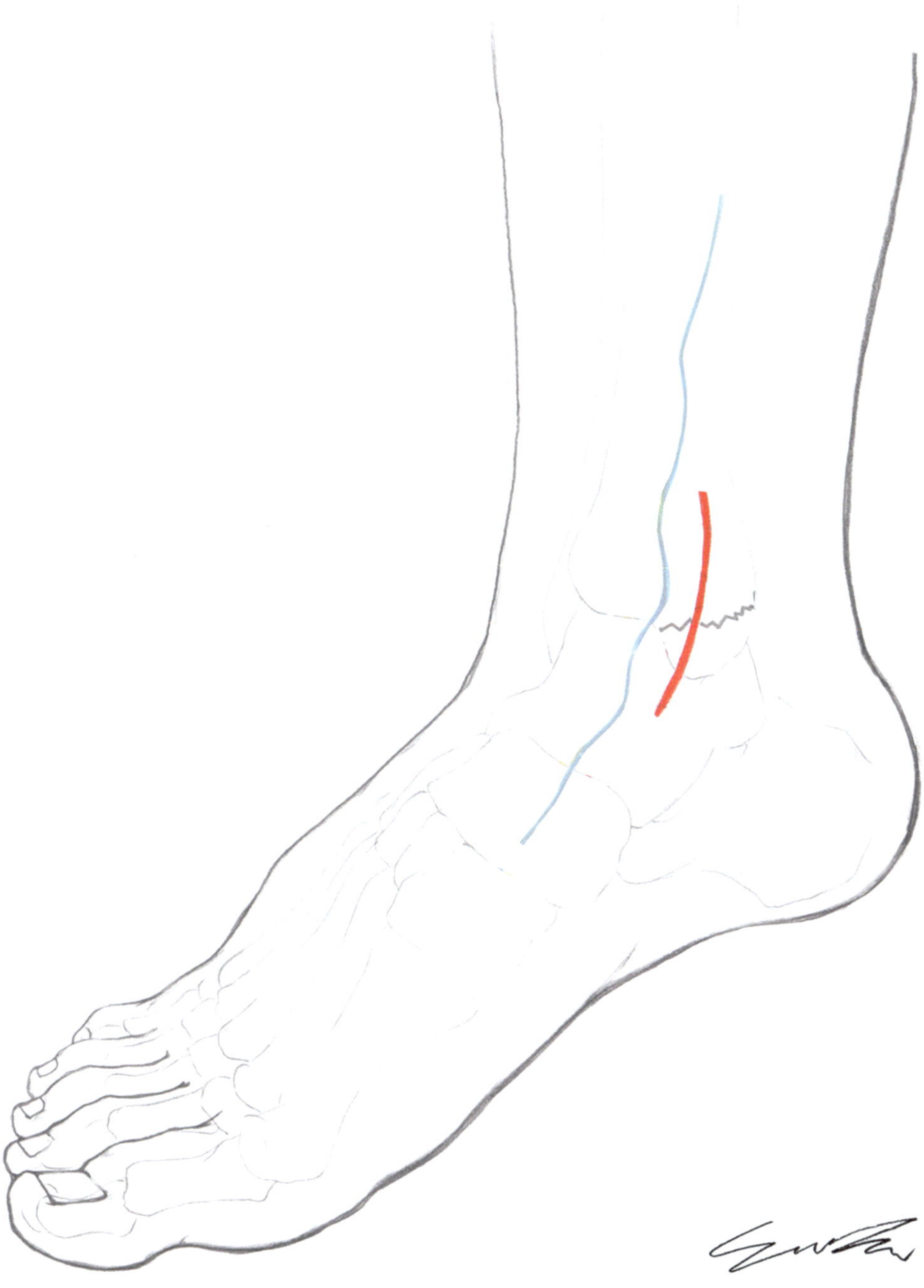

Fig. 2.3 Surgical Approach to the tibial malleolus: the skin incision is centred on the bone, being careful to protect during the dissection if possible the saphenous branch that passes on the anterior malleolus edge

allow to perform a compression synthesis in the best conditions, without any translational stress (Fig. 2.5). The compression osteosynthesis is delegated to one or two interfragmentary screws, based upon the extension and obliquity of the fracture line; it is important to use thinner screws (2.7 or 2.4 mm) than the classic 3.5 mm diameter, to avoid any secondary iatrogenic fractures, above all, when the thickness of the bone segment is limited. Regardless of the diameter, the positioning technique for this essential screw is always the same: first it requires a gliding hole in the near cortex, with the same axis as the thread hole in the far cortex; the diameter of the gliding hole is the same as the thread of the screw so that the thread gets no purchase. Then a drill sleeve is placed within the gliding hole to direct the drill bit for the threaded hole in the far cortex. A drill hole, which has the same diameter as the core of the screw, is drilled, and a depth gauge is used to determine the screw length; the screw is

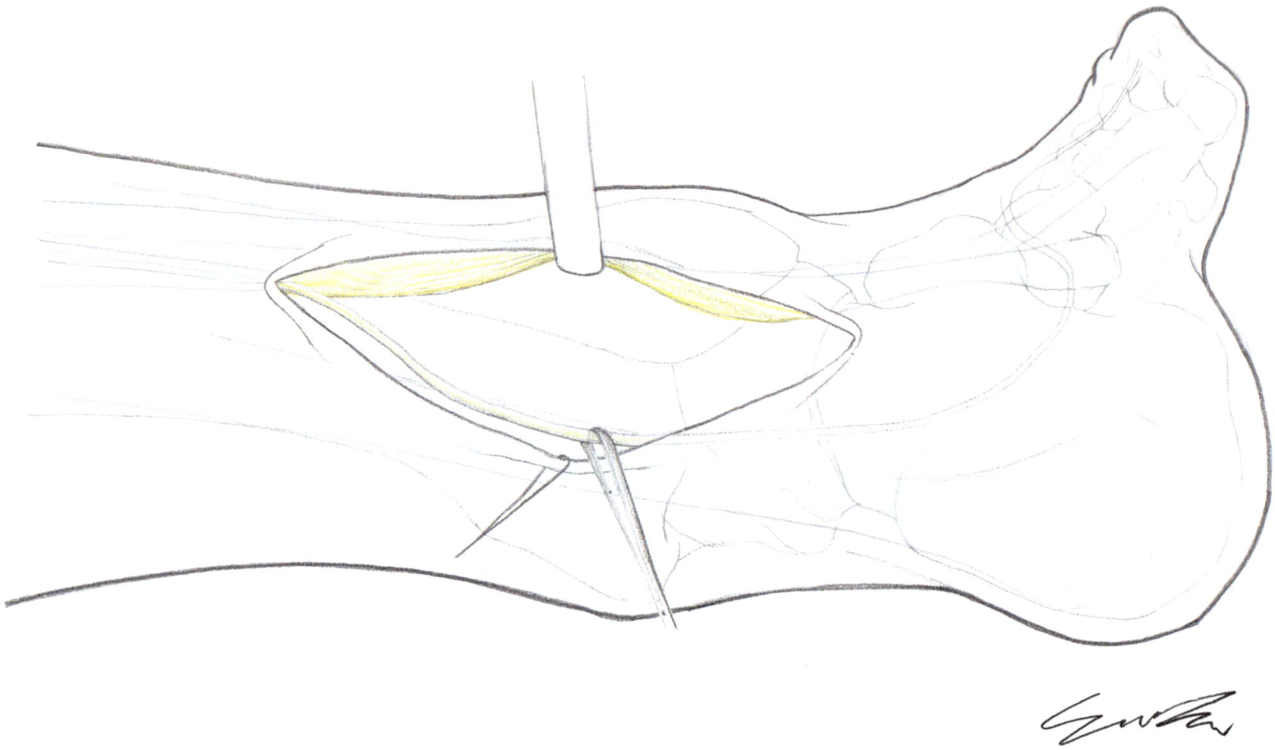

Fig. 2.4 Posterior surgical access to the posterior malleolus: the skin incision is done between the Achilles tendon and the peroneal tendons; the access to the third malleolus is granted retracting anteriorly the peroneal tendons and posteriorly protecting, after having it dissected, the sural nerve

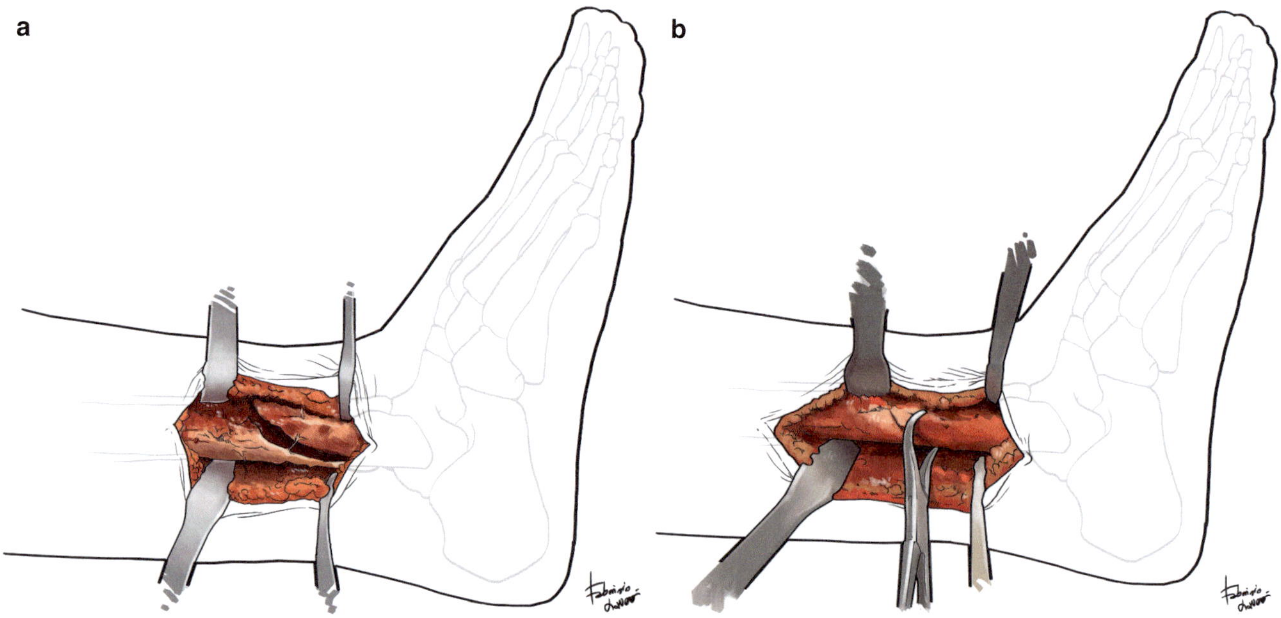

Fig. 2.5 Isolated and prepared carefully the extremities of the fracture (**a**), the reduction and temporary fixation is achieved through a pointed surgical clamp for little segments (**b**)

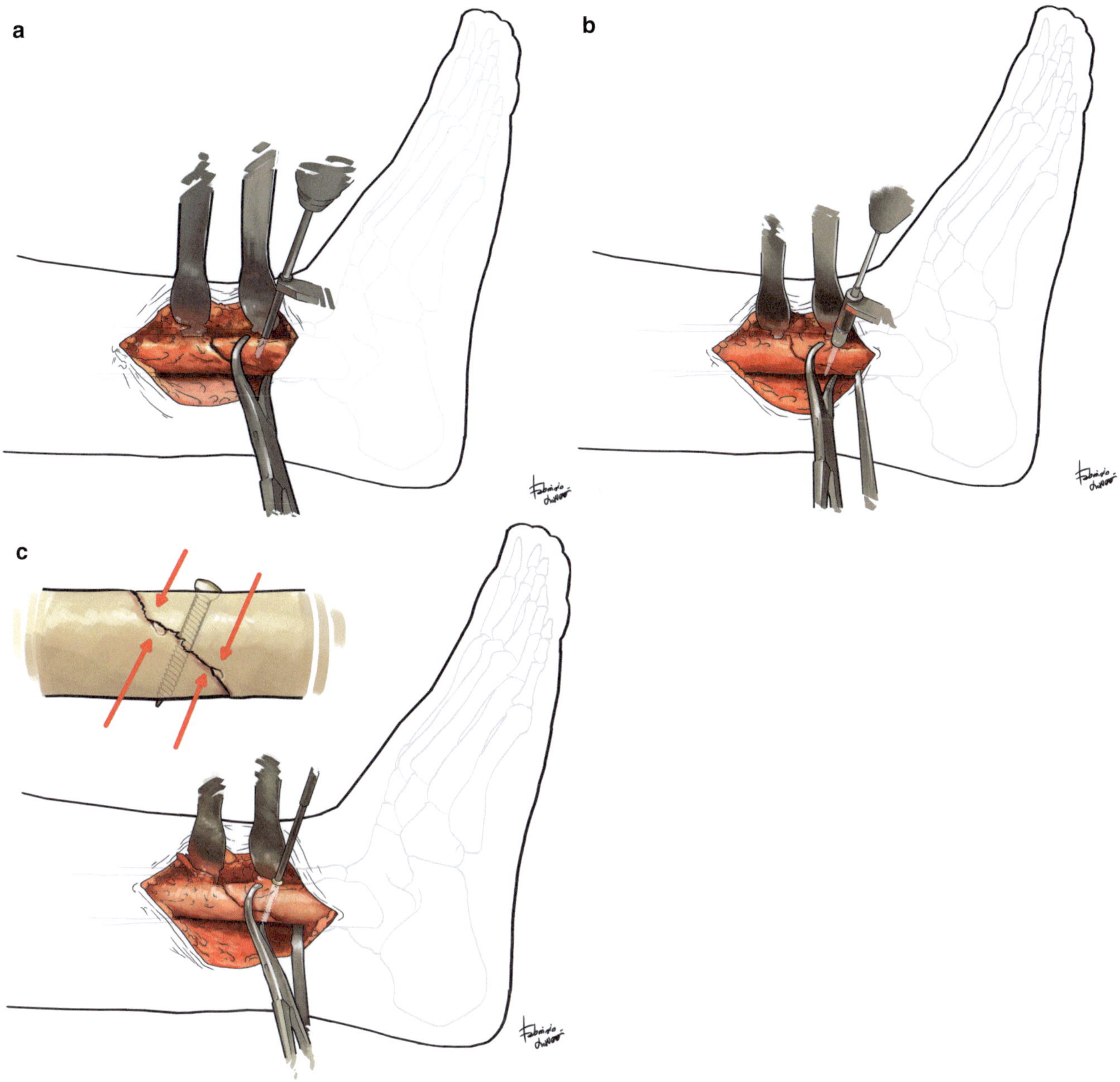

Fig. 2.6 Synthesis of the fibula with a free compression screw: (**a**) realization of the sliding hole, with a drill bit of the same diameter of the chosen screw; (**b**) the centering drill guide is inserted in the sliding hole and the hole in the opposite cortex is done with a drill bit under dimensioned; (**c**) after measuring to select the correct length, the screw is inserted, and thanks to the sliding hole, the compression of the fracture is achieved

then inserted either with motorized instrumentation or hand screwdriver. It's important that the last turns of the screw must be done with the hand screwdriver to better dose the compression effect (Fig. 2.6).

The direction of the screw is mainly perpendicular to the fracture line or along the bisector between the perpendicular of the latter and the perpendicular of the bone segment, if there is a force acting on the axis of the bone that fosters a translation of the bone segments during the tightening of the screw [13]. The synthesis with the compression screws is then protected through a neutralizing plate, generally placed on the lateral surface of the bone; with the increased solidness achieved with the locking plates, it is possible to ignore the rule of three screws for each side of the osteosynthesis to consider it stable: to grant early mobilization of the affected limb, it is considered enough the use of two screws for each side of the osteosynthesis, when at least one screw in both parts is fixed on the plate [14] (Fig. 2.7); this results particularly useful in those fractures where the fracture line extends more distally. The use of one cortical screw for each side of

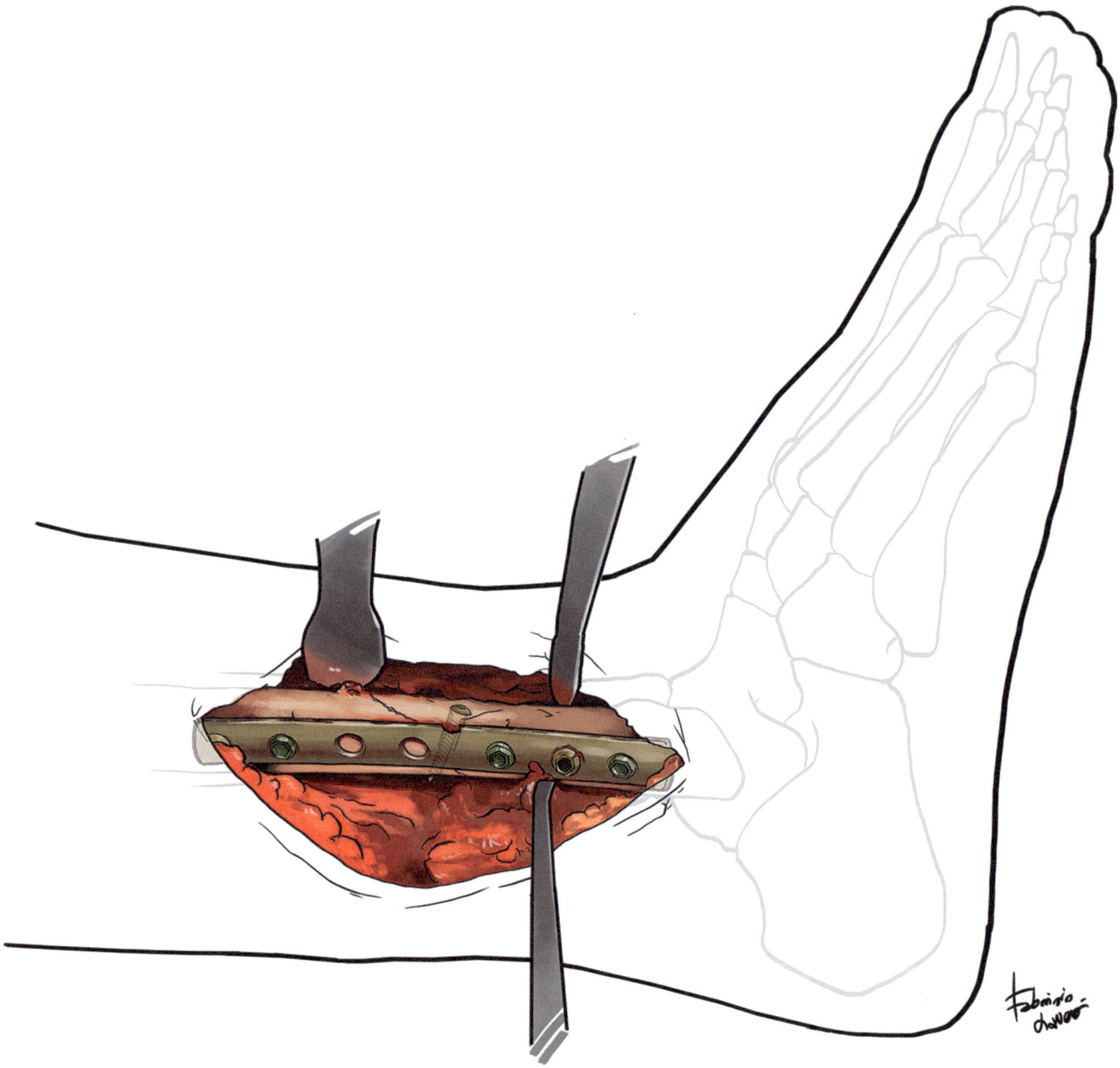

Fig. 2.7 Image obtained after the positioning of the 1/3 tubular neutralizing plate (Synthes®), protecting the synthesis of a cortical lag screw. The yellow screws are conventional, and the green are locking screws that allow to increase considerably the stability of the device

the fracture line allows to fit precisely the plate on the bone reducing the bulkiness of the plate on the soft tissues; when using different combinations of cortical and locking screws, it is essential, like in any other segment, to remember to position the latter only after that the normal screws are fixed, to avoid the loss of grip between the bone-screw interface due to mechanical stress.

If a fracture morphology that eases the posterior sliding of the fragments is present or if a surgical access that allows it has been used, the plate can be positioned posterior to the fibula, avoiding any kind of friction with the peroneal tendons that are located nearby [1, 15].

There are no substantial changes if the fracture line is complex, but there is only one butterfly fragment associated, especially if the dimensions are inferior to the diameter of the bone; but in the case of an extensive comminution and if an anatomical reduction is impossible, it is appropriate to use techniques of indirect alignment of the fracture, sliding the implants under the soft tissues to respect the biology of the injured segments and bridging the comminution with the plate. Before fixing the plate to the bone, fluoroscopy is needed to check the correct length and rotation of the segment, achievable through external manoeuvres and comparing the healthy

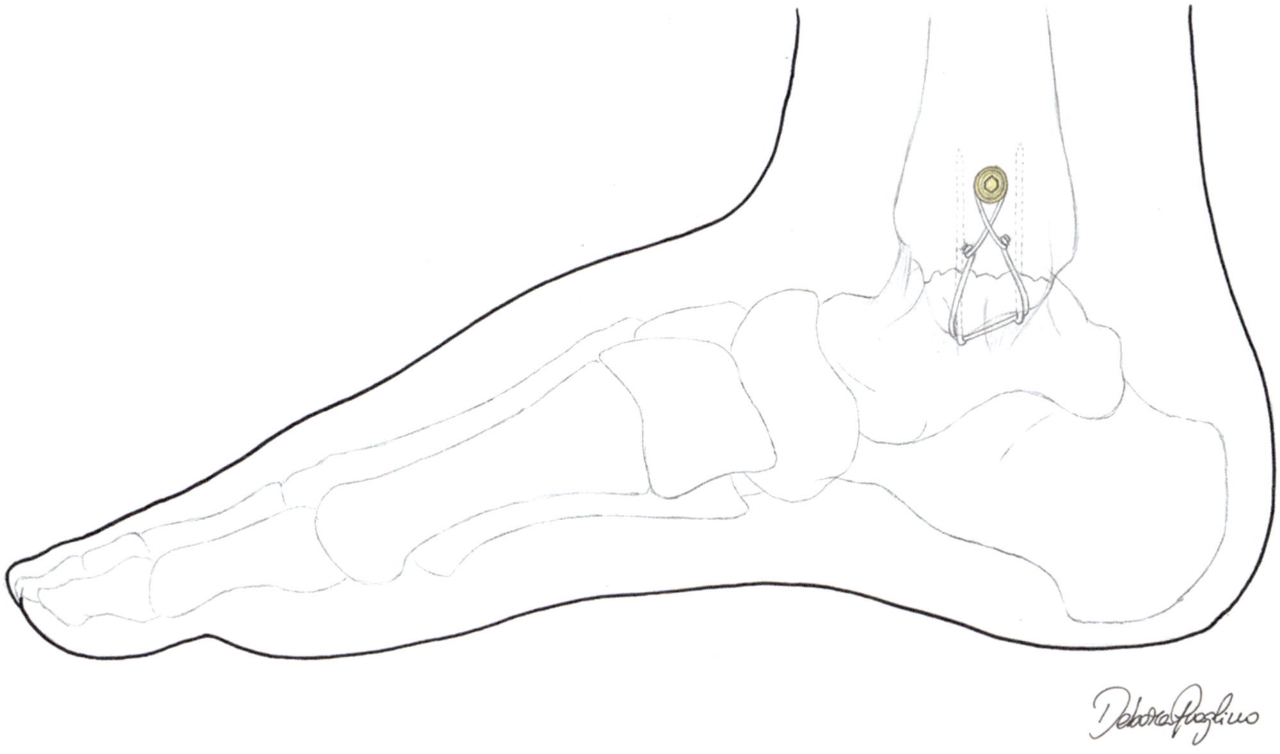

Fig. 2.8 Scheme of tension band with proximal anchoring with a metaphyseal screw, useful to synthetize highly comminuted medial malleolus fractures; the two vertical wires are bent as a hook and drowned into the bone after the tension band is tensioned

side for the length and using indirect landmarks, such as the correspondence with the lateral profile of the talus to check the rotation [2].

Tibial Malleolus

Even for the tibial malleolus, the surgical debridement of the fractured segments is mandatory, where all the single matching lines must be identified without compromising the bone, because it could threaten the reduction phase.

Once the reduction is achieved, the osteosynthesis is performed with two partially threaded screws, diameter 4.0 and 4.5 mm, which are positioned perpendicular to the fracture line with the aid of the fluoroscopy to check the correct placement.

The possibility of using cannulated screws simplifies the correct positioning; if the malleolar fragment is too little to fit two screws, it is possible to use only one, adding a Kirschner wire or a PLLA pin, left completely buried in the bone, acting as an antirotatory effect.

If there is a comminution of the malleolus, the best solution is a tension band built with wires of diameter between 1 and 1.8 mm, fixed to the main bone fragments to keep the reduction in relation to their size and anchored proximally through a free 3.5 mm screw fixed to the tibia (Fig. 2.8).

If the dimension of the third malleolus fragment requires a surgical treatment [2], this is reduced by indirect ligamentotaxis, by the action of the tibiofibular inferior posterior ligament during the reduction of the lateral malleolus or by open reduction through a posterior access to the fibula.

The decision regarding the type of synthesis influences the surgical access selected; for this reason it must be carefully studied during the preoperative planning, built on a complete radiological imaging. Once reduced, it is possible to synthetize this fragment positioning one or more free screws in a compression configuration of diameter 4 or 4.5 mm, with an anteroposterior or postero-anterior direction. In both cases the screws must be partially threaded or with a sliding hole in the bony part were the screw is inserted [2]. The more the fragment is posterior, the more it's difficult to stabilize it, and the more it is useful to have cannulated screws. The osteosynthesis option with postero-anterior direction grants an easier positioning of the entire thread of the screw overtaking the fracture line.

Once the malleoli are reduced, if there is instability of the tibiofibular syndesmosis, this must be stabilized through a trans-syndesmotic screw. If there is a doubt regarding the indication, the final decision is taken evaluating the intraoperative x-ray anteroposterior projection, showing if there is

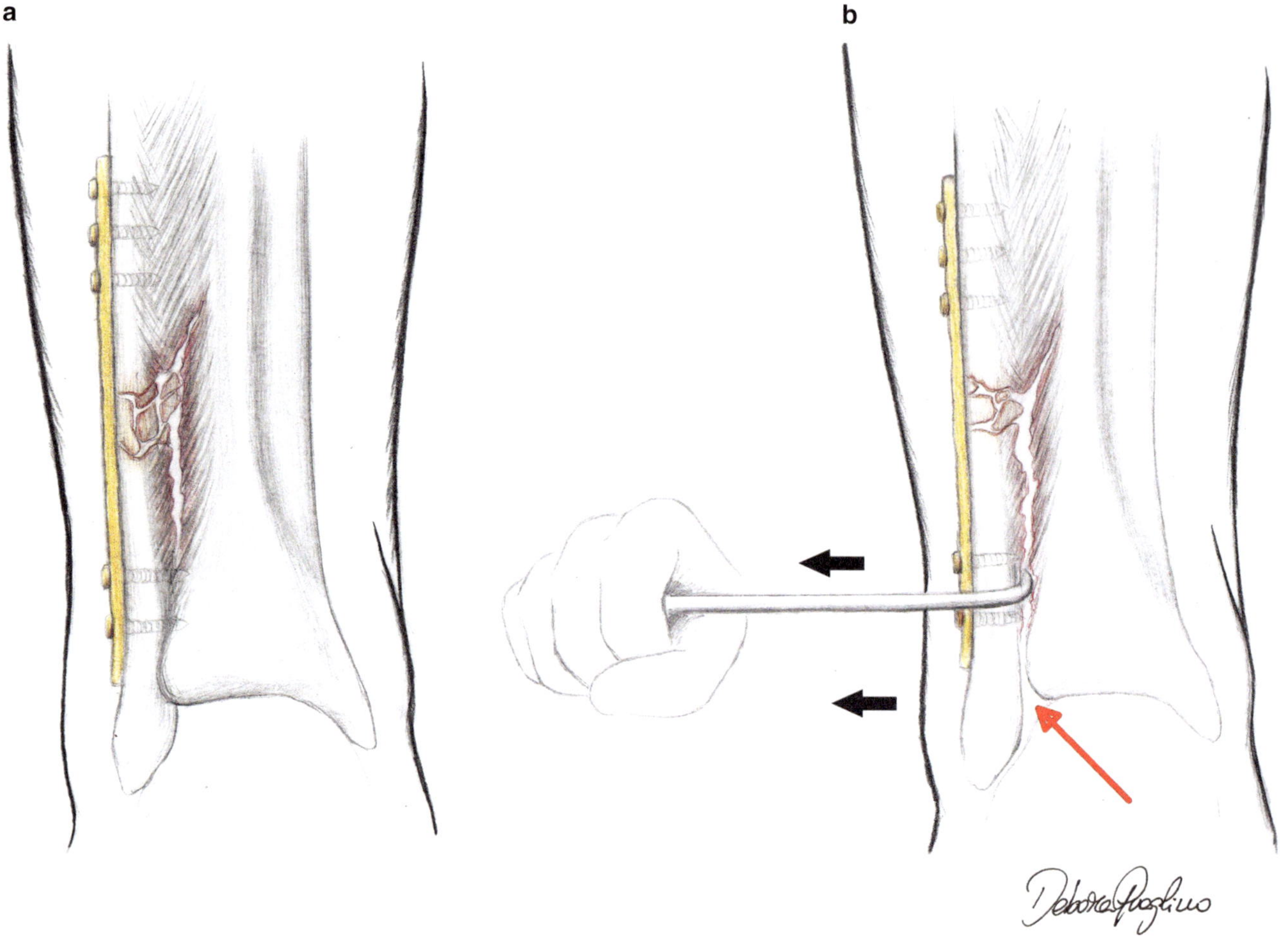

Fig. 2.9 Hook test to detect a possible injury of the tibiofibular syndesmosis: if after fibular synthesis is performed (**a**), pulling laterally the fibula with a hook (**b**), a gap of the latter with the tibia (red arrow) is seen, it means that the test is positive and that there is a lesion that needs to be treated

an asymmetry of the medial gutter, with the confirmation of the hook test: stressing in a posterolateral direction with a hook the fibula after the synthesis, it is possible to see any abnormal translation of the syndesmosis [2] (Fig. 2.9).

Many controversies are present regarding the positioning of the stabilizing synthesis at this level; considering carefully the anatomical characteristics and the goal pursued, the more rational way of proceeding seems to be the following (Fig. 2.10):

- The screw must be positioned proximal to the syndesmosis, without crossing it, to avoid the possibility of reactive ossification of the interosseous membrane.
- The direction of the screw must be parallel to the joint line with a postero-anterior inclination of about 30°, to adapt to the anatomy of the segment.
- The screw used is fully threaded and without any gliding holes, therefore not in compression, but only to stabilize the correct position of the malleolar mortise, achieved through the help of a second surgeon or the use of a tong clamp applied on the external part of the malleoli, keeping the ankle at a 90° angle to allow the correct housing of the anterior part of the body of the talus, larger, in the tibiofibular mortise and to avoid excessive narrowing of the latter [2].
- The fixation of this screw is limited to three cortices that appear to be enough to grant the maintenance of the correct positioning and has a lower grade of complications [2, 16].
- The X-ray intraoperative check must go along all the steps of this stabilizing procedure (Fig. 2.11).

2.1.4.5 Postoperative Care

The postoperative programme prescribes the non-weight bearing of the lower limb that is kept in a splint in a functional position for 2 weeks, removing the stitches simultaneously with the splint; from then a mobilization is begun keeping a non-weight bearing on the affected limb. If positioned, the supra-syndesmotic tricortical screw is removed, through a

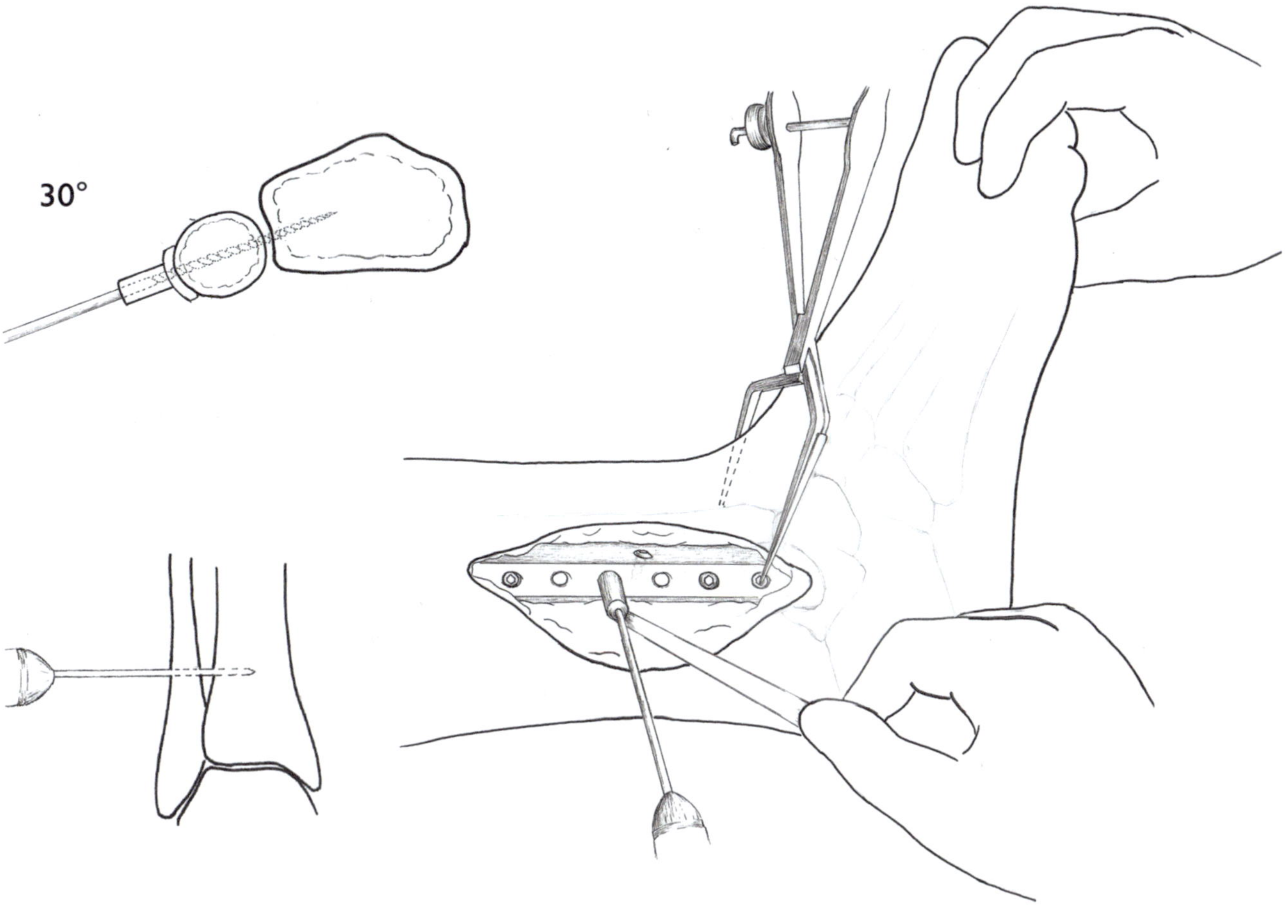

Fig. 2.10 Tibiofibular syndesmosis screw positioning procedure: the screw is positioned with the ankle flexed at 90°, tricortical, proximal to the syndesmosis, parallel to the joint line and tilted from posterior to anterior at 30°

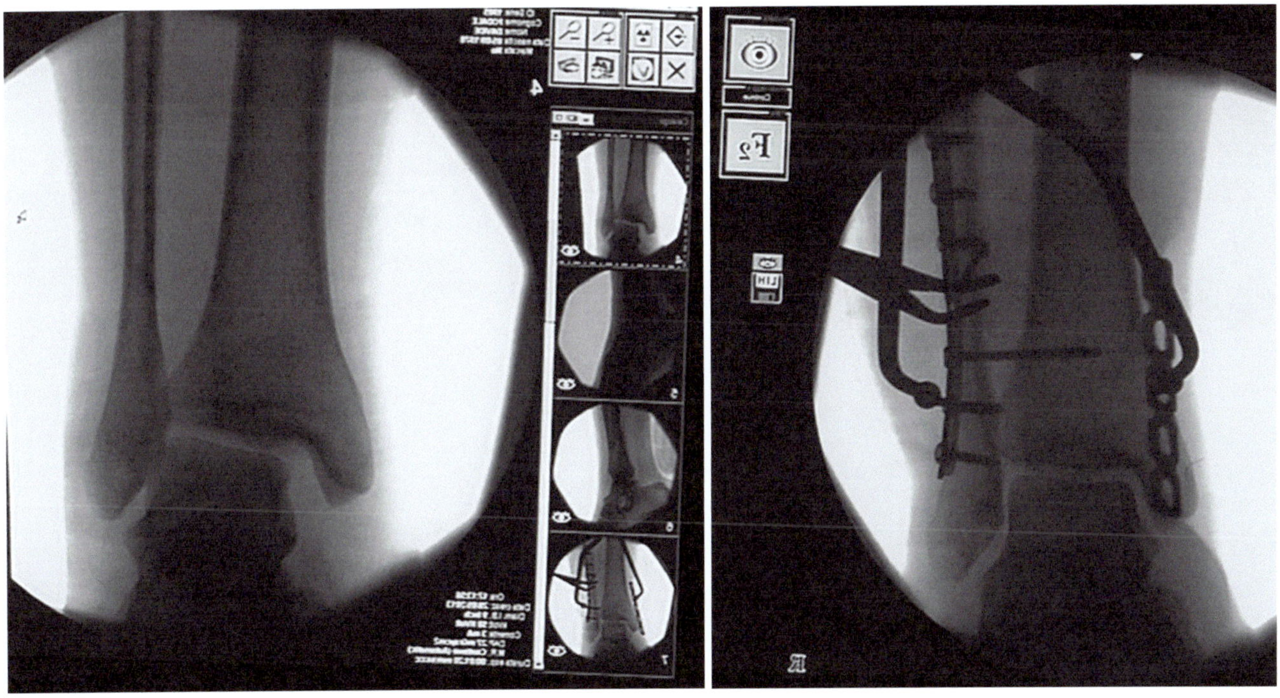

Fig. 2.11 The X-ray confirms the recovery of the correct skeletal relationships, compared to the initial diastasis, of the tibiofibular distal syndesmosis, achieved with the external reduction manoeuvres and stabilized with a tricortical screw

local anaesthesia, after 6 weeks post surgery. Checking with the X-ray imaging the correct evolution of the healing process, after 60 days, weight bearing is allowed with the use of crutches, and after 90 days the full weight bearing is allowed.

References

1. Court-Brown CM, Caesar B (2006) Epidemiology of adult fractures: a review. Injury 37(8):691–697
2. Hahn DM, Colton CL (2007) Malleoli. In: Ruedi TP, Buckley RE, Moran CG (eds) AO principles of fracture management, 2nd expanded edn. Thieme, New York, pp 871–897
3. Walling AK, Sanders RW (2007) Ankle fractures. In: Coughlin MJ, Mann RA, Saltzman CL (eds) Surgery of the foot and ankle, 8th edn. Mosby Elsevier, Philadelphia, pp 1973–2016
4. Kellam JF, Audigé L (2007) Fracture classification. In: Ruedi TP, Buckley RE, Moran CG (eds) AO principles of fracture management, 2nd expanded edn. Thieme, New York, pp 69–85
5. Schepers T, De Vries MR, Van Lieshout EM et al (2013) The timing of ankle fracture surgery and the effect on infectious complications; a case series and systematic review of the literature. Int Orthop 37(3):489–494
6. Tarkin IS, Sop A, Pape HC (2008) High-energy foot and ankle trauma: principles for formulating an individualized care plan. Foot Ankle Clin 13:705–723
7. Tarkin IS, Clare MP, Marcantonio A et al (2008) An update on the management of high-energy pilon fractures. Injury 39(2):142–154
8. Khan U, Smitham P, Pearse M et al (2007) Management of severe open ankle injuries. Plast Reconstr Surg 119(2):578–589
9. Stover MD, Kellam J (2007) Articular fractures principles. In: Ruedi TP, Buckley RE, Moran CG (eds) AO principles of fracture management, 2nd expanded edn. Thieme, New York, pp 139–153
10. Buckwalter JA (1995) Activity vs. rest in the treatment of bone, soft tissue and joint injuries. Iowa Orthop J 15:29–42
11. Mitchell N, Shepard N (1980) Healing of articular cartilage in intrarticular fractures in rabbits. J Bone Joint Surg Am 62A(4): 628–634
12. Lorich DG, Gardner MJ (2007) Plates. In: Ruedi TP, Buckley RE, Moran CG (eds) AO principles of fracture management, 2nd expanded edn. Thieme, New York, pp 227–247
13. Messmer P, Perren SM, Suhm N (2007) Screws. In: Ruedi TP, Buckley RE, Moran CG (eds) AO principles of fracture management, 2nd expanded edn. Thieme, New York, pp 213–225
14. Sommer C, Schutz M, Wagner M (2007) Internal fixator. In: Ruedi TP, Buckley RE, Moran CG (eds) AO principles of fracture management, 2nd expanded edn. Thieme, New York, pp 321–335
15. Ostrum RF (1996) Posterior plating of displaced Weber B fibula fractures. J Orthop Trauma 10:199–203
16. Wikerøy AK, Høiness PR, Andreassen GS et al (2010) No difference in functional and radiographic results 8.4 years after quadricortical compared with tricortical syndesmosis fixation in ankle fractures. J Orthop Trauma 24(1):17–23

Subcutaneous Rupture of the Achilles Tendon

3

Contents

3.1 Subcutaneous Rupture of the Achilles Tendon

It is an extremely frequent injury, with an incidence of 18 cases over 100,000 individuals per year and with a main involvement of the male gender (84%) [1].

There are two main peaks of onset, one between the age of 35 and 40 years, with injuries caused by sport trauma (more frequent in soccer, basketball and volleyball), and one in elder age, over 55 years, without any connection with the activities performed in the moment of the injury [2].

The loss of anatomical continuity takes place in a precise moment, in which the patient becomes symptomatic, usually associated with a traumatic event, but it is acknowledged that this is the final event, frequently with a low-energy involvement, that ends a degenerative chronic process that changes the normal tendon, provoking a progressive fibre laceration [3].

Considering these premises, it is understandable how the clinical presentation can be evident but in some cases less certain or even misleading, with 25% of injuries unknown at 7 days from the trauma and 15% at 3 weeks [4].

3.1.1 Injury Areas

Classically the injury involves the mid-third of the tendon, in 75% of the times; this is due to the anatomical characteristics of this segment, that is, the most distant from the vessels that supply the tendon and for this reason the less vascularized; furthermore it is the segment with the minor diameter: for these reasons the tendon in this part is mechanically less strong and with the healing process impaired [5]. Only in the 14–24% of the cases the injury interests the distal third of the tendon, with possible avulsions that need to be repaired through a reinsertion with anchors or screws connected with big diameter non-absorbable sutures (see

W. Daghino et al., *Foot and Ankle Trauma Injuries*, https://doi.org/10.1007/978-3-319-69617-1_3

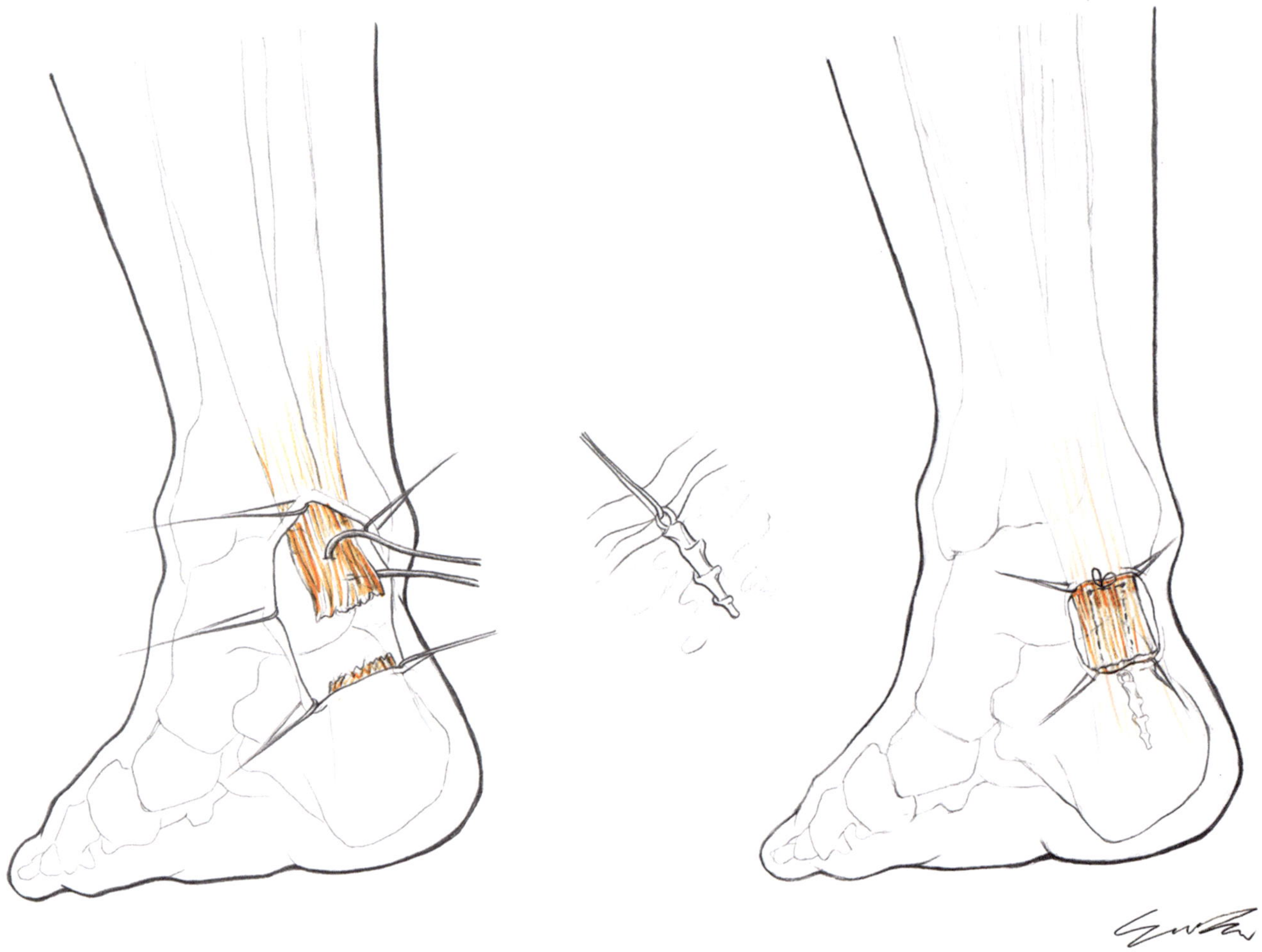

Fig. 3.1 Distal detachment of the Achilles tendon: once the tendon is isolated and the posterior tuberosity prepared, the reinsertion can be accomplished by the use of non-absorbable sutures, fixed to the bone through an anchor or a transosseous screw

Fig. 3.1). Less frequent (4–14%) are the third proximal injuries. The latter, when so near to the muscle-tendon junction to not leave sufficient tendon to achieve a direct suture, could need to be repaired through the use of a fascia grafts, like those used in the unacknowledged injuries or in the ruptures with a loss of substance [6] (see Fig. 3.2).

3.1.2 Indications

The conservative treatment has its indication only in selected cases, such as in the elderly, in people that are inactive or have low functional requests or in poor general conditions or in subjects that have serious skin or soft tissue modifications or have systemic serious illness. The foot is positioned equinus in a cast or brace for 6 weeks, later recovering the functional position gradually and allowing weight bearing after 8 weeks, with the protection of a heel or of braces that prevent the dorsiflexion of the foot, which need to be removed or switched to a 3 cm heel pad after 3 months from the injury [7].

The reconstructive surgery or the reinsertions of the tendon used in the more peripheral injuries, high or low, are performed considering every time the pathological anatomy of the specific case; instead, the tenorrhaphy is the actual gold treatment for the mid-third injuries, above all, for the proven capacity to reduce the re-rupture rate in comparison with the conservative treatment [8–10]. Furthermore it is reported that the patient satisfaction after surgical treatment is clearly more stable than the conservative option, judged unsatisfactory by one patient every three [1].

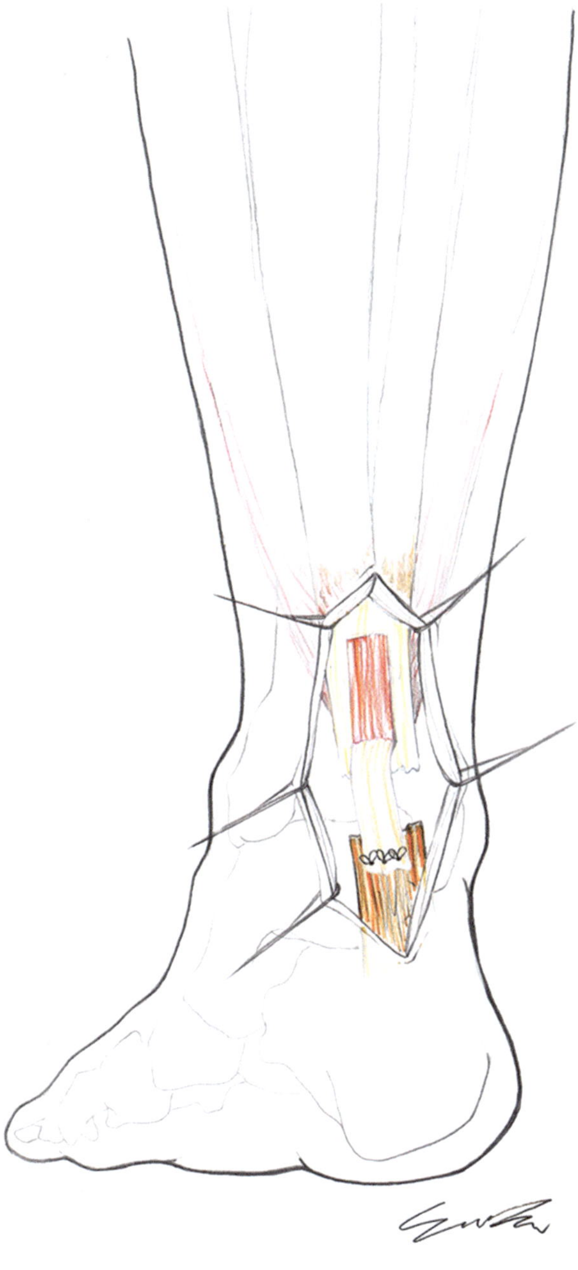

Fig. 3.2 The fascia grafting to repair a high or inveterate injury of the Achilles tendon: a rectangular graft is sculptured on the mid-third of the triceps fascia; once it is tipped over, it grants the correct amount of tissue to repair the injury and restore continuity with the distal stump

3.1.3 Goals

To achieve the goal of obtaining a lower rate of re-rupture after suture, preserving the function of the injured segment, surgery of the subcutaneous Achilles tendon lesion must be able to restore the tendon continuity and above all maintain it in a sufficiently stable way to allow early mobilization, because it is one of the main factors that can improve the outcome of the treatment [11].

3.1.4 Surgical Technique

Independently from the technique chosen, the surgical access is performed with the patient prone, raising the affected limb with a support on the ankle or keeping the feet hanging out from the table, to allow the equinus positioning; a soft cushion under the opposite iliac crest is very useful to nullify the normal tendency to external rotation of the interested foot. With a dermographic pen, after clinical identification, the injured area is marked (Fig. 3.3) and a Thompson test is performed (Fig. 3.4) after anaesthesia, to have a comparable clinical parameter and to evaluate the functionality of the tendon suture that will be performed. At this point the following manoeuvres and cares vary on the base of the used technique. Many different surgical techniques are described, but every one, even with its peculiar characteristics, is placed in one of these three fundamental types: open suture, percutaneous or mini-invasive.

3.1.4.1 Open Tenorrhaphy

It is the more classic way to perform a tendon suture, the first described and still actual and largely appreciated for the solidity that it is able to grant. Unfortunately the large surgical exposure needed generates a high risk of complications on the soft peritendinous tissues, with the possibility of skin suffering or necrosis and the formation of scar adhesions between the tendon and the overlying tissues that can spoil the outcome [12]. Such complications are more frequent if associated with other risk factors such as smoke, steroid use, diabetes, female gender and age over 50 years old [13], and the patient must be adequately informed of these facts before signing a written consent.

Preoperative Preparation

It is necessary to position a tourniquet on the thigh, because it is advisable to perform the surgery without blood to have a better view of the tissues that need to be repaired.

Instrumentation

For this surgery, sutures are needed to suspend the soft tissues; besides braided, non-absorbable and of high diameter sutures to perform the tenorrhaphy (e.g. Flexidene® 2), braided or monofilament absorbable sutures of lower diameter (3-0, 4-0 and 5-0) can be useful after the ana-

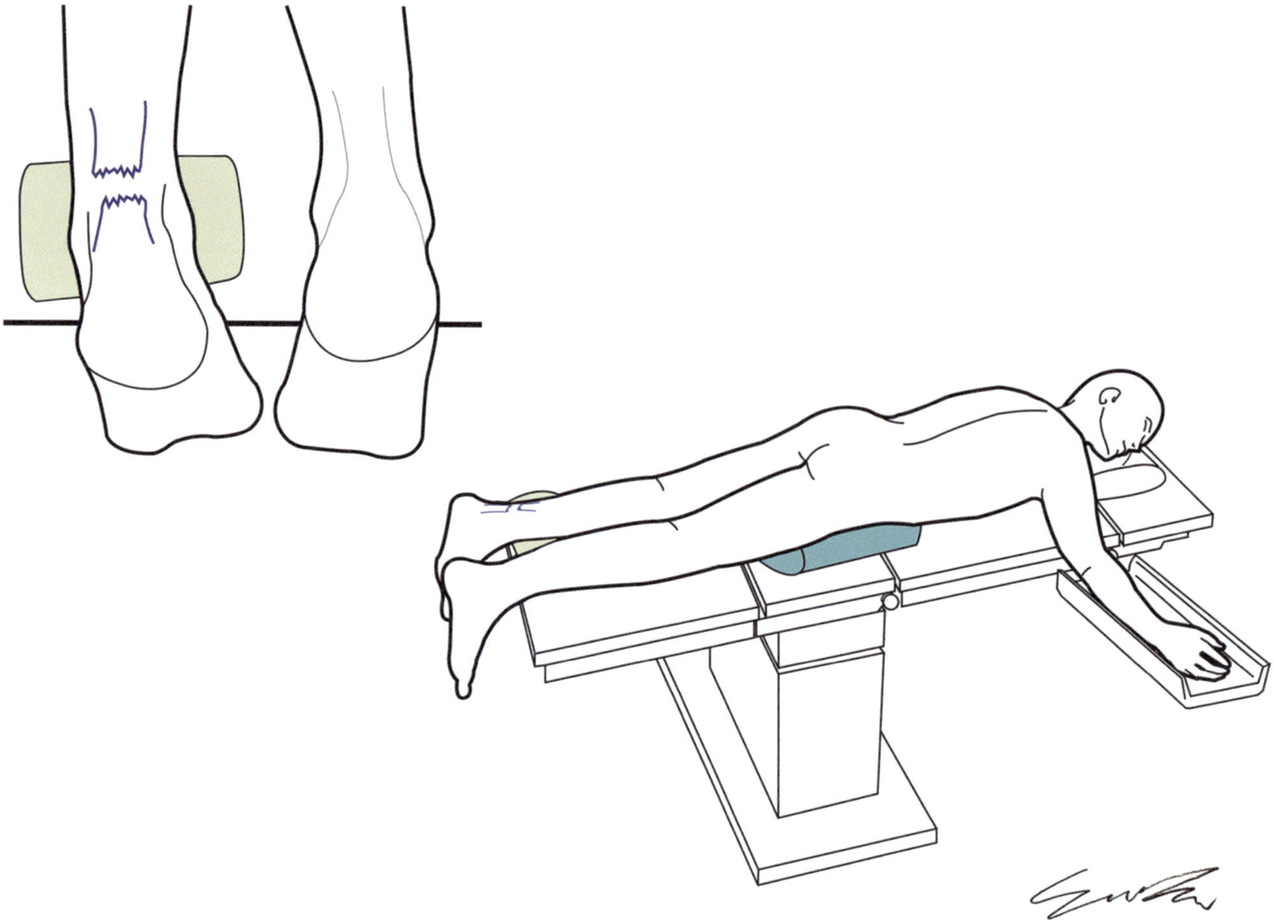

Fig. 3.3 Achilles tenorrhaphy: the patient is positioned prone on the table; a cushion is positioned under the iliac crest on the opposite side granting a reduction of the lower limb rotation

tomical continuity is restored to achieve a tubular shape of the tendon, to perfect the tendon and to reconstruct the peritenon.

Surgical Access

A longitudinal incision, directly medial to the tendon, is performed, to protect the sural nerve that lies just by the lateral border of the Achilles tendon; it is extended proximally and distally until a healthy tendon is spotted, resulting usually of many centimetres.

The peritenon is identified and separated from the subcutaneous tissues, with highly delicate manoeuvres to preserve its integrity and to avoid iatrogenic injuries to this important structure that represents the main barrier against the formation of tendon adhesions. Once it is isolated, it is incised longitudinally showing the underlying tendon.

Restoration of Continuity

The tendon distally and proximally is freed from all the area with the typical fibrillar degeneration that led to the rupture of the tendon until healthy tissue is exposed; afterwards the two tendon stumps are captured with sutures.

Many different techniques are described: the more known and used are outlined in the Fig. 3.5. The continuity of the tendon is restored closing the sutures with the end of the wire that point out the tendon stumps, if needed with the foot held in slight equinism to facilitate the contact of the two parts; if the latter is not enough or the resulting tension is excessive or the suture isn't adequately stable, a reinforcement with the gracilis tendon is advocated (Fig. 3.6). These techniques, through the detachment of the proximal or distal part of the gracilis tendon, can be useful, but they increase the aggressiveness of the procedure [14]. Once the main procedure is ended, some sutures are used to tubulize the reconstructed tendon, with continuous stitches or with single stitches, performed through the use of a low-calibre absorbable suture; the restoration of a tubular shape of the tendon, in addition to the reorientation of the injured fibres, grants the best reconstruction of the overlying peritenon, which is essential for the best outcome, even if it is

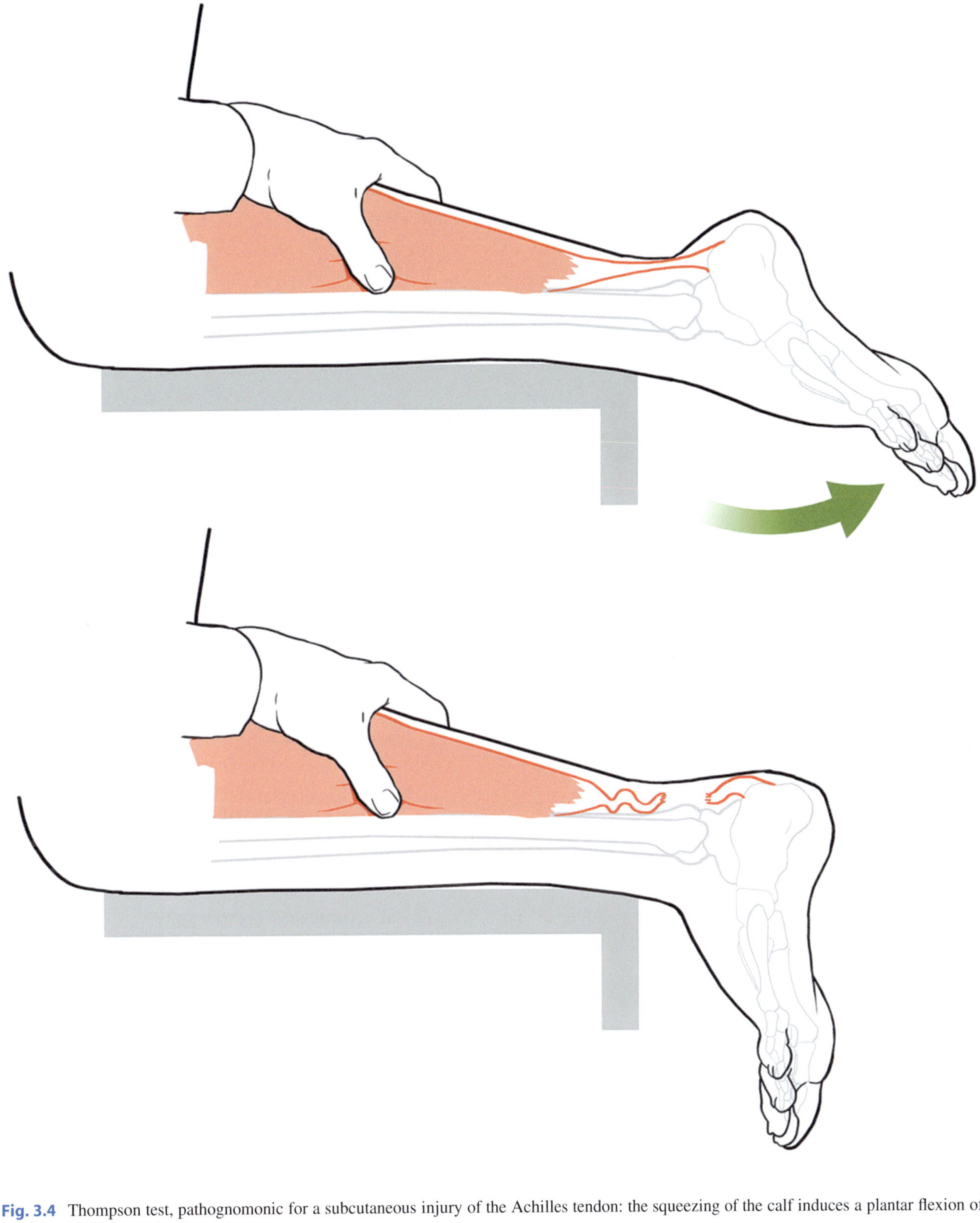

Fig. 3.4 Thompson test, pathognomonic for a subcutaneous injury of the Achilles tendon: the squeezing of the calf induces a plantar flexion of the foot only if the tendon is continuous

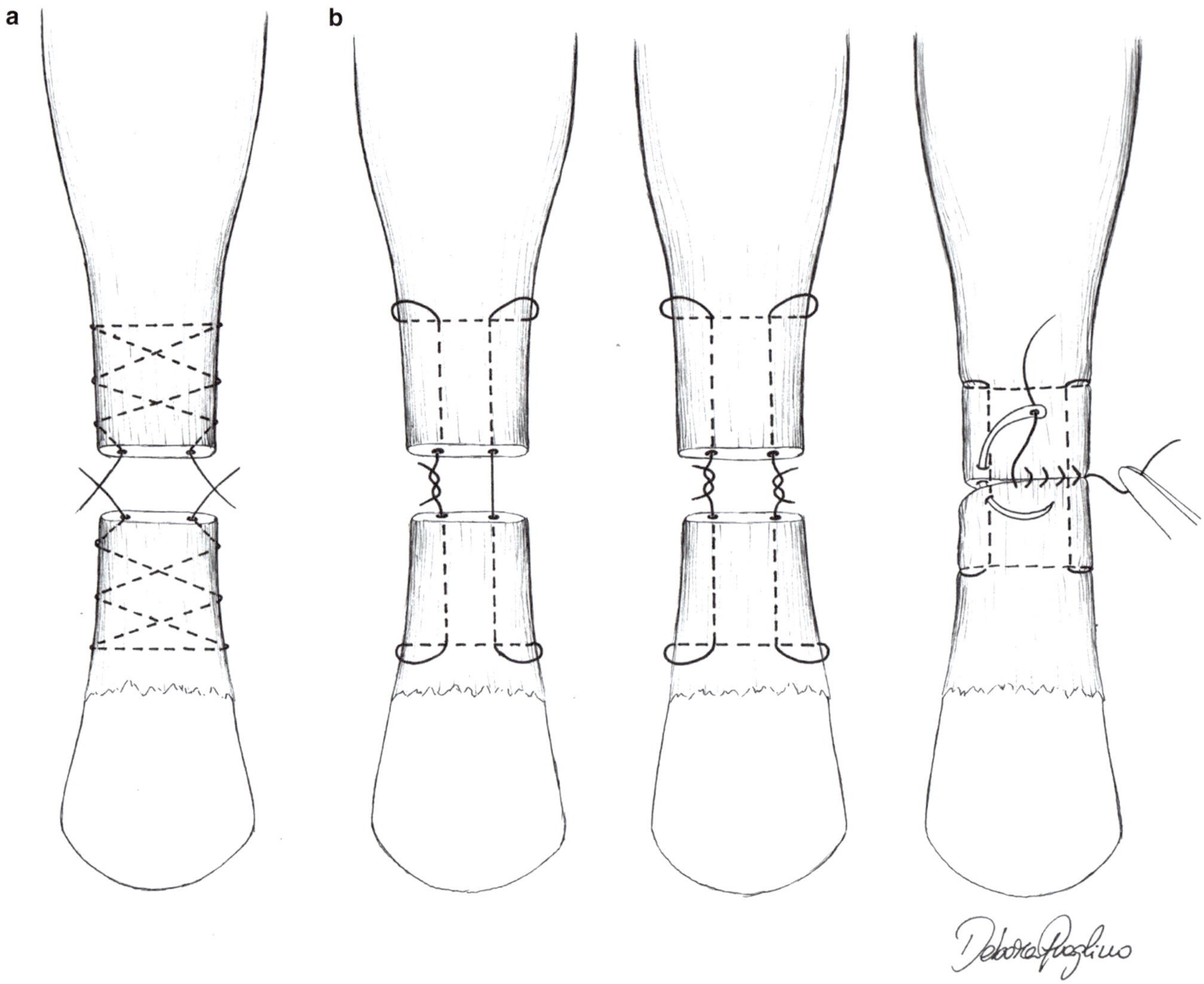

Fig. 3.5 Open tenorrhaphy: Bunnell type (**a**); Kessler type (**b**), with the one thread or two threads and with continuous suture for tubulization

very difficult to obtain. In this manner the sliding of the tendon is granted, reducing the risk of adhesions after surgery [15].

Postoperative Care

Considering the high aggressiveness on the soft tissues typical of this technique, a proper resting period is needed to foster the healing process. For this reason the foot is kept in slight equinism through the use of a plaster cast or brace for 4 weeks, following a period of a progressive recovery of the functional position of the foot that needs to be done in the following 4 weeks; the full weight bearing is allowed after 12 weeks, with a 2 cm insole that grants a slight equinism of the foot in the shoes. Any kinds of functional solicitations (jumping, running, leaping) are avoided for 5–6 months after surgery.

3.1.4.2 Percutaneous Tenorrhaphy

Described for the first time in 1977 by Ma and Griffith [16], the percutaneous tenorrhaphy aims to obtain the fixation of the two stumps through a strong suture that is advanced from the outside with a straight needle and free needles, without touching the injured site (see Fig. 3.7): the closure and stabilization of the sutures with the foot in equinism is the mechanism that provides the nearing of the stumps, which is noticeable only through direct palpation from the skin because the injured site is not viewable. This procedure can be performed in local anaesthesia and without the use of a tourniquet, resulting very quick to be accomplished; furthermore, it is clearly very respectful of the soft tissues, and for this reason the complication and infectious rates reported are significantly lower than any classic open technique. On the other side, it has to be said that the literature published shows

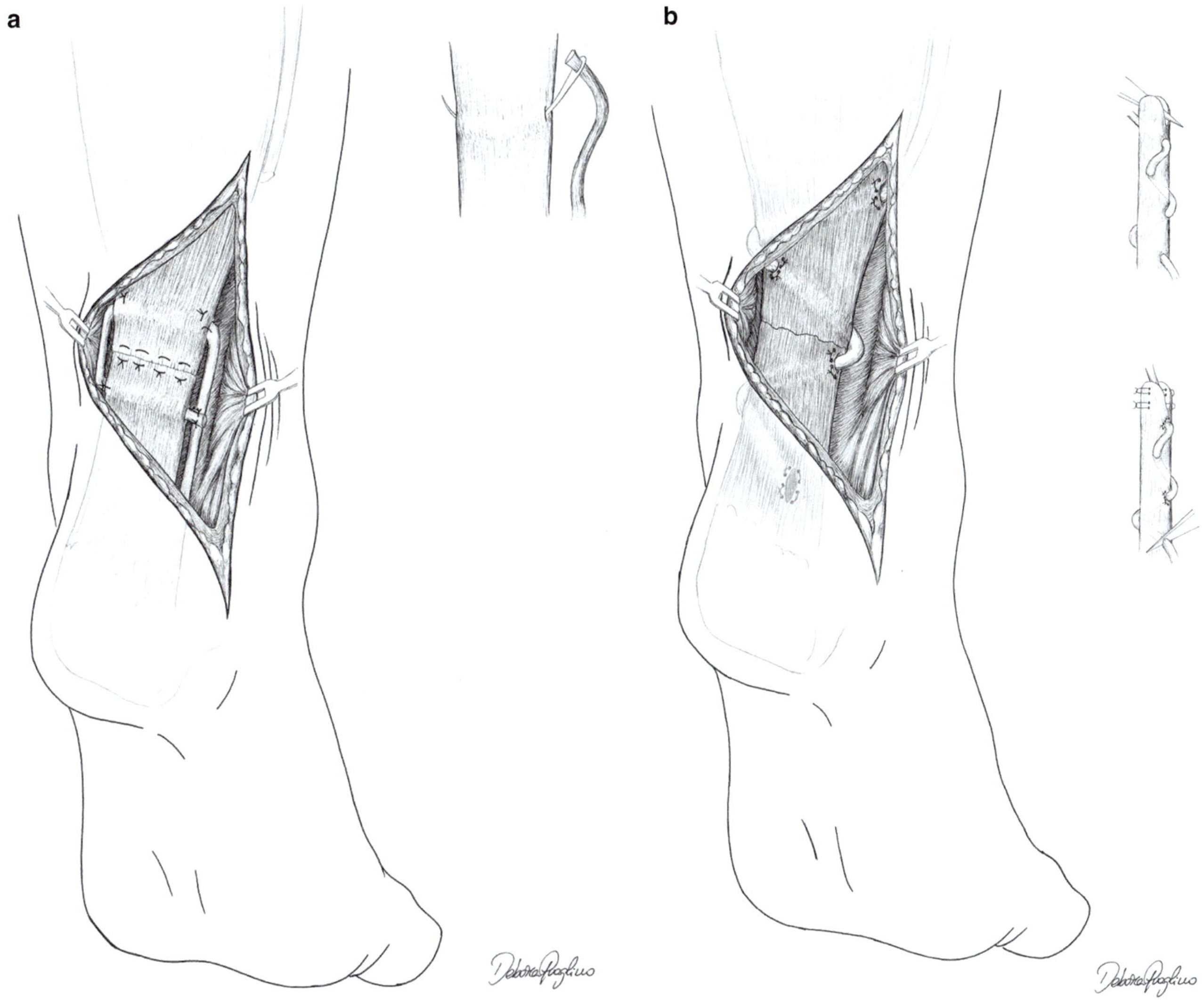

Fig. 3.6 Plantaris reinforcement graft of the Achilles tenorrhaphy: simple square type (**a**) and Pulvertaft type (**b**)

reports with a low number of patients, and a higher number of re-ruptures are reported, beyond cases of trapping and strangling of the sural nerve in the suture, mainly when crossed stitches are used [17].

Postoperative Care

Considering the preservation of the soft tissues, typical of this technique, it is possible to reduce the period of interruption of solicitations to promote the healing process; consequently, after a period of casting or bracing of the foot in equinus for 4 weeks, it is possible to allow active mobilization in the following 4 weeks, with the aim to restore more rapidly and with less functional impairment the 90° position of the ankle; the restoration of the weight bearing protected through the use of a cast or brace in a functional position is allowed after 8 weeks and the full weight bearing after 12 weeks, with a 2 cm insole that grants a slight equinism of the foot in the shoe. Any kinds of functional solicitations (jumping, running, leaping) are avoided for 5–6 months after surgery.

3.1.4.3 Minimally Invasive Tenorrhaphy

These techniques have been developed with the aim to achieve stable sutures like the ones obtained through open surgery, but avoiding all the soft tissue complications like in the percutaneous sutures [18]. One of the most known techniques is the one developed by Assal in 2002, and it needs a specifically designed device named Achillon® [19, 20]. Such procedure has its unique application in the injuries of the mid-portion of the tendon, with the limits that

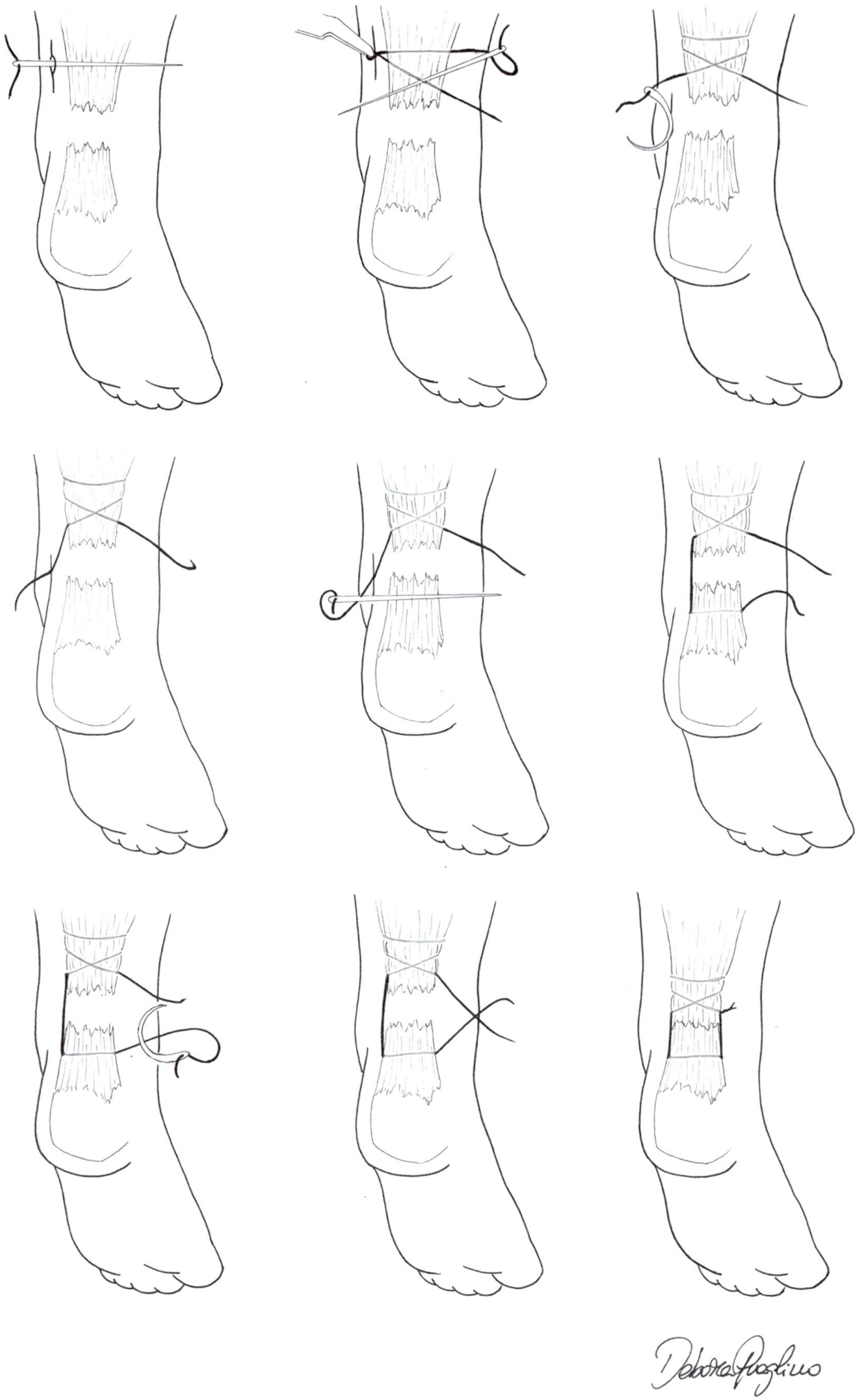

Fig. 3.7 Percutaneous suture positioning for the Achilles tendon following the Ma and Griffith technique

lay in an area between 2 and 8 cm from the calcaneal tuberosity and time passed since trauma at the most 10 days [20].

Preoperative Preparation

Even if the skin incision is notably reduced, it is necessary to position a tourniquet on the thigh, because it's best to perform the surgery without blood to better see all the different layers and structures that need to be addressed.

Instrumentation

Beyond the wires needed for the suspension of the skin and peritenon planes, there are three couples of measure 0 wires, one of them is monofilament, non-absorbable suture and the other two are braided with long absorbability; it is very important that each couple of sutures are of different colours, to foster the reckoning of the single ends during surgery and allowing the accuracy of the sutures.

Surgical Access

The skin incision is straight longitudinal, immediately medial to the tendon, aimed on the defect of the tendon, and 3 cm long (see Fig. 3.8). Once the two skin flaps are suspended through sutures or retractors, carefully the peritenon is isolated and separated from the subcutaneous tissue, and then it is incised longitudinally at the centre of the sheath, in the area where the interruption of the tendon is palpated, and the two flaps are then fixed on a 3.0 braided absorbable suture, to grant an easy book-type opening of the peritenon and obtaining the access to the injured area (see Fig. 3.9).

Restoration of Continuity

The two stumps of the tendon are found, checking their retraction and mobility after they are grabbed with an Allis clamp; the plane between the tendon and the peritonon is delicately sectioned proximally and distally to the incision of the latter. This will grant the way to the introduction in the sheath of the wire-positioning instrument.

The insertion of the diapason device is performed proximally, with the two arms introduced by blunt dissection between the peritenon and the tendon; then the instrument is pushed in a retrograde way and simultaneously opening the two middle arms through an opening screw, to better adapt to the shape of the tendon (see Fig. 3.10).

Once the instrument is positioned reaching the maximal proximal progression, the two middle arms are completely opened, and the three diameter 0 sutures of different colours are introduced through the proper straight needle that is included in the kit and pushed through the

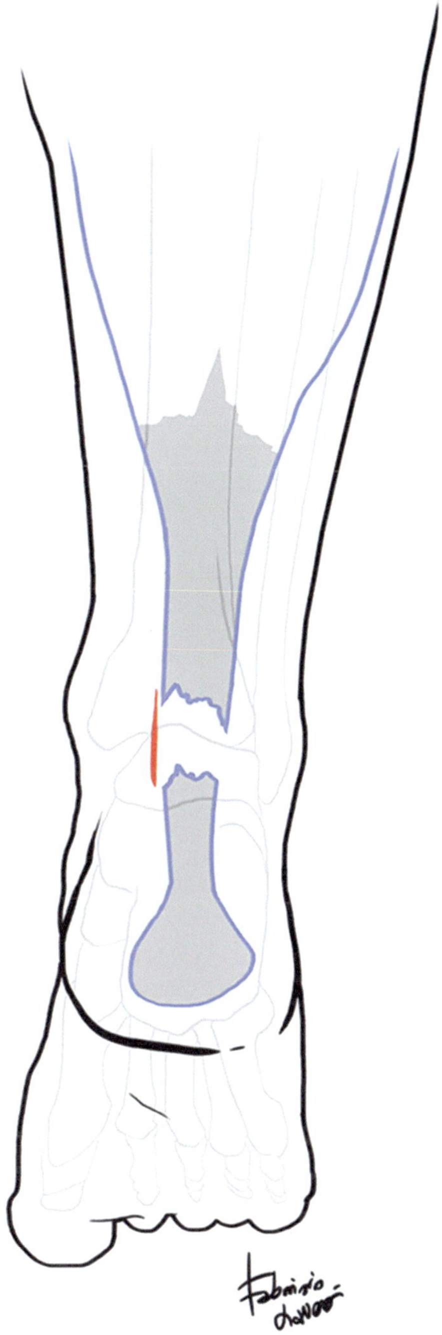

Fig. 3.8 Achilles tenorrhaphy with Achillon®: medial incision aimed on the tendon defect

holes of the devices' arms with an out-in-out direction (see Fig. 3.11), keeping checked the sequence and level of introduction of the threads thanks to the different colours of the latter.

The diapason device is retracted while the mid-arms are closed to facilitate the removal: the pulling out of the

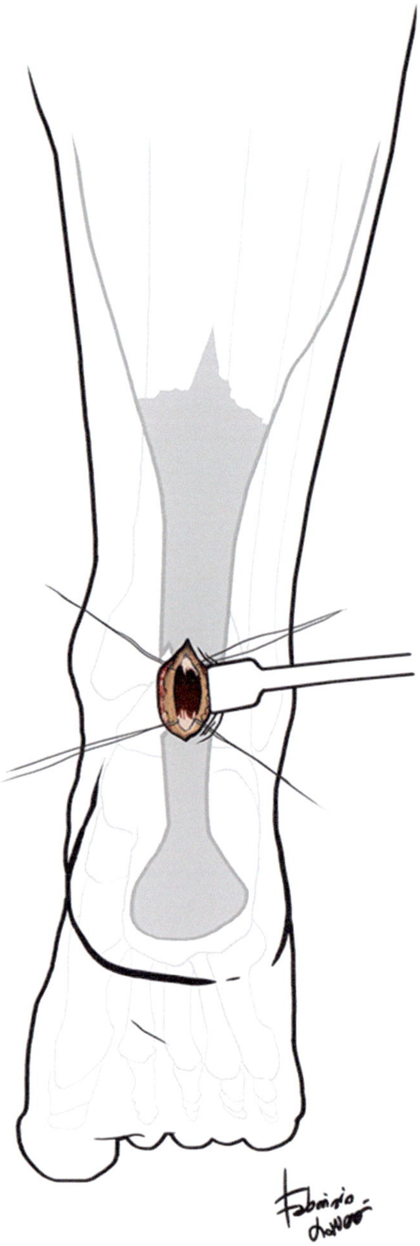

Fig. 3.9 Achilles tenorrhaphy with Achillon®: once the two peritenon flaps are opened, fixed on absorbable 3.0 sutures, the two tendon stumps are identified

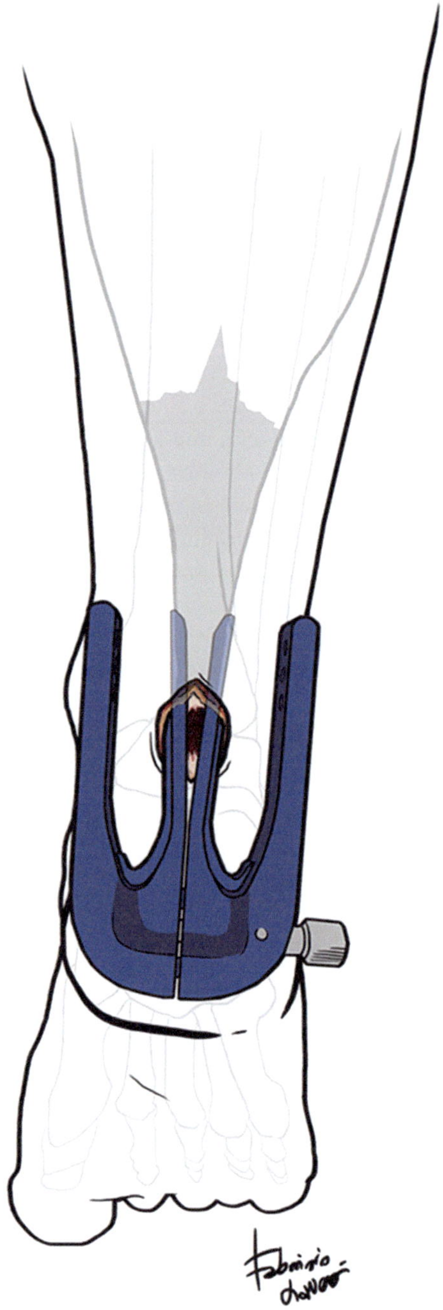

Fig. 3.10 Achilles tenorrhaphy with Achillon®: insertion of the diapason device, with the two arms introduced by blunt dissection between the peritenon and the tendon; the opening screw allows the spreading of the two middle arms that grant a better adaptation of the device to the shape of the tendon

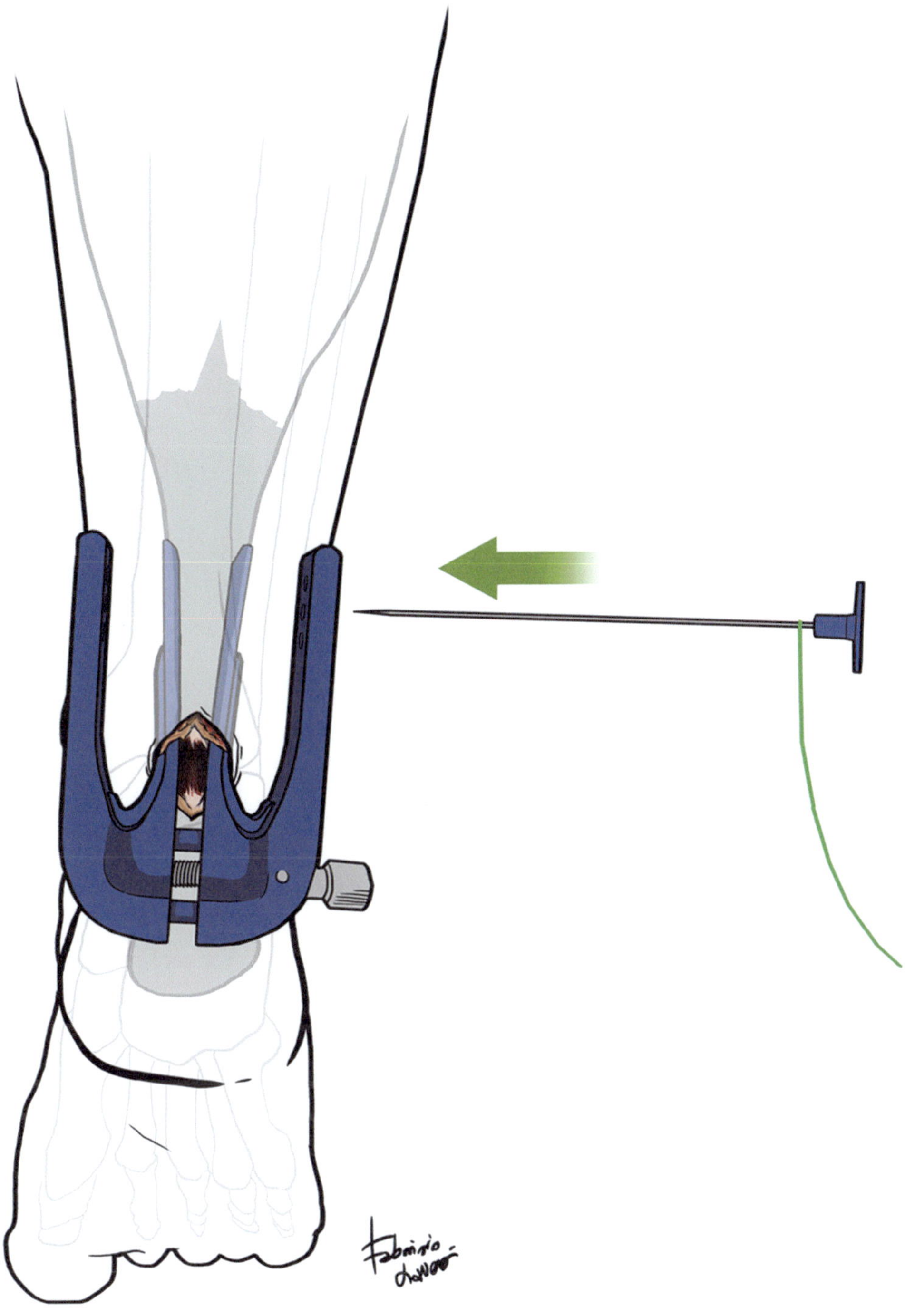

Fig. 3.11 Achilles tenorrhaphy with Achillon®: with a needle, provided in the kit, the differently coloured threads are passed through the three holes of the device, the soft tissues and tendon

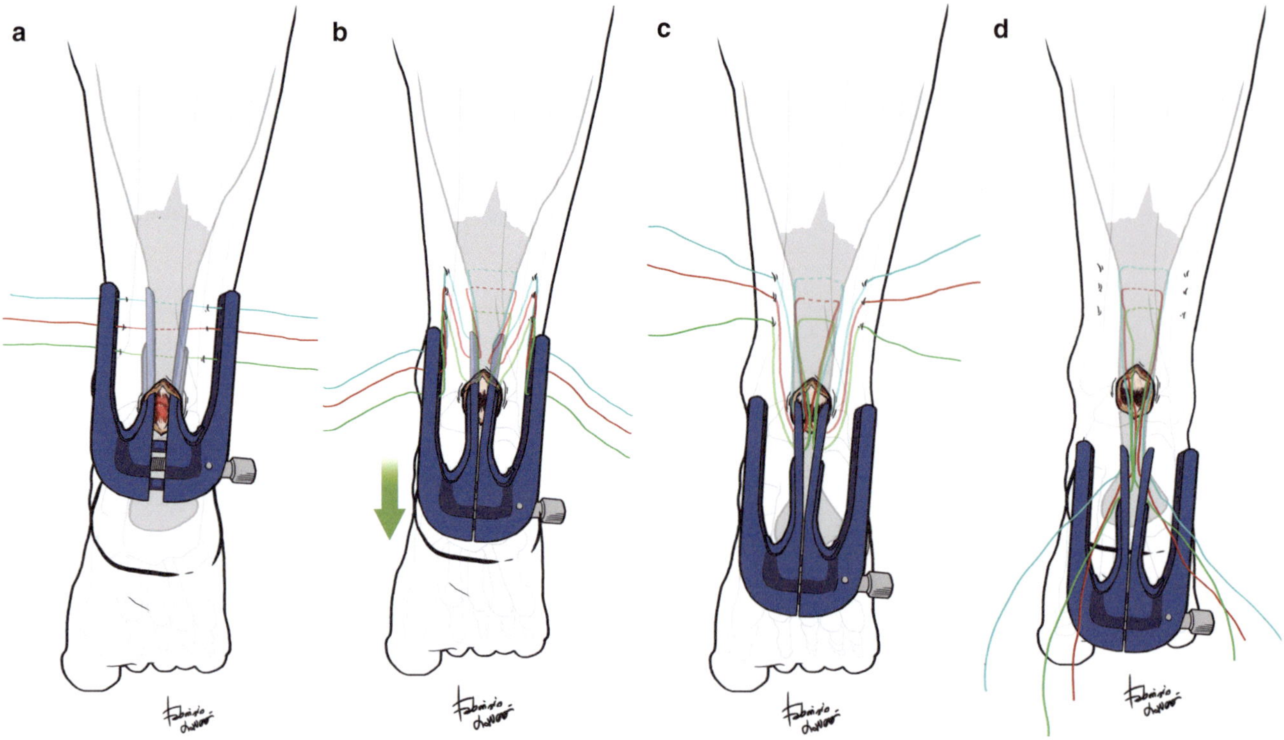

Fig. 3.12 (**a–d**) Achilles tenorrhaphy with Achillon®: the removal of the device permits the migration of the suture wires that will become intratendinous and stay under the paratenon, exiting from the proximal stump, insuring a solid fixation

device produces the migration of the wires previously positioned; consequently the sutures are under the peritenon, and the only anchoring point is the proximal tendon (see Fig. 3.12).

The same procedure is performed for the positioning of the distal sutures, being careful to perform the same sequence of steps; in this way the sutures should match the colours in the different areas of the tendon, distant, intermediate and proximal to the injury.

Then the two stumps are correctly put in contact under direct sight through a slight equinus positioning of the foot, and the three rectangular sutures are completed between the three couples of threads of the corresponding colour, performing a first knot in one way and the closing knot in the opposite way (see Fig. 3.13). During every tightening of the knots, it is possible to check through direct vision the best matching of the tendon stumps, which is stabilized by the completion of the sutures.

Postoperative Care

Considering the low impact on the soft tissues and the simultaneous great tightness of the tenorrhaphy obtained [18], the postoperative care protocol allows a more early rehabilitation, with a equinus positioning of the foot in a cast or bracing for only 3 weeks, followed by an active mobilization without weight bearing for 3 weeks, where the bracing is kept only for protection when walking and during the night, with a progressive dorsiflexion of the foot through the bracing modification of the ROM: this allows to keep and stabilize the improvements achieved during the day; after 6 weeks the weight bearing is allowed always through bracing with the foot in a functional position. The full weight bearing without any bracing is allowed after 8 weeks, with an insole that grants a 2 cm equinus of the foot in the shoes. Any kinds of functional solicitations (jumping, running, leaping) are avoided for 5–6 months after surgery.

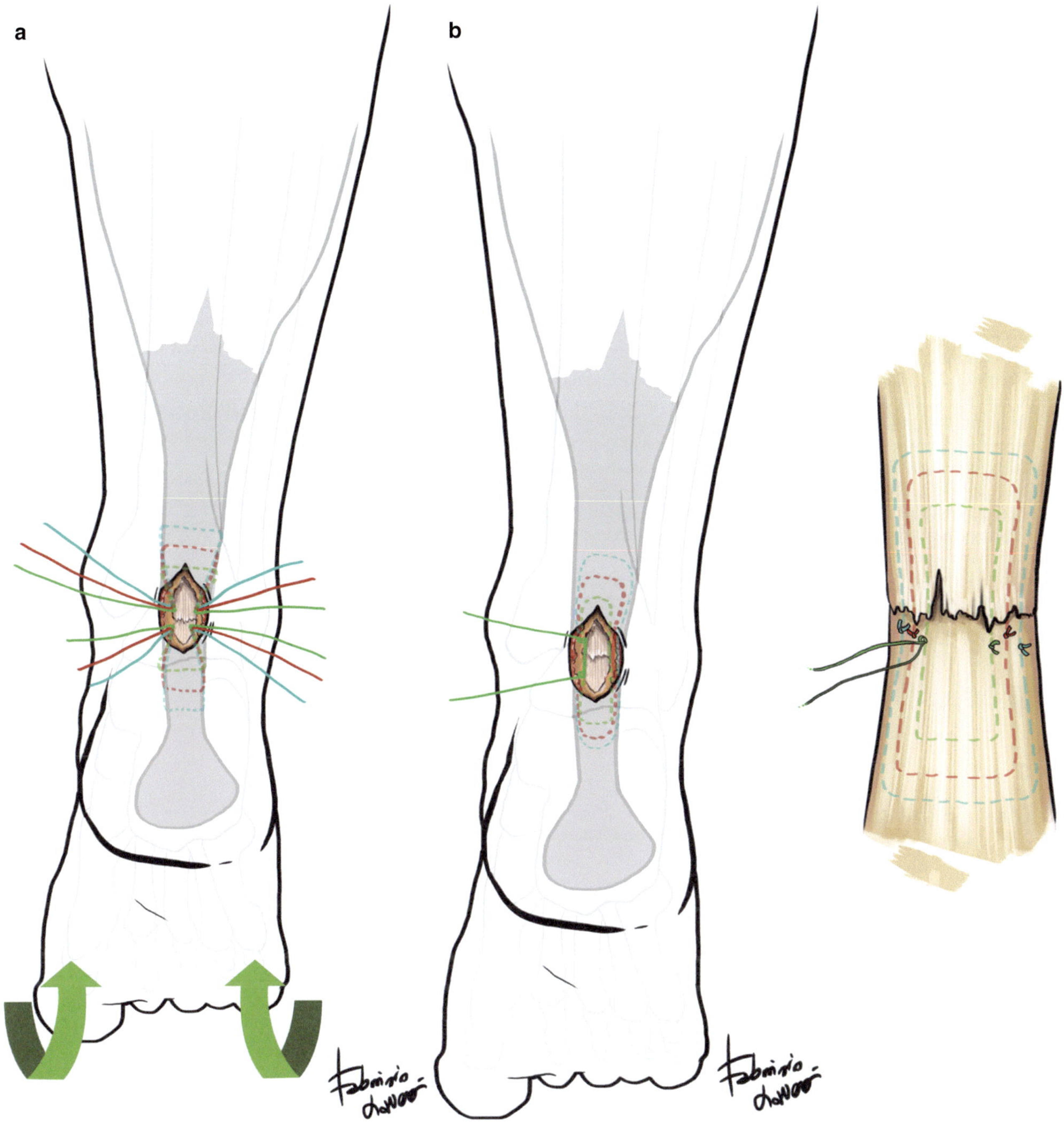

Fig. 3.13 Achilles tenorrhaphy with Achillon®: accomplished the suture positioning on the distal stump and keeping the foot plantar flexed to grant the correct contact between the tendon stumps (**a**); the sutures of the corresponding colour are completed, closed with two knots for each couple (**b**)

References

1. Kellam JF, Hunter GA, McElwain JP (1985) Review of the operative treatment of Achilles tendon rupture. Clin Orthop Relat Res 201:80–83
2. Leppilahti J, Puranen J, Orava S (1996) Incidence of Achilles tendon rupture. Acta Orthop Scand 67(3):277–279
3. Thomopoulos S, Parks WC, Rifkin DB et al (2015) Mechanisms of tendon injury and repair. J Orthop Res 33(6):832–839
4. Scheller AD, Kasser JR, Quigley TB (1980) Tendon injuries about the ankle. Orthop Clin North Am 11(4):801–811
5. Hattrup SJ, Johnson KA (1985) A review of ruptures of the Achilles tendon. Foot Ankle 6(1):34–38
6. Coughlin MJ, Schon LC (2007) Achilles tendon rupture. In: Coughlin MJ, Mann RA, Saltzman CL (eds) Surgery of the foot and ankle, 8th edn. Mosby Elsevier, Philadelphia, pp 1237–1261
7. Greenberg RC, Saltzman CL (2004) Disfunzioni del tendine di Achille. In: Brotzman SB, Wilk KE (eds) La riabilitazione in Ortopedia, 2nd edn. Excerpta Medica, Italia, pp 405–412
8. Popovic N, Lemaire R (1999) Diagnosis and treatment of acute ruptures of the Achilles tendon. Current concepts review. Acta Orthop Belg 65(4):458–471
9. Riedl S, Sandberger L, Nitschmann K et al (2002) Suture of fresh Achilles tendon rupture. Comparison of open with percutaneous suture technique. Chirurg 73(6):607–614
10. Khan RJ, Fick D, Brammar TJ et al (2004) Interventions for treating acute Achilles tendon ruptures. Cochrane Database Syst Rev 3:CD0036749
11. Strauss EJ, Ishak C, Jazrawi L et al (2007) Operative treatment of acute Achilles tendon ruptures: an institutional review of clinical outcomes. Injury 38(7):832–838
12. Rippstein PF, Jung M, Assal M (2002) Surgical repair of acute Achilles tendon rupture using a "mini-open" technique. Foot Ankle Clin 7(3):611–619
13. Bruggeman NB, Turner NS, Dahm DL et al (2004) Wound complications after open Achilles tendon repair: an analysis of risk factors. Clin Orthop Relat Res 427:63–66
14. Kelly IP, Stephens M (2000) Rottura acuta e cronica del tendine d'Achille. In: Encyclopédie Médico-Chirurgicale. Elsevier, Paris
15. Clanton TO, Waldrop NE III (2007) Athletic injuries to the soft tissues of the foot and ankle. In: Coughlin MJ, Saltzman CL, Anderson RB (eds) Surgery of the foot and ankle. Elsevier, Philadelphia, pp 1531–1688
16. Ma GW, Griffith TG (1977) Percutaneous repair of acute closed ruptured achilles tendon: a new technique. Clin Orthop Relat Res 128:247–255
17. Khan RJ, Fick D, Brammar TJ et al (2004) Interventions for treating acute Achilles tendon ruptures. Cochrane Database Syst Rev 3:CD003674
18. Ismail M, Karim A, Shulman R et al (2008) The Achillon achilles tendon repair: is it strong enough? Foot Ankle Int 29(8):808–813
19. Śliwa M (2014) Percutaneous and minimally invasive Achilles tendon repair—review of surgical techniques. Pol Orthop Traumatol 79:92–96
20. Davies MS, Solan M (2009) Minimal incision techniques for acute Achilles repair. Foot Ankle Clin 14(4):685–697

4 Surgical Treatment of Traumatic Injuries of the Talus

Contents

4.1 Traumatic Injuries of the Talus

The talus fractures, with or without dislocation of the peritalar joints, are injuries relatively infrequent that represent less than the 1% of all the fractures and only the 3–5% of the fractures of the foot [1]. The anatomical peculiarity of this bone, covered by cartilage for its 60% and with an ending-type vascularization, explains the highly frequent problems with this type of fracture and how the prognosis for the more complicated injuries is unlucky [2, 3]; for these reasons the treatment is a real challenge for the orthopaedic surgeon [4].

4.1.1 Classification

Considering only the descriptive part of the talus fractures, they are divided into three categories: of the neck, which represents the more frequent site (50% of the total), even because anatomically it is the part of the bone with the smaller diameter that explains its fragility, of the body (30%), and of the head (20%).

Briefly and to keep homogenous the evaluations, it has to be specified that the limit between the body injuries and the neck injuries must be considered as the lateral process of the talus, evaluating the distal fracture line and the latter: all the fractures that end anteriorly to the lateral process, leaving unharmed the posterior subtalar joint, without considering their proximal origin, must be defined as fractures of the neck, while the fractures that end with their line posteriorly to this process are to be considered as body fractures [5].

The Hawkins classification is the most famous classifying system with connected prognostic indications [2], but it considers only the fractures of the neck that are the most frequent, but they include only half of the total injuries of this segment. For this reason we prefer to use the Marti-Weber classification [3] equally well known that unites the value of gathering all prognostic indications with the advantage of including all the injuries of the talus, even the less frequent (see Fig. 4.1).

In this classification the fractures of group I include all the injuries that do not interrupt the anatomical continuity of the

W. Daghino et al., *Foot and Ankle Trauma Injuries*, https://doi.org/10.1007/978-3-319-69617-1_4

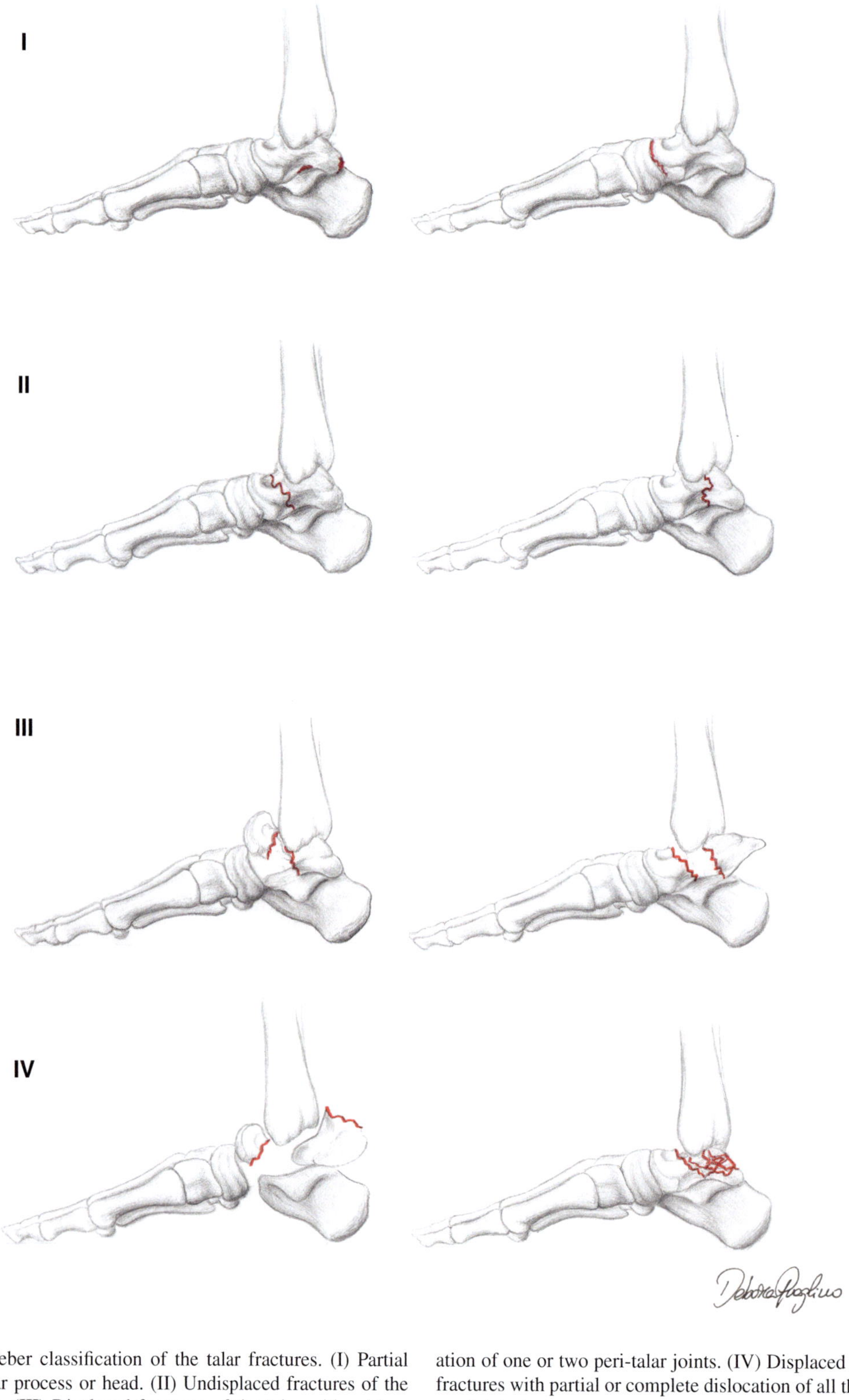

Fig. 4.1 Marti-Weber classification of the talar fractures. (I) Partial injuries of the talar process or head. (II) Undisplaced fractures of the talar neck or body. (III) Displaced fractures of the talar with subluxation of one or two peri-talar joints. (IV) Displaced talar neck or body fractures with partial or complete dislocation of all the peri-talar joints/crush injuries

bone, such as the ones including the lateral or posterior process, and the osteochondral lesions and the injuries of the head; these are all injuries that have a good prognosis regarding the worse complication of these fractures; the osteonecrosis complication is not present in these groups of fractures.

The fractures of group II include injuries of the body and the neck without any displacement, for which the osteonecrosis is theoretically possible, but very rare in the clinical practice. The fractures of group III are the ones of the body and the neck where there is both a displacement of the fracture and a partial or complete dislocation of some peri-talar articulations (tibio-talar, subtalar and talo-navicular), in which the evolution in osteonecrosis is highly recurrent. At last the injuries of group IV that include the displaced fractures with dislocation of all the peri-talar joints or crush syndromes with complete destruction of the main part of the body, for which the osteonecrosis is considered constant and unavoidable [4].

4.1.2 Indications

4.1.2.1 Diagnostic Procedures

The diagnostic process starts from the traditional radiology, in the classic two projections anteroposterior and lateral, which are the basis for the classification that suggests the type of treatment. The CT is performed mainly not for the diagnosis but for the study of the morphology of the injury, needed for the surgical planning. Even for the follow-up, the main exam is the plain X-rays in two projections, reserving the MRI in the cases in which an osteonecrosis is suspected and needs to be diagnosed.

4.1.2.2 Surgical Treatment

In absence of general contraindications about the surgery, it is considered appropriate an open reduction and internal fixation every time that after CT or X-ray a significant, more than 1mm, dislocation of the fracture or osteochondral fragments are spotted.

4.1.3 Objectives

The aim of the surgical treatment of the injuries of the talus is dual: reconstruct precisely the bony anatomy and achieve a stable osteosynthesis that allows an early joint mobilization.

4.1.3.1 Anatomical Reconstruction

The anatomical conformation of the talus is not simple, with the anatomical axis of the three parts that result orientated in all the dimensions; the correct disposition of these angular correlations leads the spatial stance of the segment and consequently influences the positioning of the hindfoot and the relationship with the rest of the foot.

The main anatomical aspect that is nodal for the reconstruction is the neck-body angle, inclined on all the spatial planes (see Fig. 4.2), and is a possible cause of abnormal foot stance if the angles aren't correct [6].

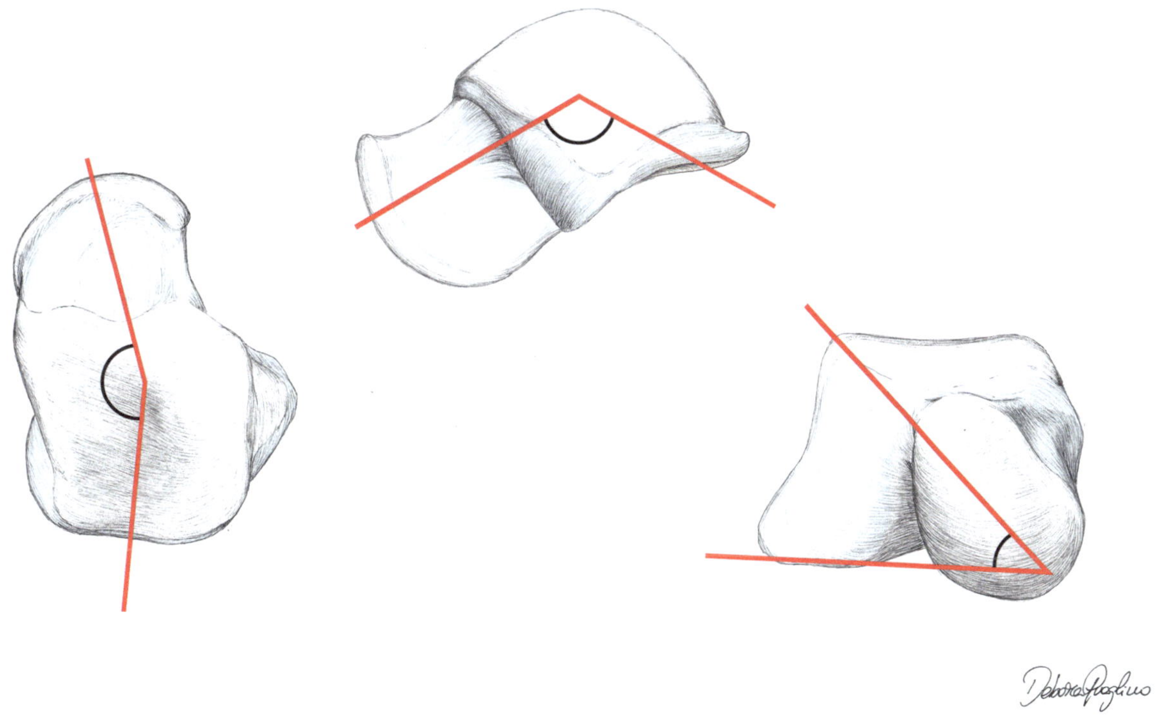

Fig. 4.2 The surgical anatomy of the talus has as a key point the exact reconstruction of the angle between the neck and the head, which is sloping in all the three dimensions, and it guides the positioning of the hindfoot and the consequent relationship with all the proximal and distal bone segments

The precise reconstruction of such crucial element is complicated by the fact that frequently on the medial portion of the neck, a bony fragmentation is found and by the limited vision achievable during surgery, because combined medial and lateral surgical accesses are very dangerous.

As a matter of fact the monolateral access limits the risk of iatrogenic injuries that may lead to a complete disruption of the vascular support that is already compromised by the trauma and by the type of terminal blood supply that the body of the talus receives [7].

These difficulties must not be excuses to accept compromises in the reduction of the fracture that must always be the more precise as possible, eventually using both bony fragments correspondence and radiological imaging during surgery to indirectly confirm the correct reduction.

4.1.3.2 Stable Osteosynthesis

To achieve a stable fixation of the talus is not simple, because of its anatomical complex conformation, with a great part of it made of cartilage surface and considering all the angular inclinations and the precariousness of the surrounding soft tissues that impede the use of screws and blade systems.

Besides this, because of the proven weakness of the percutaneous Kirschner wire fixation to prevent malunions [8] and simultaneously restricting the early mobilization, essential for the best functional recovery, achieving a stable fixation is mandatory.

To achieve the latter, the use of free screws, of diameter 4 mm, fully or partially threaded, usually cannulated to ease the correct positioning, is needed. Such screws must be able to stabilize the fragments and keep safe the achieved reduction, granting simultaneously an active mobilization of the tibio-talar and midtarsal joints. Many theories, based upon refined biomechanical concepts, suggest the positioning of the screws through an anterograde approach rather than retrograde [8, 9]; in the common clinical practice, the polymorphism of the injuries and the exiguity of the bone fragments force more frequently the positioning of the screws in obligated ways; the screw direction should adapt always to the pathologic anatomy of the fracture and should be considered always good if long as a stable fixation is achieved.

4.1.4 Surgical Technique

4.1.4.1 Positioning

A radiolucent surgical table is used; the tourniquet is positioned at the thigh; because the surgical approach used is usually medial, the surgeon frequently stays on the opposite side of the injured limb, and the best positioning of the patient is supine, with the healthy limb elevated and kept in position with the hip and knee flexed on a support (see Fig. 4.9); in this way the surgical procedures and the intraoperative imaging are granted.

Even in this case, the positioning of the patient is concluded, before the surgical field is prepared, by the execution of plain X-rays of the ankle with the image intensifier. This allows achieving the correct vision of the segments that need to be treated on the surgical table and to keep them in the memory of the intensifier granting the possibility to compare them during the surgery and to confirm the correct reduction of the fracture during the procedure.

4.1.4.2 Surgical Access

Theoretically the talus is accessible in all the directions; for this reason dorsal, medial, anterolateral, posterolateral and postero-medial accesses have been described, isolated or variably combined.

To use simultaneously more than one surgical access is dangerous, both for the proximity of the incisions, that if with a distance inferior of 5 cm can lead to a vascular injury of the skin flap, but mainly because it's possible to produce a iatrogenic vascular injury at the bone in consequence of the bilateral access; that said, the best surgical approach and the more used is certainly the medial [4, 7, 10], with a skin incision extended from the apex of the medial malleolus to the navicular bone, eventually enlarged proximally and with a tibial malleolus osteotomy if there is a fracture of the talus body (see Fig. 4.3).

This surgical approach is developed between the anterior tibial tendon dorsally and the posterior tibial tendon in the plantar part, giving the best exposure of the medial portion of the talar neck: this is a critical area, because frequently comminuted, with a possible high risk of malreduction and consequent varus deformity of the body-neck angle, caused by the relative bone loss.

In the situation of a proximal extension of the surgical access to control the fracture of the talus body, a malleolar osteotomy is necessary, and it must be performed keeping a vascular pedicle on the distal fragment, where the deltoid ligament is attached, to grant the blood supply. A trick very useful to grant an optimal execution of the osteotomy can be to perform the holes for the screws before the osteotomy is performed and to fulfil the latter in a delta shape (see Fig. 4.4).

Furthermore it is advisable to proceed with a motorized saw only to accomplish the first part of the bony cut, finishing it with a chisel, avoiding to create chondral injuries from the high temperature generated by the saw and simultaneously creating surfaces that help the correct matching during the synthesis.

During the execution of this extended access, it can be useful to isolate the tibialis posterior neurovascular

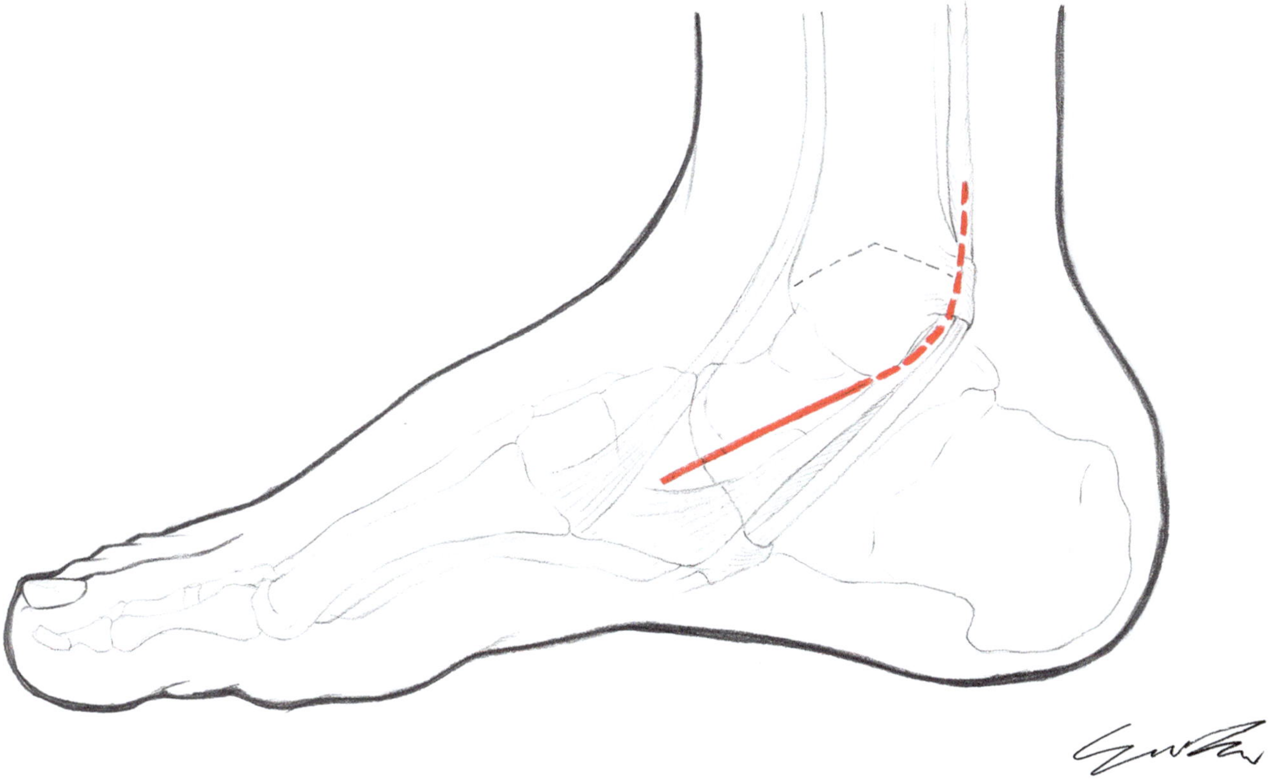

Fig. 4.3 Surgical access to the medial side of the talus: in red the skin incision, extended from the tip of the medial malleolus to the navicular bone; the dotted lines depict the extension of the skin incision proximally and the course of the malleolus osteotomy that could be needed if a fracture of the body needs to be addressed

bundle, to avoid any iatrogenic injuries during the reduction manoeuvres, especially when a body fragment is present, which can modify the normal route of the bundle (see Fig. 4.5).

4.1.4.3 Reduction and Osteosynthesis Manoeuvres

The reduction must be carefully planned preoperatively, considering the CT images performed in the three spatial planes, eventually integrated by three-dimensional reconstructions to grant a more easy understanding of the fracture and to plan precisely all the reduction sequences needed and all the anatomical landmarks useful to obtain the best anatomical restoration.

The planning must include the recognition of all the main bony segments, the evaluation of the displacement of the latter and of eventual articular portions that are displaced, the best surgical access to ease the procedure, the sequence of all the manoeuvres needed to achieve the best result and finally all the instrumentation needed to obtain the best anatomical reduction and the less invasive procedure possible.

During the surgical procedure, a useful manner to spot in the best way the anatomical landmarks, which will allow to confirm a good reduction, is to proceed to free and clean the fractured bone only with the scalpel, avoiding to rub the bone with a periosteal chisel that could lead to an increase of a comminution of the fragments, because of the fragility of the latter and the thin cortical of the involved bone, mainly cancellous; this advice is even more useful when the comminution of the fracture rises, especially on the medial side of the neck, more exposed to this event [11].

Once the bone is exposed and the injured segments prepared, the constant visualization of the preoperative planning, which must be exhibited in front of the surgeon, allows to identify precisely in the surgical field nature and position of the fragments, granting the reduction only after the latter is completed following the planned sequence (see Fig. 4.6).

The reduction achieved is temporarily stabilized with some Kirschner wires, and the intraoperative X-ray check allows to see the correct positioning of the single segments and the peri-talar joint, completing the limited surgical view due to the unilateral access used.

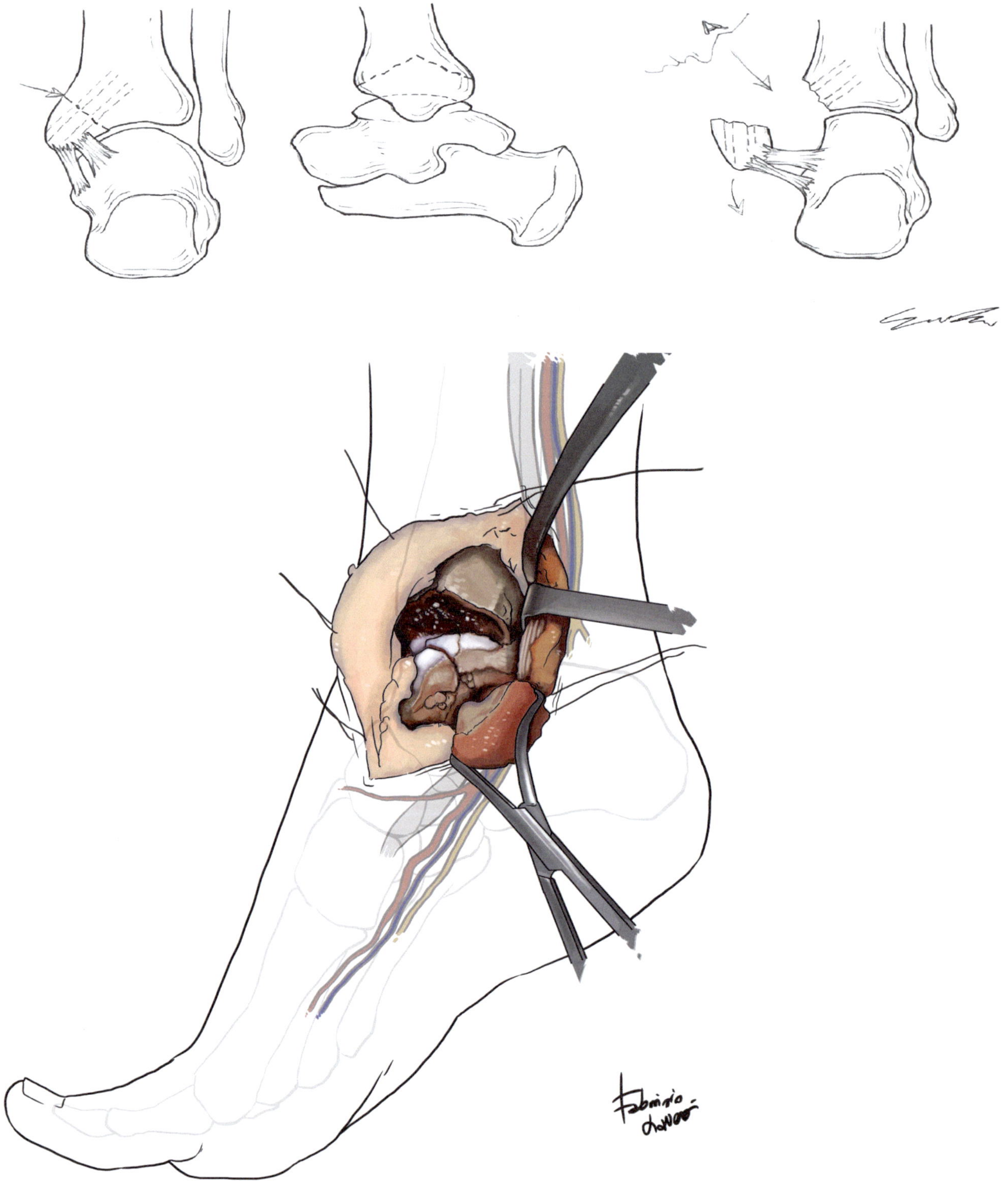

Fig. 4.4 Surgical access with osteotomy of the malleolus to grant the exposure of the talar body; the posterior tibial tendon and the corresponding neurovascular bundle are retracted posteriorly and inferiorly; the tibial malleolus must be kept safe with its vascular peduncle and inferiorly tipped over. It is very useful to perform the holes for the screws, which will be used afterwards for the bone synthesis, before performing the malleolus osteotomy

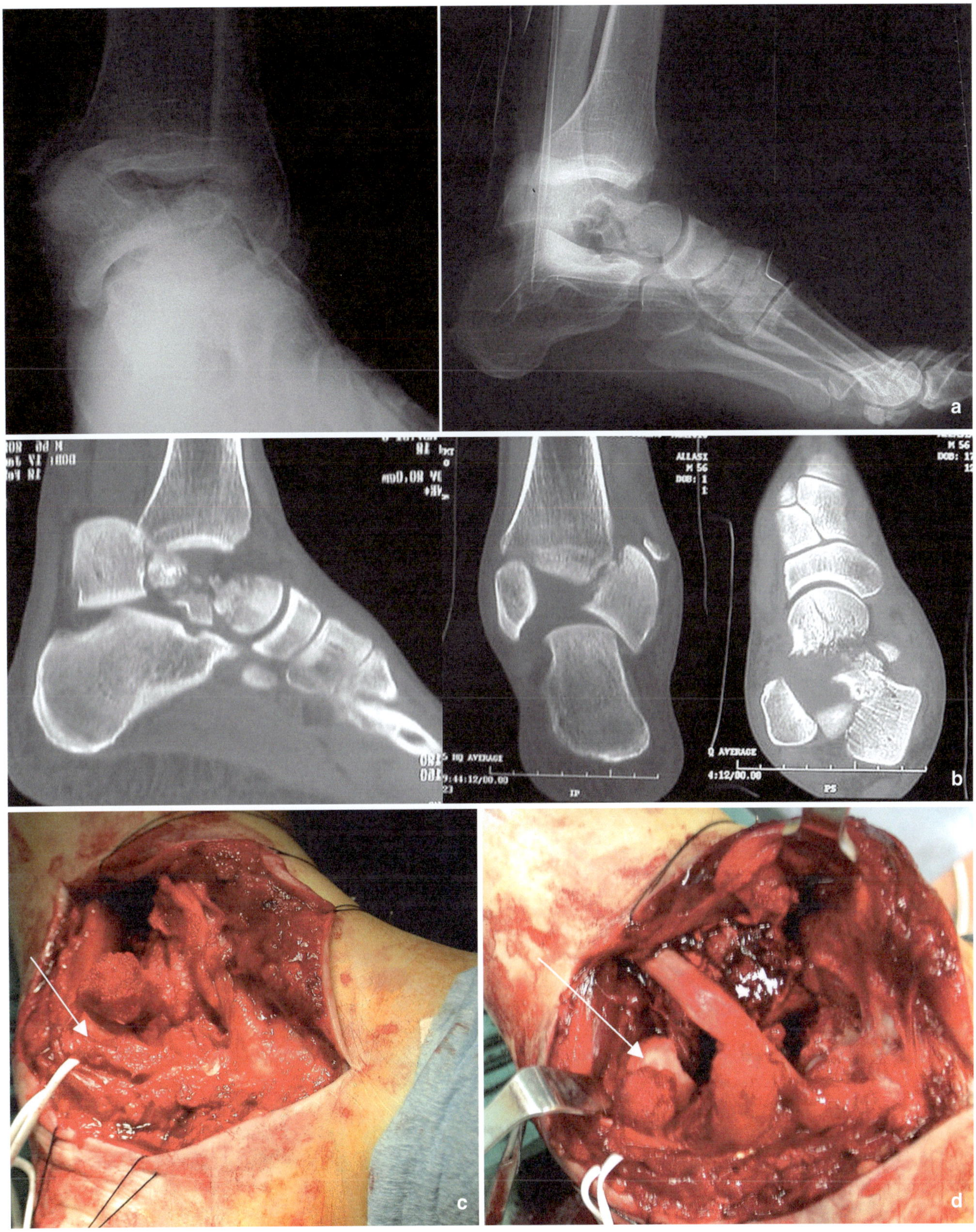

Fig. 4.5 Clinical case: complex fracture of the talus and the medial malleolus, with medial dislocation of the talar body; (**a**) X-ray evaluation; (**b**) the CT shows the entity and the extension of the dislocation; (**c**) intraoperative image, where it is possible to understand the compression of the dislocated body (white arrow) on the retracted neurovascular bundle (protected by a white lace), isolated and protected during the dissection; (**d**) once that the surgical preparation is completed, the compressive effect carried out by the dislocated body on the posterior tibial neurovascular bundle is more evident

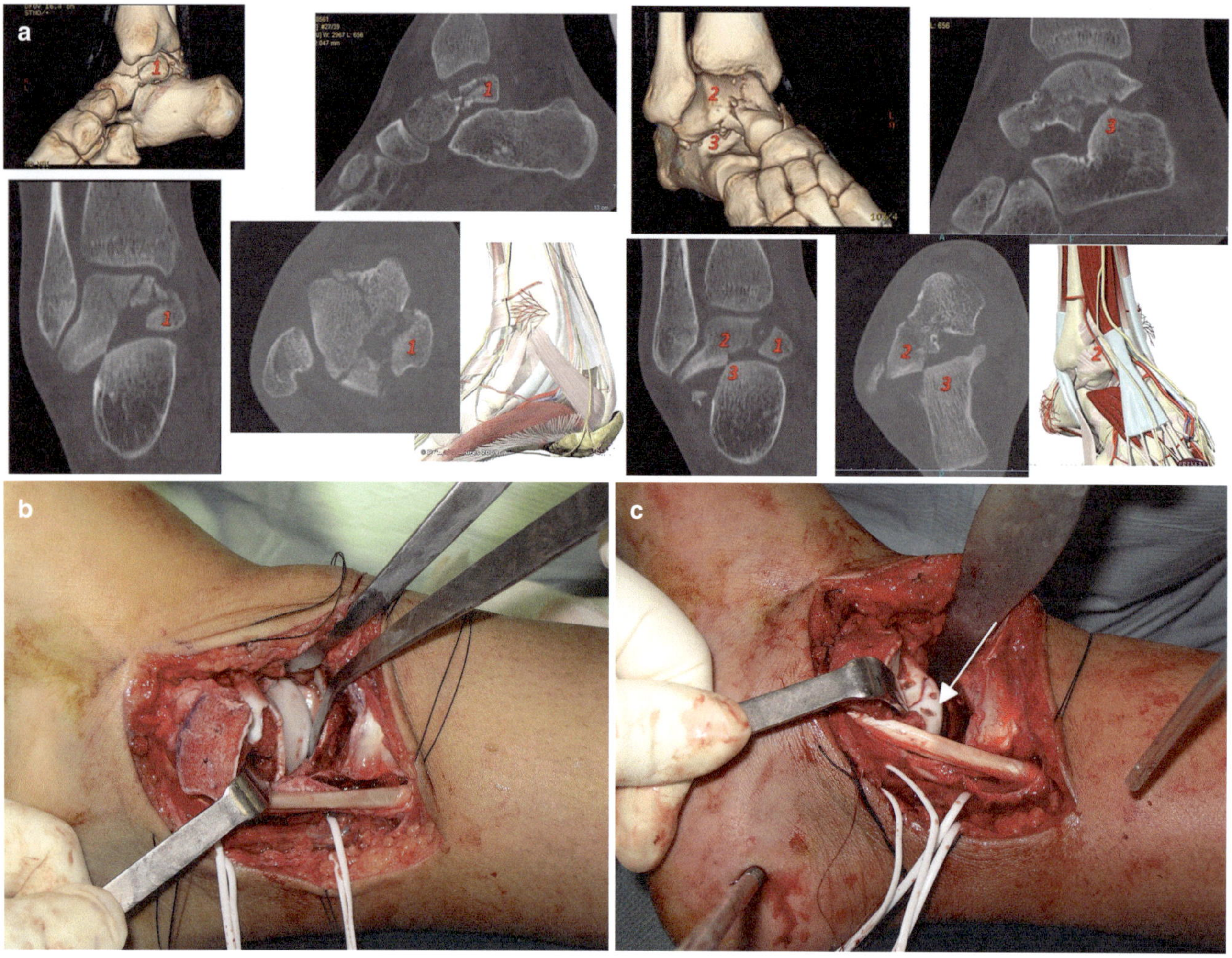

Fig. 4.6 Importance of the preoperative planning (**a**) that allows to program the timing of the surgical manoeuvres to find all the main fragments in their dislocated spot (**b**). Once all the dislocated parts have been identified, it is possible to proceed to the reduction restoring the normal anatomy: in the picture (**c**) it is possible to see the fragment enlightened as n.1 in the preoperative planning (indicated by the arrow), repositioned in its natural site

Two free-handed screws are used to obtain an osteosynthesis of the main fragments that need to be positioned parallel, if an interfragmentary compression is searched, or intersected (see Fig. 4.7), with an anteroposterior or posteroanterior direction, avoiding any cartilage portions or using double-threaded screws if they need to be fully buried in the chondral surface if it isn't possible to avoid it. These screws are made of titanium, to allow more reliable MRI images if a specific follow-up is needed when osteonecrosis is suspected.

The choice of using fully or partially threaded screws is bound on the morphology of the fracture, selecting the first if there are big and stable fragments, instead choosing the latter when the fragments are little, because the medial comminution of the talar neck could be deformed in varus by a high compression generated by the fully threaded screw.

Even if less mechanically performing and more difficult to position due to the surgical technique that request the threading of the hole before the screws are inserted, absorbable poly-L-lactic acid (PLLA) screws can ease the follow up through MRI and are precious if the bony or chondral fragments are in difficult to access positions (see Fig. 4.8), allowing an easier management of complications that could lead to further surgeries.

4.1.4.4 Postoperative Care

A cast is kept for 3–6 weeks, depending on the stability of the synthesis; the removal of the stiches is done after 3 weeks; after 6 weeks from surgery, the first X-ray check is performed; the following radiological check is done after 3 months, time in which, if no complications developed, the partial weight bearing is allowed. After 4 months,

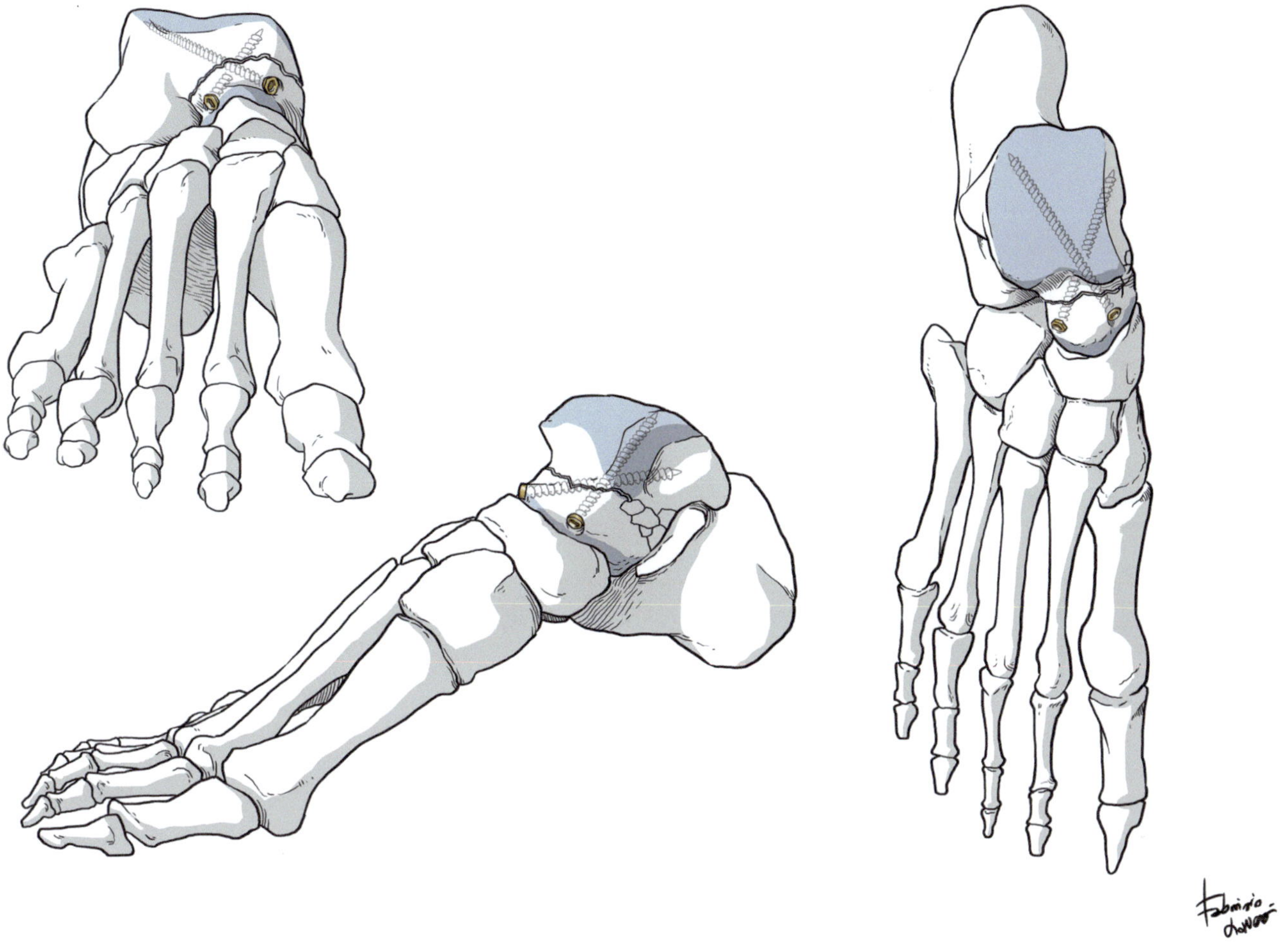

Fig. 4.7 Osteosynthesis with screws of a talar fracture: aiming to have crossed screws and not parallel, the compression is achieved only by the first screw

if everything is correctly proceeding, full weight bearing is allowed, and an appropriate hydro-kinesis therapy program is started to restore as much as possible muscular strength and volume and joint range of motion.

Because the most feared complication, the osteonecrosis of the talus, is more frequent between 3 and 12 months but can occur even after 2 years, the follow-up consists of clinical and radiological checks at 6, 12 and 24 months, undergoing MRI if any alterations of the bone depict a possible bone avascular necrosis, in which it could be advisable to further avoid weight bearing on the affected limb to foster an eventual recovery [4].

4.1.4.5 Specific Cases

Even if the talar fractures are rare, there is the possibility to encounter during the clinical practice many different injuries, of which a peculiar management can be needed.

Snowboarder's Talus

The so-called snowboarder's talus is a fracture of the lateral process, caused by an impact of the hindfoot kept in pronation, typically when a snowboarder falls after a jump.

It is a type of injury that can be misdiagnosed or underestimated with the normal radiology, for this reason the CT is imperative. The coronal reconstruction of the CT scan can reveal a central sinking of the bone that would be other way unrecognizable, very dangerous for the consequence on the subtalar joint (see Fig. 4.9).

The management of these fractures is based on an overturning of the lateral fractured process to gain access to the central part of the talus that needs to be reduced checking the cartilage surface and eventually using some bone autologous or synthetic graft to fill the defect, use with a mechanical value. Only when a correct reduction is

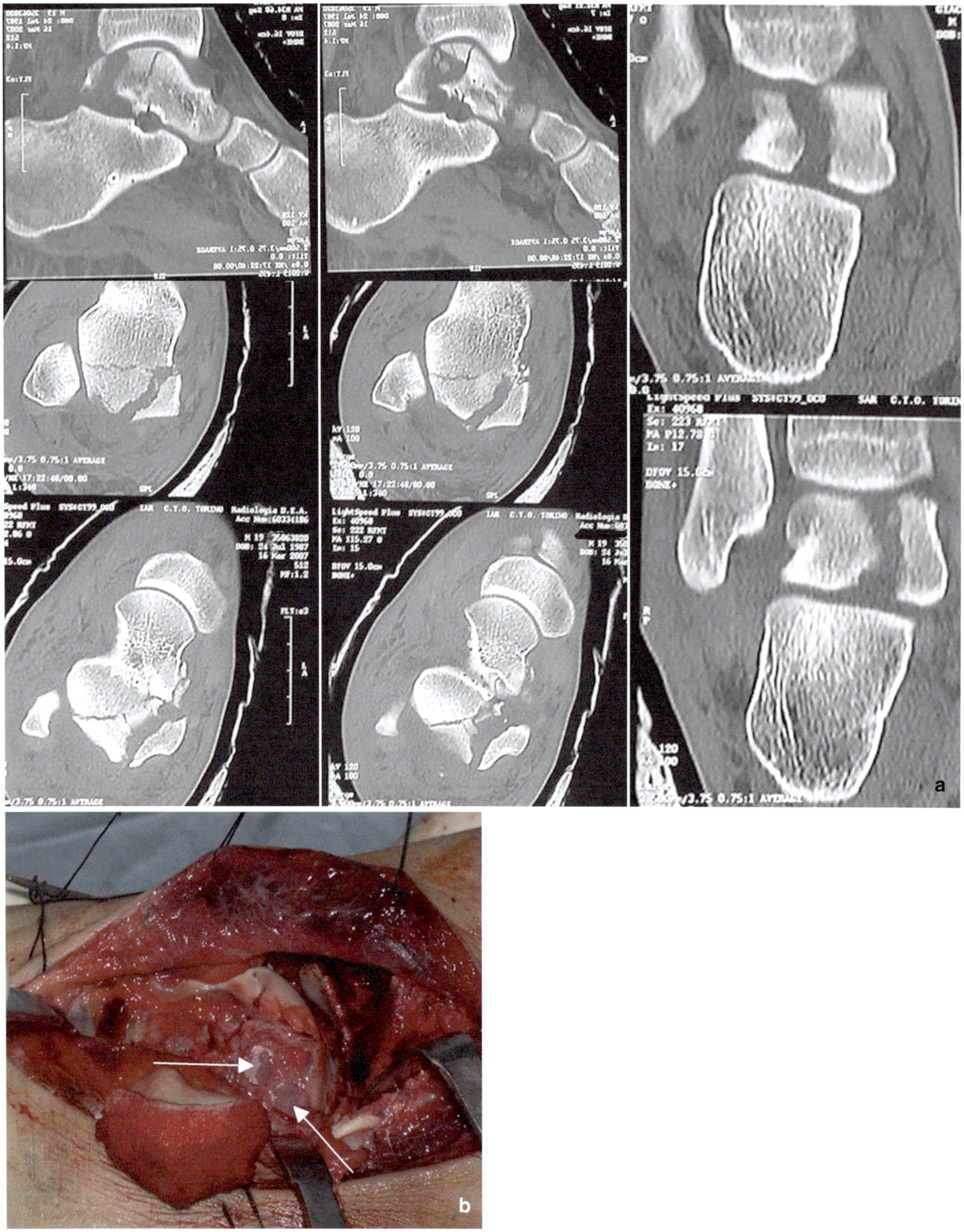

Fig. 4.8 Case of a dislocated fracture of the postero-medial body part of the talus: the CT scan (**a**) shows the important dislocation of the fragments. (**b**) Intraoperative imaging after reduction and osteosynthesis with PLLA screws (arrows) after an osteotomy of the medial malleolus is performed. (**c**) CT scan after 5 months, where it is still possible to see the screws (arrows), but the healing of the fracture is demonstrated

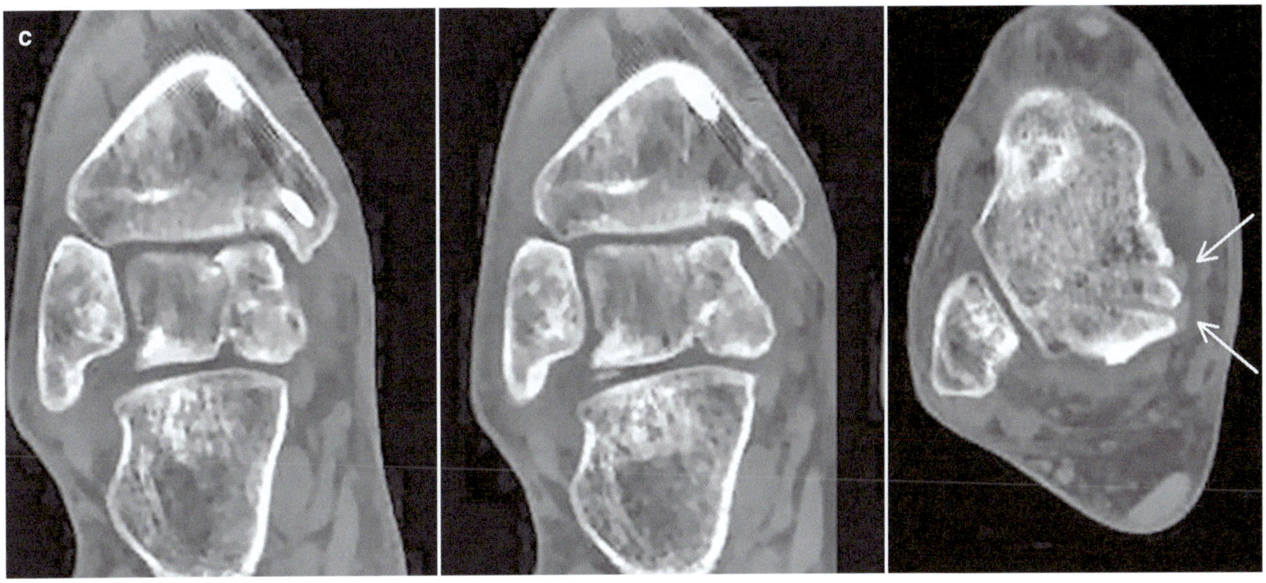

Fig. 4.8 (continued)

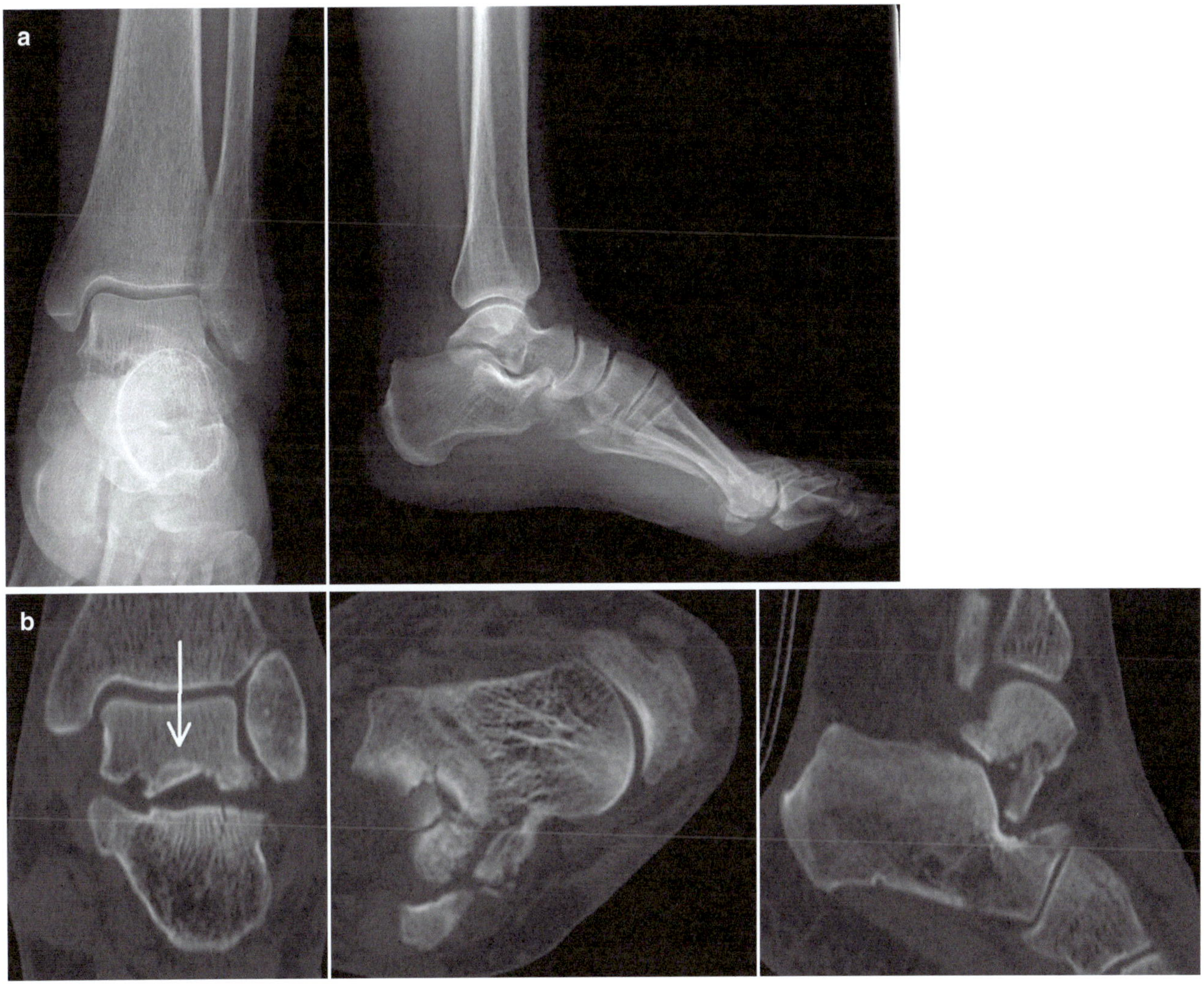

Fig. 4.9 Fracture of the lateral process with partial sinking of the subtalar joint, usually indicated with the acronym "snowboarder's talus fracture": in the standard X-ray projections (**a**) it is not possible to understand the real entity of the injury, which is more clear during the CT scan (**b**), where it is possible to appreciate the amount of sinking of the central part of the subtalar joint (arrow)

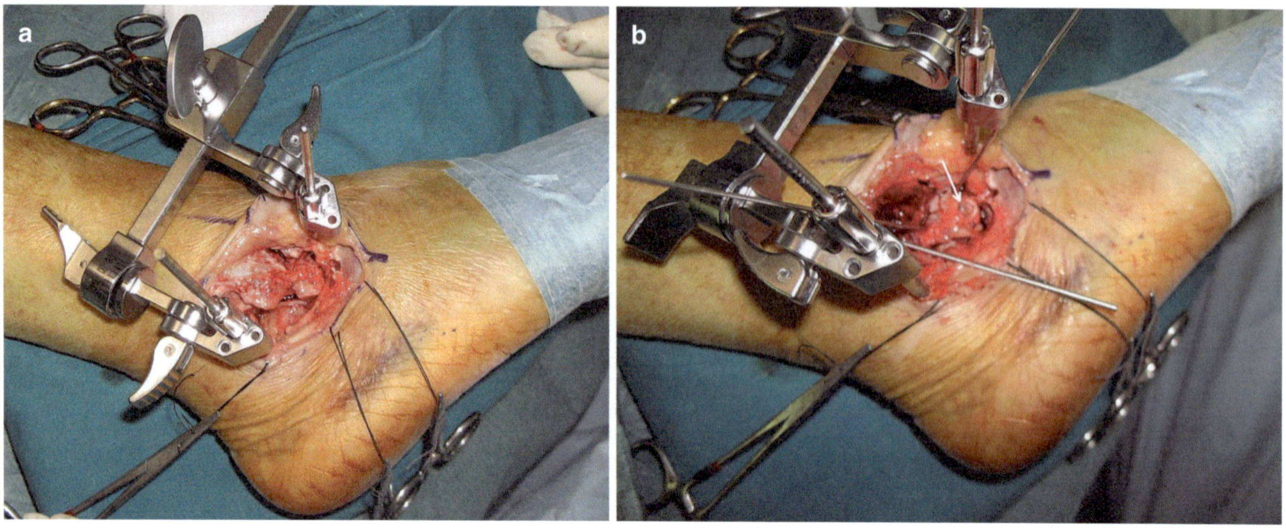

Fig. 4.10 (**a**) Intraoperative imaging after the peroneal osteotomy, where it is possible to clearly depict the dislocation of the lateral process; (**b**) once the subtalar joint has been reduced and a central graft to avoid the dislocation of the osteochondral fragment has been positioned, the lateral process is reduced at its correct height and synthetized with PLLA screws (arrow)

achieved it is possible to recompose the lateral process and synthetize it with titanium or PLLA screws (see Fig. 4.10).

Crush Injuries

They represent the more serious injuries that can occur at the talus; usually they include the body of the bone and they have a highly invalidating prognosis [12, 13].

The treatment options for these fractures are extremely demanding: tibio-calcanear arthrodesis or combined, salvage procedures such as the Blair procedure [14] or substitution of the body of the talus with "custom made" prosthesis [15] have been all reported in literature, because an open reduction and osteosynthesis are common opinions to have a negative prognosis [16].

Only in very young and motivated patients, osteosynthesis is possible to offer as an option, as a propaedeutic surgery that will be followed by a pantalar arthrodesis, to try to avoid the tibio-calcanear fusion, which is the only possible solution in the more severe cases [17, 18].

In our personal experience in these cases, we advise to approach the injury through a single surgical access, avoiding combined routes that have higher risk of iatrogenic damage to the blood supply that needs to be preserved to help the healing of the fractured segments.

Furthermore great attention must be paid to obtain the better anatomical restoration, to foster the best articular recovery or at least to grant the best morphology to allow a successful fusion, if the synthesis succeeds. The osteosynthesis with absorbable materials such as poly-L-lactic acid (PLLA) has proven to achieve sufficient stability of the fractured elements to maintain the reduction (see Figs. 4.11, 4.12, 4.13, 4.14, 4.15, 4.16), and the removal has the undeniable advantage of being unnecessary if any other fusion surgeries are needed.

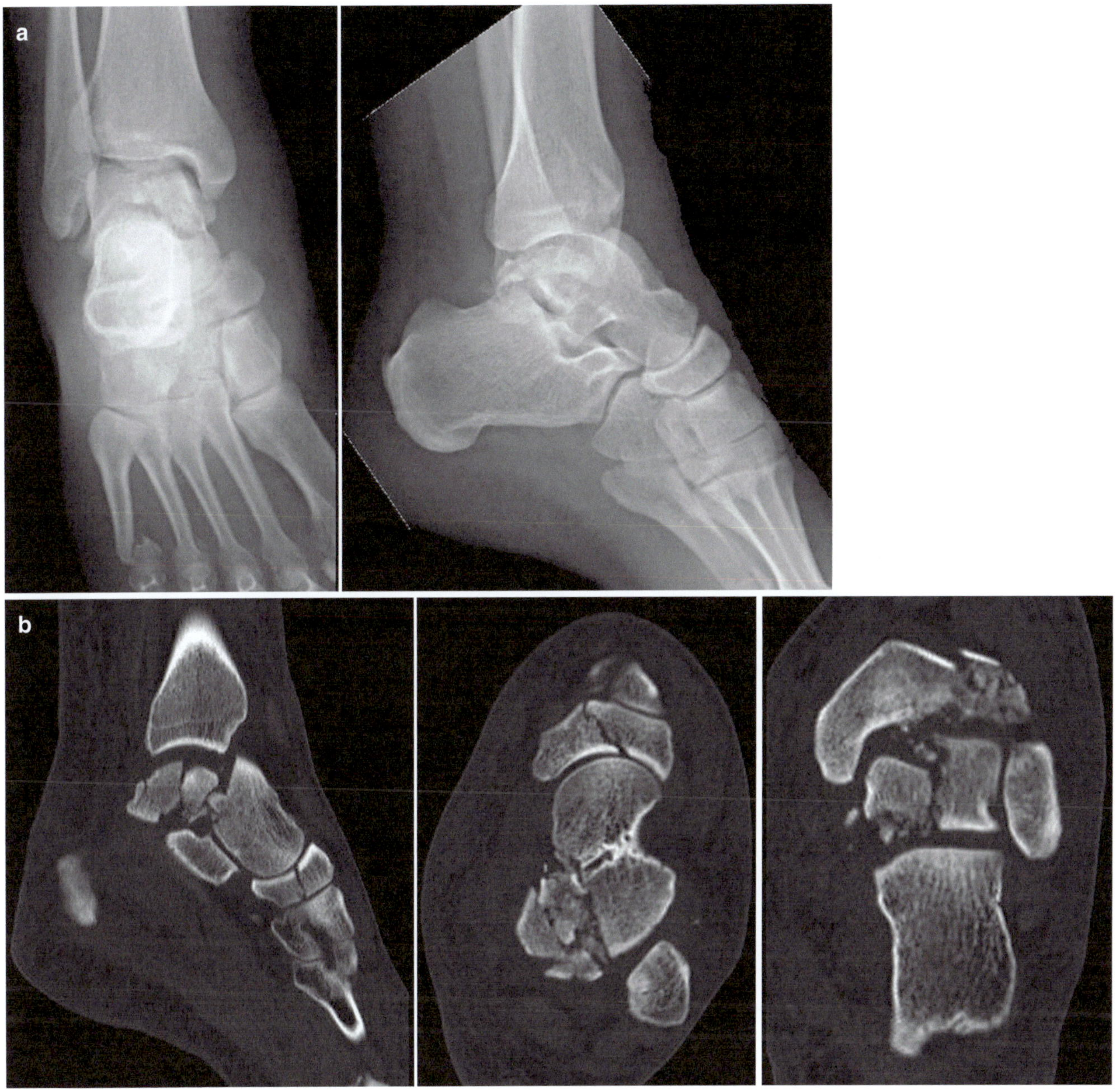

Fig. 4.11 Crush fracture of the body of the talus, coexisting with a navicular fracture: X-ray evaluation in 2 projections (**a**) and morphologic definition through CT scan (**b**)

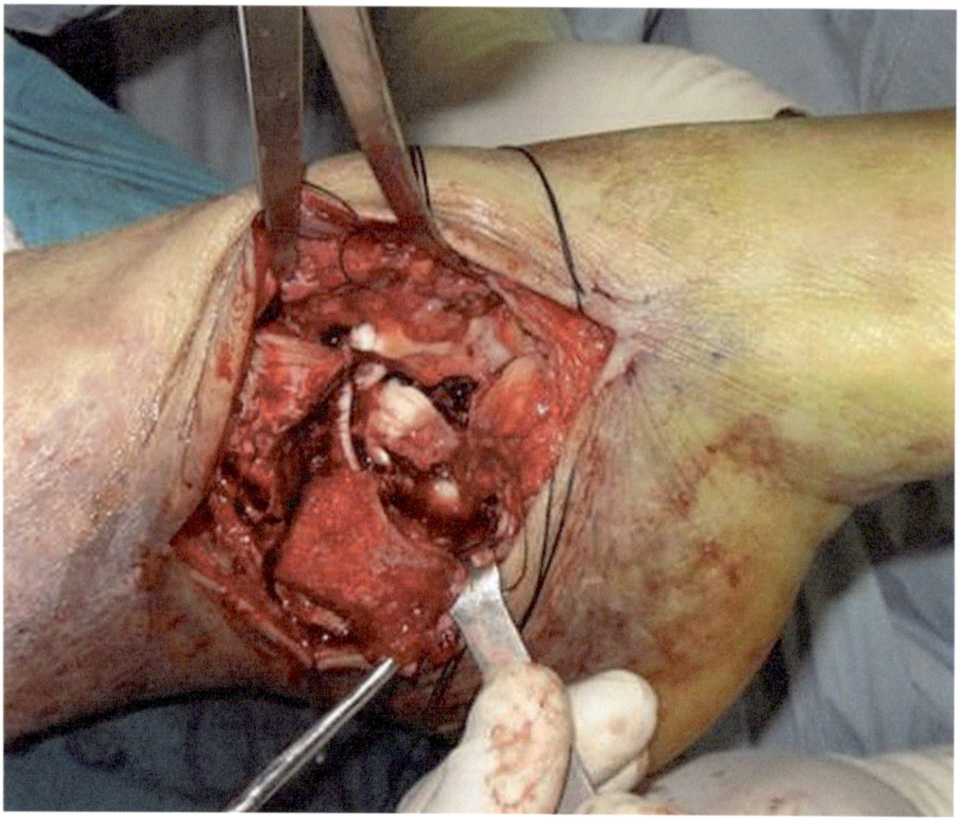

Fig. 4.12 Intraoperative image after medial malleolus osteotomy that shows the pathologic anatomy of the injury with a broad fragmentation of the body

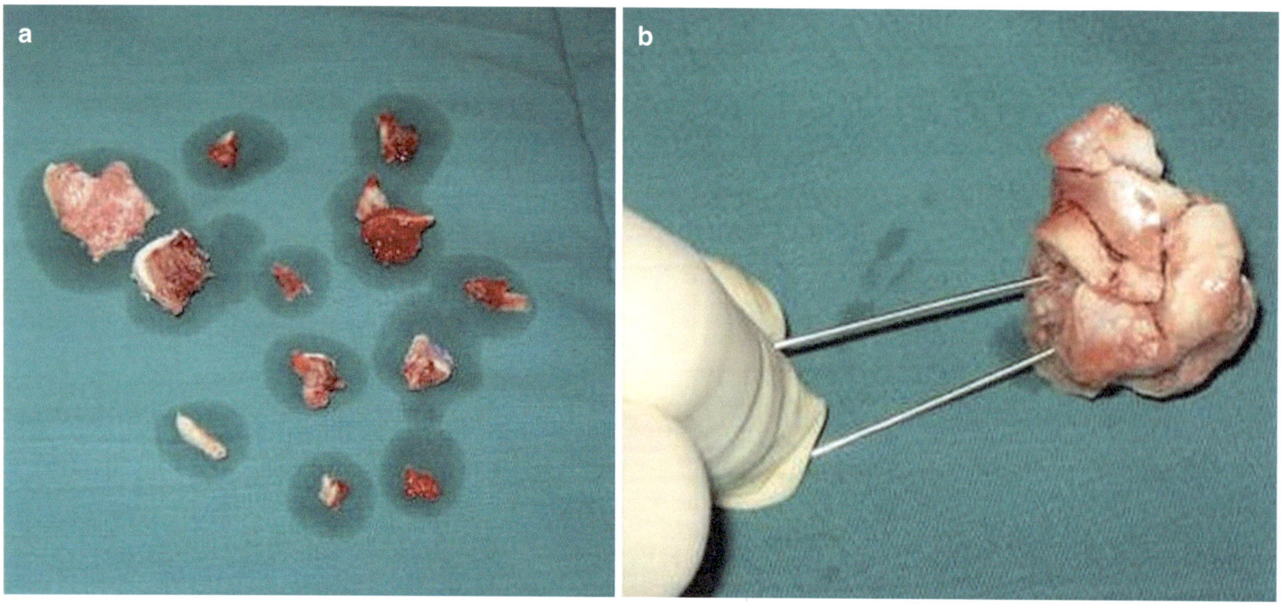

Fig. 4.13 (**a**) Main removed fragments and (**b**) body segment restored at the end of the reconstruction with PLLA pins and screws (sight of the subtalar facet)

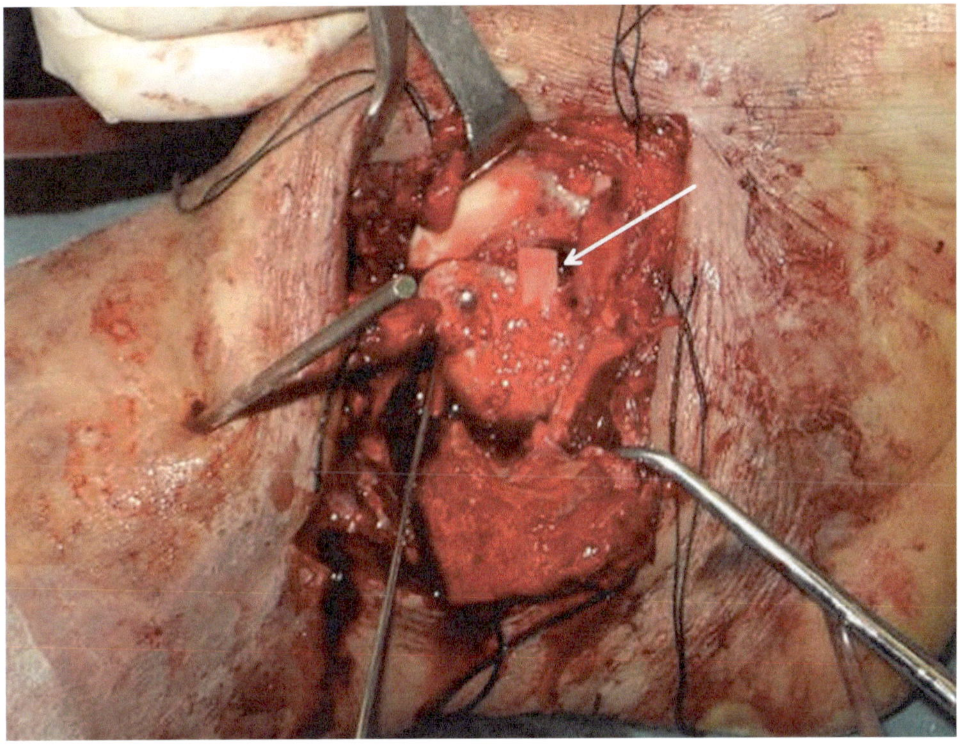

Fig. 4.14 Intraoperative imaging of the restored bone continuity after the talar fragment is reduced. The white arrow enlightens the synthetic bone graft that fills the extra-articular central bone defect

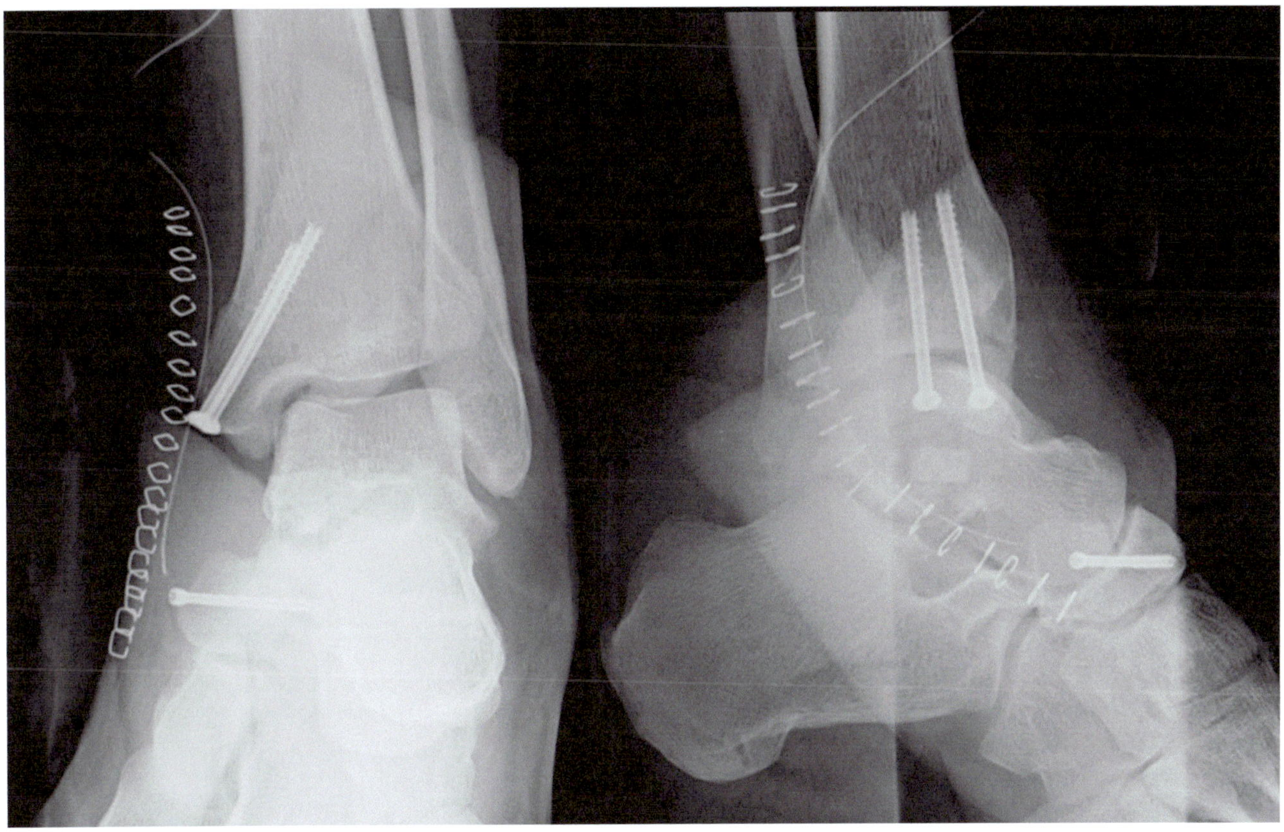

Fig. 4.15 Postoperative X-ray check

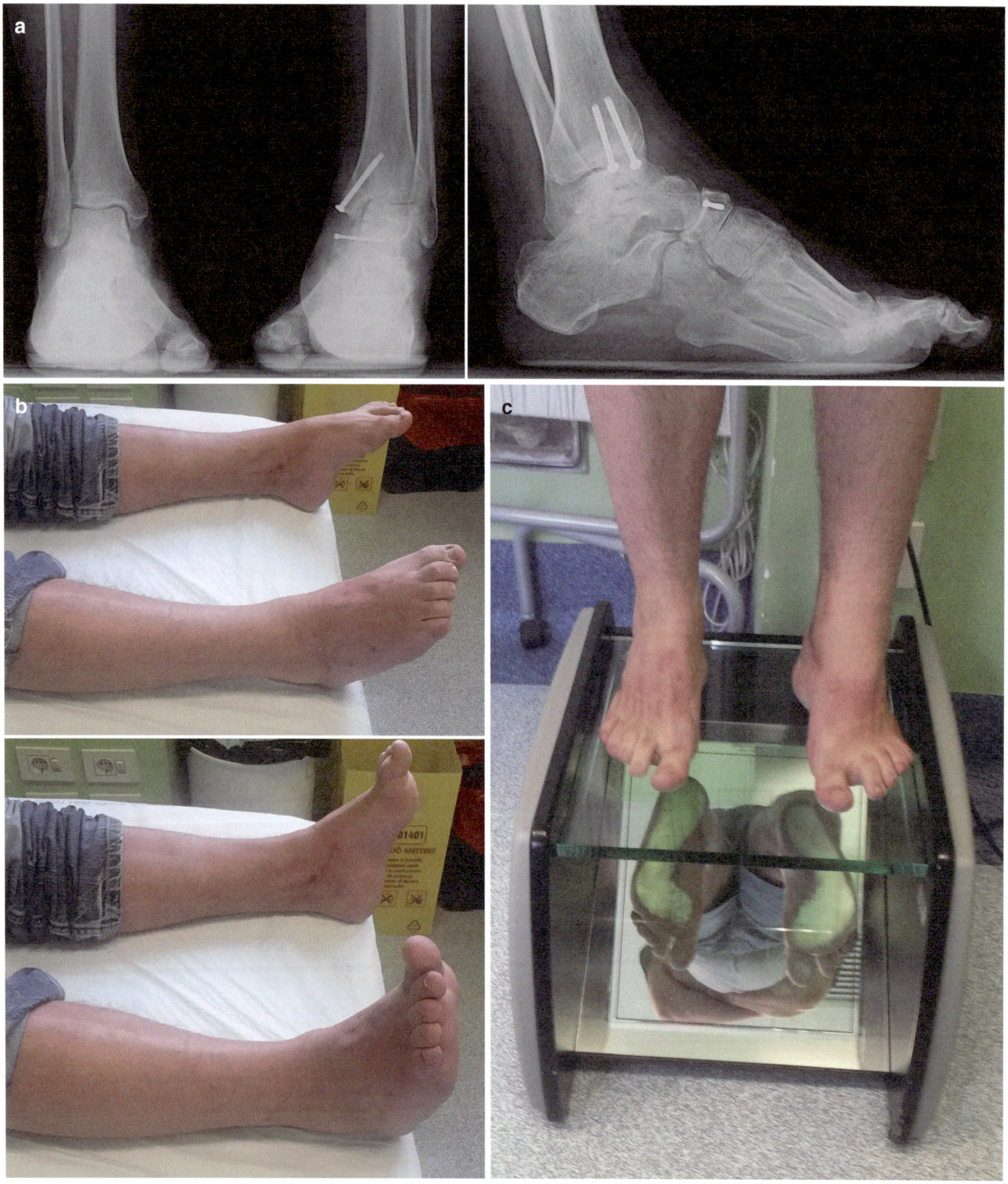

Fig. 4.16 12-month follow-up: (**a**) the X-ray shows the conservation of the anatomical continuity, even if a deterioration of the tibio-talar and subtalar joints and a tendency in supination of the hindfoot are present; clinically it is possible to observe a good dorsiflexion range of motion maintenance (**b**) and a foot stance plantigrade even if an equine tendency is present (**c**)

References

1. Fournier A, Barba N, Steiger V et al (2012) Total talar fracture—long-term results of internal fixation of talar fractures. A multicentric study of 114 cases. Orthop Traumatol Surg Res 98(4 Suppl):S48–S55
2. Hawkins LG (1970) Fractures of the neck of the talus. J Bone Joint Surg Am 52(5):991–1002
3. Marti R (1978) Talus und Calcaneusfrakturen. In: Weber BG, Brunner C, Freuler F (eds) Die Frakturenbehandlung bei Kindern und Jugendlichen. Springer, Berlin, pp 373–384
4. Sanders RW, Lindvall E (2007) Fractures and fracture-dislocations of the talus. In: Coughlin MJ, Mann RA, Saltzman CL (eds) Surgery of the foot and ankle, 8th edn. Mosby Elsevier, Philadelphia, pp 2075–2136
5. Inokuchi S, Ogawa K, Usami N (1996) Classification of fractures of the talus: clear differentiation between neck and body fractures. Foot Ankle Int 17(12):748–750
6. Daniels TR, Smith JW (1993) Talar neck fractures. Foot Ankle 14(4):225–234
7. Mayo KA (1987) Fractures of the talus: principles of management and techniques of treatment. Tech Orthop 2:42–54
8. Swanson TV, Bray TJ, Holmes GB Jr (1992) Fractures of the talar neck. A mechanical study of fixation. J Bone Joint Surg Am 74(4):544–551
9. Ebraheim NA, Mekhail AO, Salpietro BJ et al (1996) Talar neck fractures: anatomic considerations for posterior screw application. Foot Ankle Int 17(9):541–547
10. Schatzker J, Tile M (1993) The management of fractures and dislocations of the talus. In: Tscherne H, Schatzker J (eds) Maior fractures of the pilon, the talus, and the calcaneus. Springer, Berlin, pp 87–104
11. Dunn AR, Jacobs B, Cambell RD (1966) Fractures of the talus. J Trauma 6:443–444
12. Ebraheim NA, Patil V, Owens C et al (2008) Clinical outcome of fractures of the talar body. Int Orthop 32:773–777
13. Thordarson DB (2001) Talar body fractures. Orthop Clin North Am 32:65–77
14. Hantira H, Al Sayed H, Barghash I (2003) Primary ankle fusion using blair technique for severely comminuted fracture of the talus. Med Princ Pract 12:47–50
15. Harnroongroj T, Harnroongroj T (2014) The talar body prosthesis: results at ten to thirty-six years of follow-up. J Bone Joint Surg Am 96(14):1211–1218
16. Vallier HA, Nork SE, Benirschke SK et al (2003) Surgical treatment of talar body fractures. J Bone Joint Surg Am 85:1716–1724
17. Daghino W, Di Gregorio G, Cerlon R (2011) Surgical reconstruction of a crush injury of the talar body: a case report. J Bone Joint Surg Am 93(14):e80. https://doi.org/10.2106/JBJS.J.01358
18. Noda M, Yoshino K, Honda H et al (2004) A comminuted talar body fracture osteosynthesized with bioabsorbable screws: a case report. J Trauma 56:709–712

Surgical Treatment of Calcaneal Fractures

5

Contents

5.1 Calcaneal Fracture

The fracture of the calcaneus is a relative frequent injury, including about 2% of all fractures [1, 2]. Mostly they are displaced fractures that include the subtalar joint and/or the calcaneocuboid joint, while the open injuries, which have the worst prognosis, are luckily only 8% of the total [3].

About 90% of the calcaneal fractures happen in adult males, causing for their consequences a partial or complete inability to work [4–6]; this explains how these injuries have a serious impact on the society.

5.1.1 Classification

During the acute phase, the imaging allows to formulate a diagnosis and to define a classification that has the task to guide the treatment.

A first division is to define the injuries that affect the joints from the extra-articular ones; such distinction is frequently possible through the classic X-rays in the three planes, which need to be integrated with an axial view of the calcaneus when the fracture becomes evident.

In the doubtful situations, the CT is the second level exam that will depict the diagnosis; the CT is mandatory and irreplaceable in the articular or displaced fractures, because it allows to classify the injury pattern and to plan the surgical treatment if needed [7]. The more used and shared classification system is the one proposed by Sanders; it describes four types of fracture patterns [8] that are shown through the CT coronal scans.

To allow uniform considerations, it is important to consider only images that are achieved through techniques that are reproducible and homogeneous; to standardize the procedure, it is possible to use a reconstruction plane, the one perpendicular to the line conjoining the extremities of the subtalar joint surface, considering it on a central lateral projection (see Fig. 5.1). Considering the coronal scans achieved

W. Daghino et al., *Foot and Ankle Trauma Injuries*, https://doi.org/10.1007/978-3-319-69617-1_5

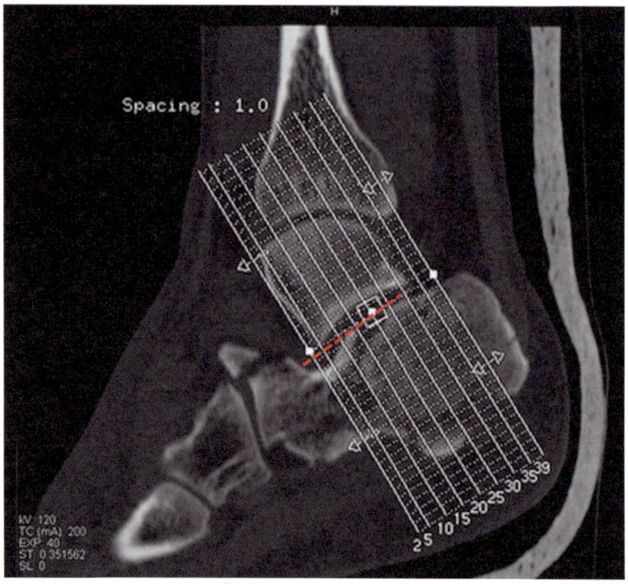

Fig. 5.1 Sanders classification of calcaneal fractures: to achieve reproducibility of the study, it is necessary to consider the only coronal scans that are perpendicular to the line that connects the extremities of the subtalar joint in the talar part (red line)

through the previous method, the study of the fracture is performed where the subtalar joint surface is larger.

Spotted the scan that needs to be examined, the surface of the posterior subtalar joint of the calcaneus is ideally divided in three portions of same extension, one lateral (A), one central (B) and one medial (C) (see Fig. 5.2); then the number of fracture lines is counted and their position is defined [8].

All the undisplaced injuries, independently from the number of fracture lines spotted, are considered type I fractures (see Fig. 5.3). When only one fracture line is recognizable, which generates two articular fragments, the injury is classified as type II, which is further divided into the A, B and C subgroups depending on the part of joint surface the fracture line lies (see Fig. 5.4); when the fracture lines that cross the joint are two, it is possible to spot three articular fragments, and the injury is classified as type III, with the subgroups AB, AC and BC, even in this case depending on the positioning of the fracture lines (see Fig. 5.5); if it is possible to depict three or more fracture lines, with consequently four or more articular fragments, the injury is always classified as type IV (se Fig. 5.6).

5.1.2 Type of Treatment and Indications (Planning)

Many different types of treatments have been proposed during this time to treat the calcaneal fractures, mainly divided into four subgroups: percutaneous pinning, external fixation

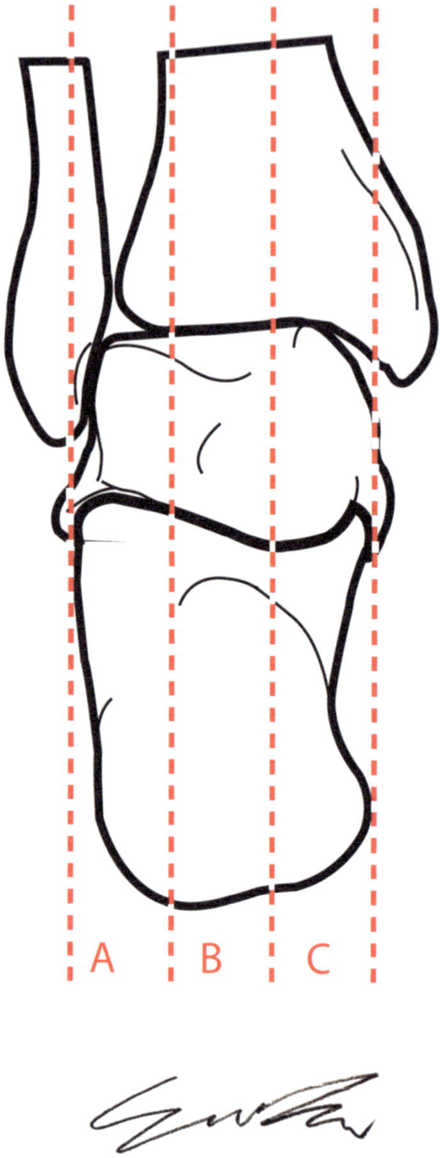

Fig. 5.2 Sanders classification of calcaneal fractures: on the coronal scan perfectly selected, the joint surface of the calcaneal posterior subtalar joint must be ideally divided into three areas: lateral (A), central (B) and medial (C)

through previous minimally invasive fracture reduction, open reduction and internal fixation and subtalar acute fusion. Each of these treatments is unable to deal with all the possible circumstances that are related with the fractures, but all of them can have a role in the management in some types of calcaneal fractures, granting the best result possible and limiting the complications.

For this reason, we suggest that the surgeon who is going to approach the treatment of a calcaneal fracture, besides being specifically trained and having performed the demanding learning curve needed for the treatment of these injuries [9], needs to know and master all these types of treatments,

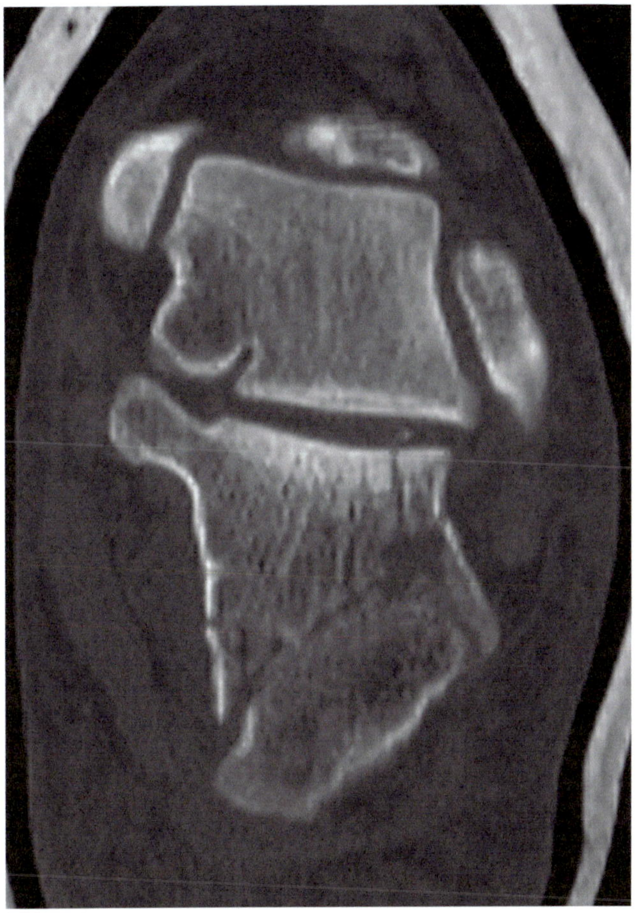

Fig. 5.3 Multifragmentary fracture of the calcaneus involving the articular surface without displacement: type I for the Sanders classification

being able to choose the best option for every single case, on the basis of the morphology of the fracture, the characteristics of the patient and the scientific evidence.

Thus it is very useful to build a treatment protocol that will help in the decisional process, to allow having a logical system, reproducible in every time a calcaneal injury is approached.

An example of the latter is reported in Fig. 5.7, and it contemplates a first distinction between open and closed fractures, foreseeing in the first case a unique type of treatment, that is, the external fixation.

In the absence of skin injuries related to an open fracture, it is mandatory to enlighten any other absolute contraindications to open surgery, represented by interval from injury longer than 20 days, impairment of the soft tissue along the incision line, severe peripheral vasculopathy, diabetes type 1, severe infirmity and immunosuppression [1].

For this purpose, it is advisable to consider part of this category even drug addiction, which could generate some kind of immunosuppression and could predispose to a higher risk of infectious-inflammatory complications.

In the case any of the latter are present, the treatment choice falls on low-impact techniques, such as mini-invasive surgery and stabilization with an external fixator; if none of the listed risk factors are present, the second step is to further classify the fracture pattern to choose the best treatment.

For this purpose, a first distinction has to be done between fractures that involve the articular surface of the posterior subtalar joint from the ones that don't include it. If the injury is not articular, the fracture patterns that need a surgical

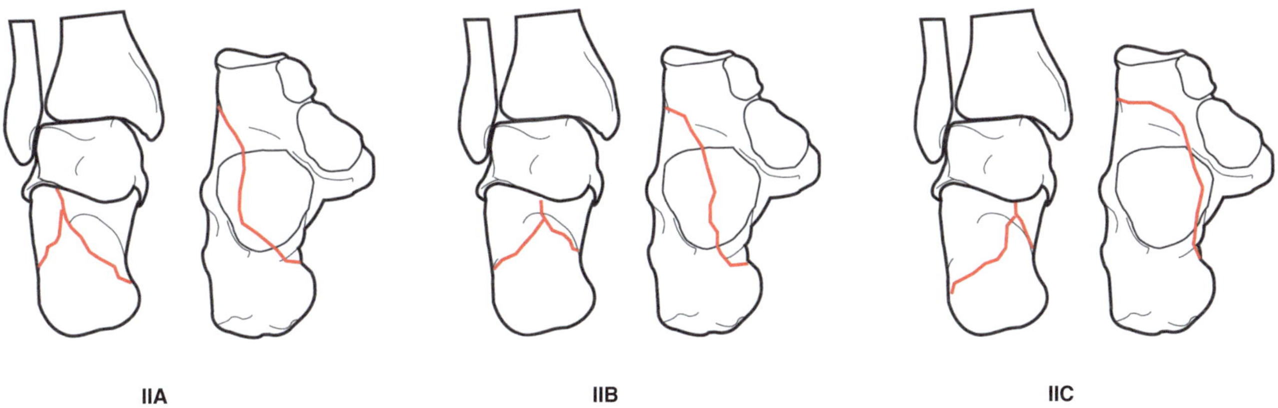

Fig. 5.4 Sanders classification: two fragments articular fracture, depending on where the fracture line falls lateral, central or medial in the subtalar joint it is defined the subgroup IIA, IIB and IIC

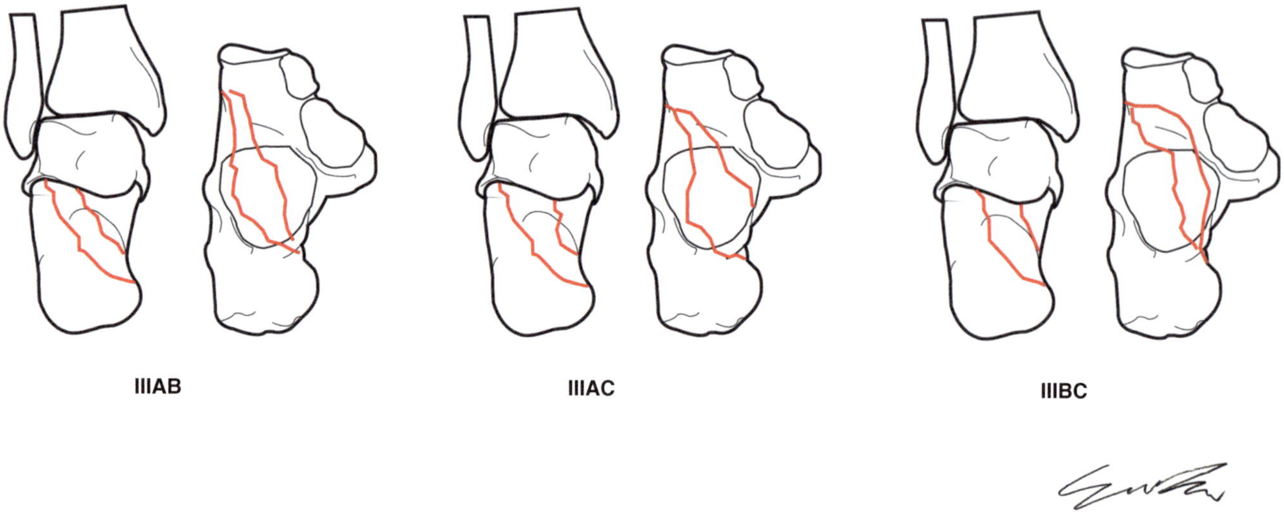

Fig. 5.5 Sanders classification: fractures that produce three joint fragments, depending on where the two fracture lines lay, the subgroups IIIAB III AC and III BC are defined

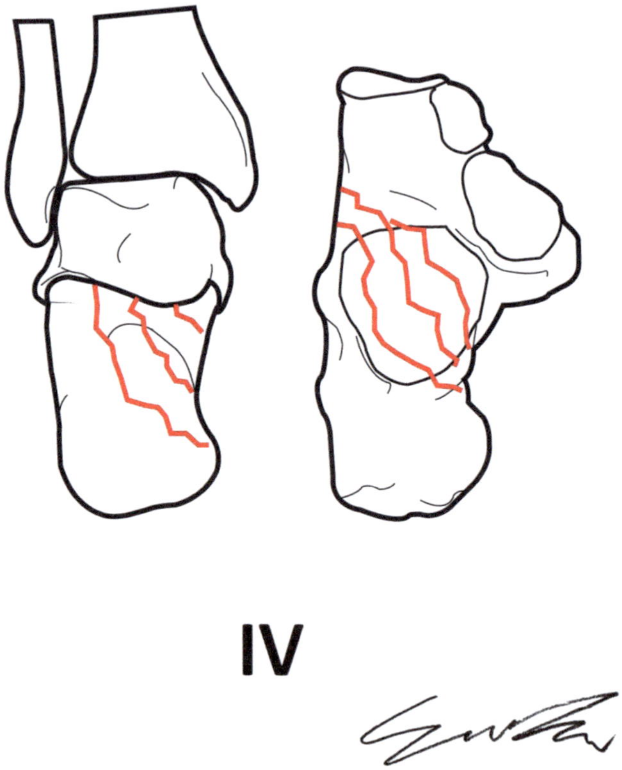

Fig. 5.6 Sanders classification: the fractures that include four or more articular fragments define the type IV, independently from where the fracture lines lay

treatment are the ones named as "tongue" fractures, where there is a complete loss of height of the entire posterior subtalar joint, which can be easily handled through percutaneous surgery and stabilization with Steinmann pins or Kirschner wires, and then both the fractures that have a complete loss of height of the sustentaculum tali and the fractures with a proximal translation of the posterior tuberosity are treated through a percutaneous reduction and osteosynthesis, usually through free screw fixation (see Fig. 5.8).

When the injury is articular and if there is an undisplaced fracture type I, the treatment is conservative, through the positioning of a plaster cast for 6 weeks and no weight bearing for 3 months; if there are fractures that have two or three articular fragments, that is, Sanders types II and III, the treatment of choice is open reduction and internal fixation. If a fracture Sanders type IV is present, some authors suggest to perform a subtalar joint fusion as the first option [8–10]; since such procedure is more complicated and risky to be performed as a first option [11], a more cautious and safe behaviour is to perform a nonsurgical approach or a percutaneous approach to achieve a reduction and stabilization of the fracture, with the aim to leave the injury heal, reserving a fusion in a second step, and to treat any consequences.

Anyhow the treatment choice must be taken on a CT planning, where the number of fragments and their spatial

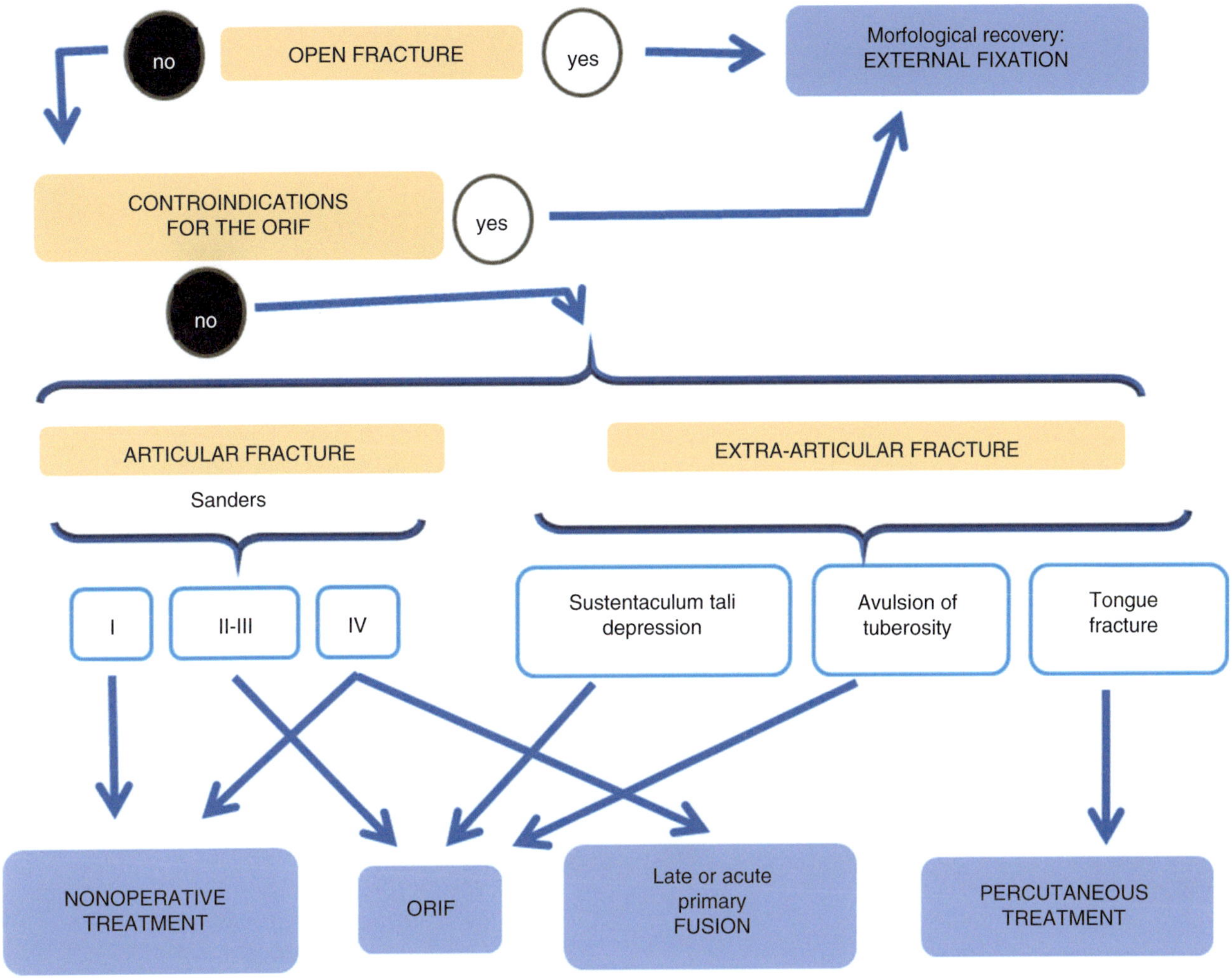

Fig. 5.7 Example of decision flow chart for calcaneal fractures

disposition, the modality of displacement and the necessary reductions manoeuvres, which are going to define the type of surgery and the best devices to achieve stabilization/osteosynthesis, must be carefully evaluated (see Fig. 5.9).

5.1.3 Percutaneous Techniques

5.1.3.1 Goals

The main indication for this technique is when the entire posterior subtalar joint, usually united with the posterior tuberosity, is tilted and sunken plantarly: the aim of the reduction and stabilization is to reposition the articular part in its natural place through indirect lever manoeuvres, restoring the bony anatomy and contemporarily lowering the surgical aggression.

5.1.3.2 Surgical Technique

Positioning

The patient is positioned on a lateral or better prone decubitus, with the extremity of the injured limb free to move and hanging out the bed and with the contralateral knee flexed through a support, allowing to obtain easily a lateral view with the X-ray image intensifier (see Fig. 5.10).

The fluoroscopy check ends this procedure, because it allows to see if the necessary views are obtainable and cor-

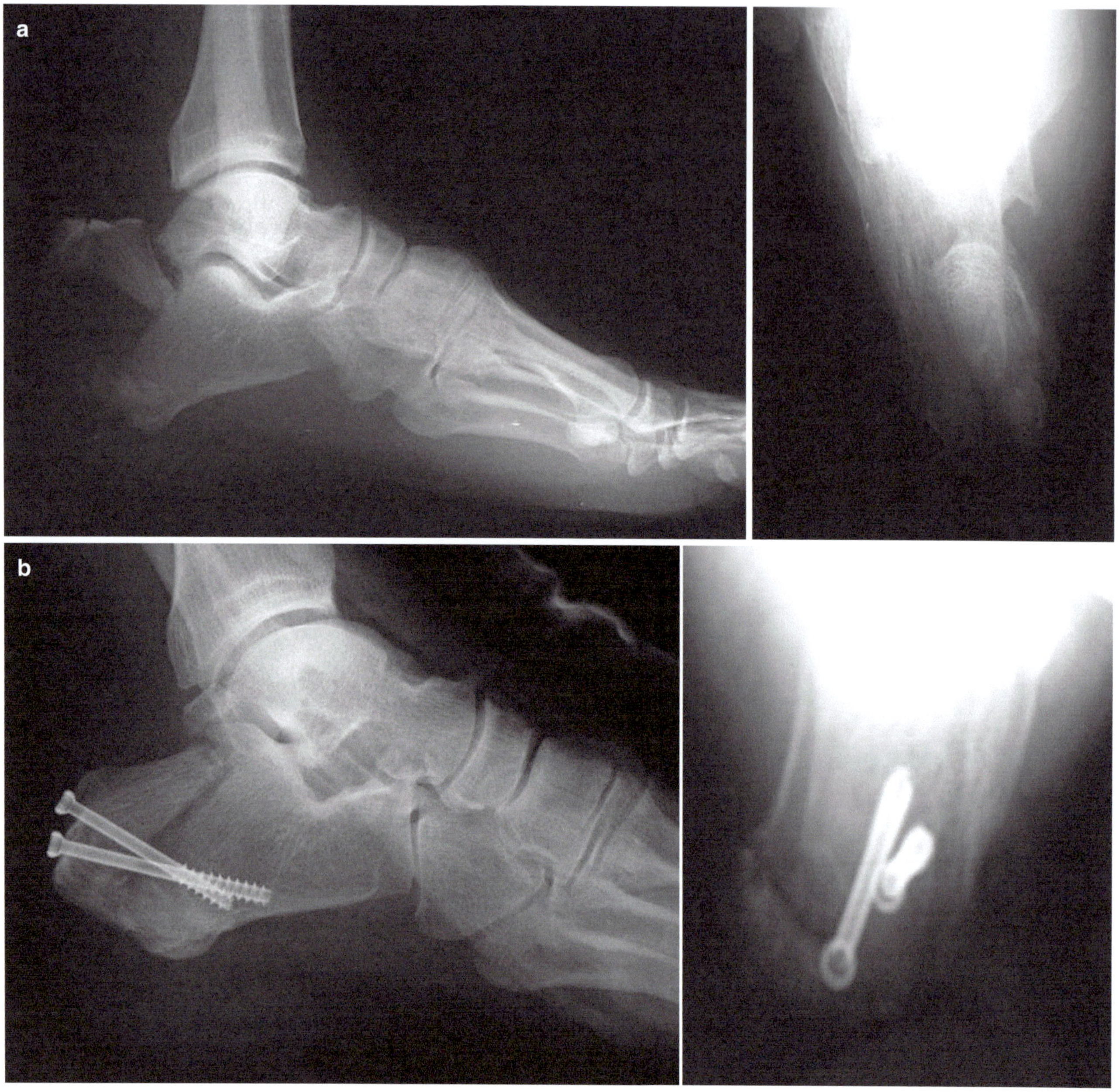

Fig. 5.8 Fracture case with proximal displacement of the posterior tuberosity: preoperative planning (**a**) and postoperative check after reduction and osteosynthesis with free-handed screws (**b**)

rect and they represent a starting point that can be confronted with the images performed during surgery. Once the latter is ended, the surgical field is prepared.

Reduction and Stabilization Manoeuvres

To grant the reduction, a surgical access with Steinmann pins through the posterior tuberosity is performed, guiding two pins to the subchondral area of the subtalar joint that is sunken (see Fig. 5.11). Using as a lever one of these pins and with the foot plantar flexed, the so-called Essex-Lopresti manoeuvre is performed [12], shifting proximally and rotating the sunken fragment until the Gissane angle is restored, which is essential to check it under fluoroscopy; when this step is achieved, while an assistant maintains the reduction, the second pin is advanced with the same direction through the talus, using the latter as a support to maintain the reduction; if the fluoros-

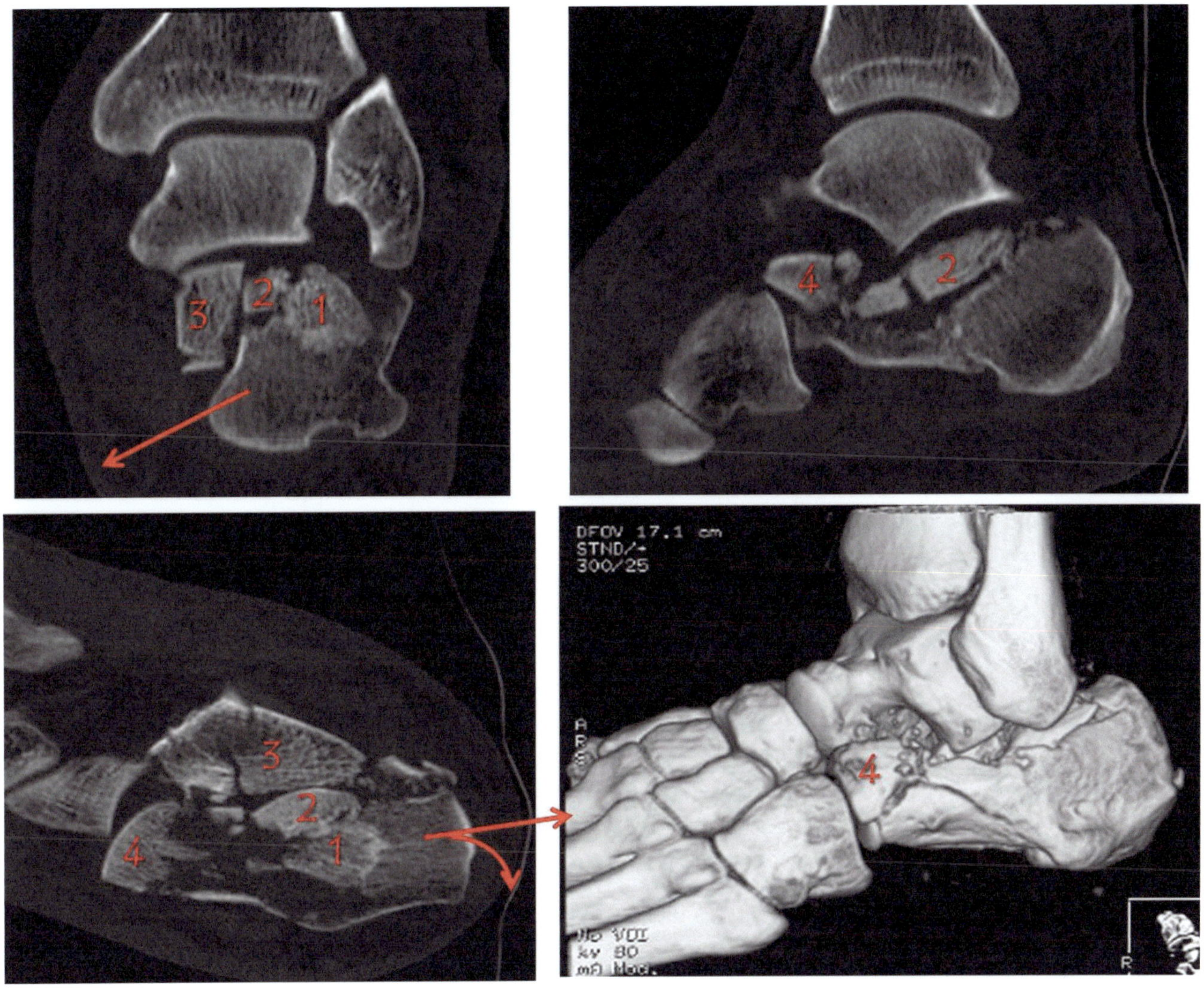

Fig. 5.9 Example of preoperative planning of a multifragmentary displaced fracture of the calcaneus (Sanders IIIAB): the main fragments are identified and numbered; the necessary proceedings are indicated through arrows indicating the movement that needs to be applied on the bony parts to achieve the reduction

copy check is satisfying, the stabilization is completed advancing the first pin directly in the talar bone (see Fig. 5.12), then the external extremities of the pins are cut and bended, and a plaster cast is done to keep the foot in neutral position.

Postoperative Care

The plaster cast is kept for 6 weeks, the moment in which the Steinmann pins are removed, after an X-ray is performed to check if the reduction has been kept. From this moment, the movement of the foot is allowed without any weight bearing, which must be avoided for a total of 3 months from the surgery; after this period, a full weight bearing is allowed gradually, initially protected with two crutches.

5.1.4 External Fixation

5.1.4.1 Goals

This option is used if open surgery is contraindicated, usually when the soft tissues are compromised. As this procedure allows to achieve reduction manoeuvres through minimally invasive techniques, and therefore granting a low impact on the soft tissues and a lower risk of infections, it is clear that in certain situations, this surgical option is an inevitable choice. In these situations, the goal is not to achieve an anatomical reduction of the fracture but only the morphology of the bone, through the restoration of possible height and length and consequently the spatial volume of the bone [13].

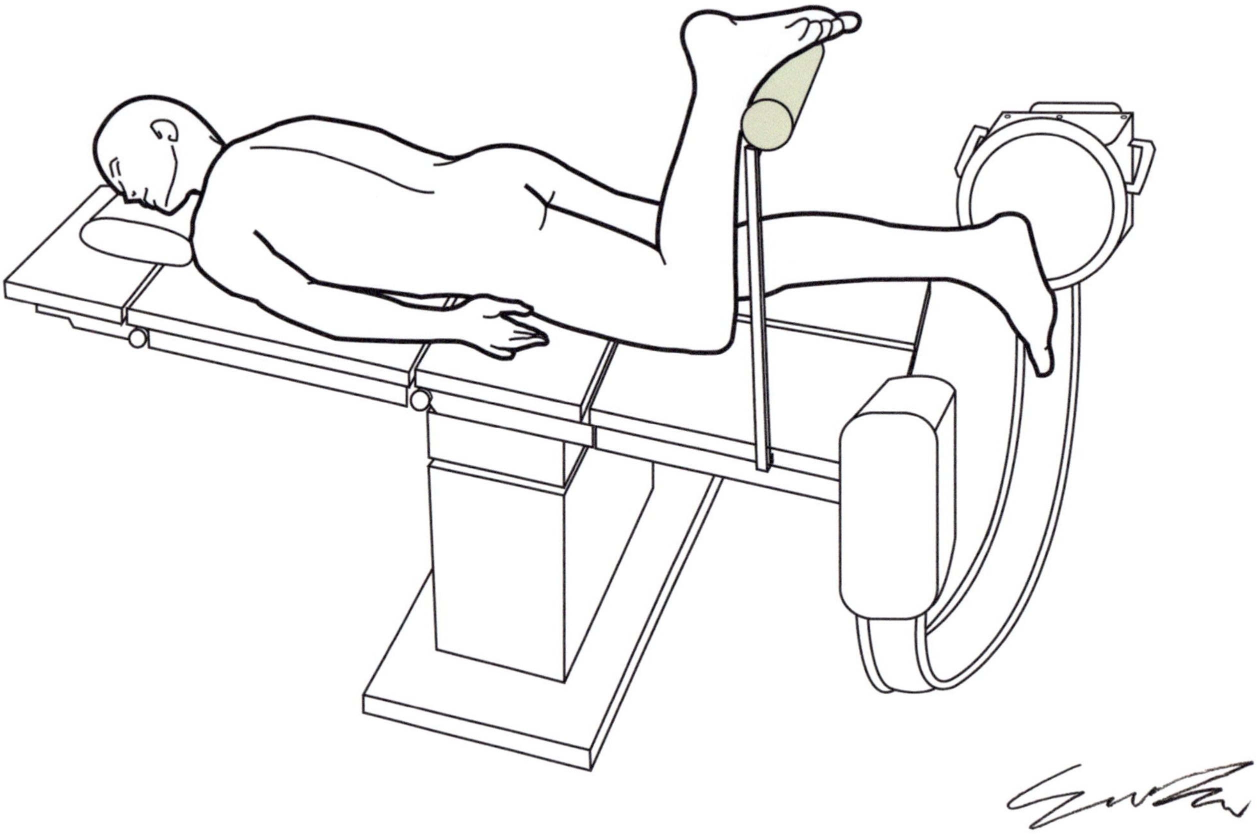

Fig. 5.10 Percutaneous fixation of a calcaneal fracture: the prone positioning of the patient can ease the reduction manoeuvres and the execution of the necessary X-ray imaging

5.1.4.2 Surgical Technique

Positioning

The patient is usually positioned on a lateral decubitus, with the lower limb that needs treating raised from the contralateral and rested over a cushion (see Fig. 5.13).

Even in this case, a fluoroscopy check is appropriate, to confirm if the correct vision of the foot is correctly obtained and adequately defined and also to generate an image of the injury that will be compared to the next images during the reduction manoeuvres. Finally the surgical field is prepared.

Surgical Access

To do a minimally invasive reduction, a lateral 2–3 cm length incision is performed, placed just under the lateral malleolus, with an oblique development to avoid crossing the line of the peroneus tendons. The best spot for the incision that will allow inserting the instrumentation to gain the reduction is chosen during the preoperative planning considering the direction of the forces used through levers (see Fig. 5.14).

Reduction and Stabilization Manoeuvres

Once the access to the bone is granted to allow the reduction manoeuvres, levers of increasing width are introduced, under fluoroscopy evaluation, the nearest as possible to the portion of the bone that needs to be elevated. Through the applicable force achieved with the instrumentation and simultaneously keeping the foot in equinus position to reduce the Achilles tendon tension and ease the translation manoeuvres, mobilization of the sunken fragments is started, using the talar part of the posterior subtalar joint as a pattern which moulds the elevated fragments (see Fig. 5.15).

Once the reduction is achieved, stabilization is performed through an external fixator, positioning the pins into the subchondral bone of the posterior subtalar joint, into the posterior and anterior tuberosity or, in case of an excessive fragmentation of the latter, into the cuboid.

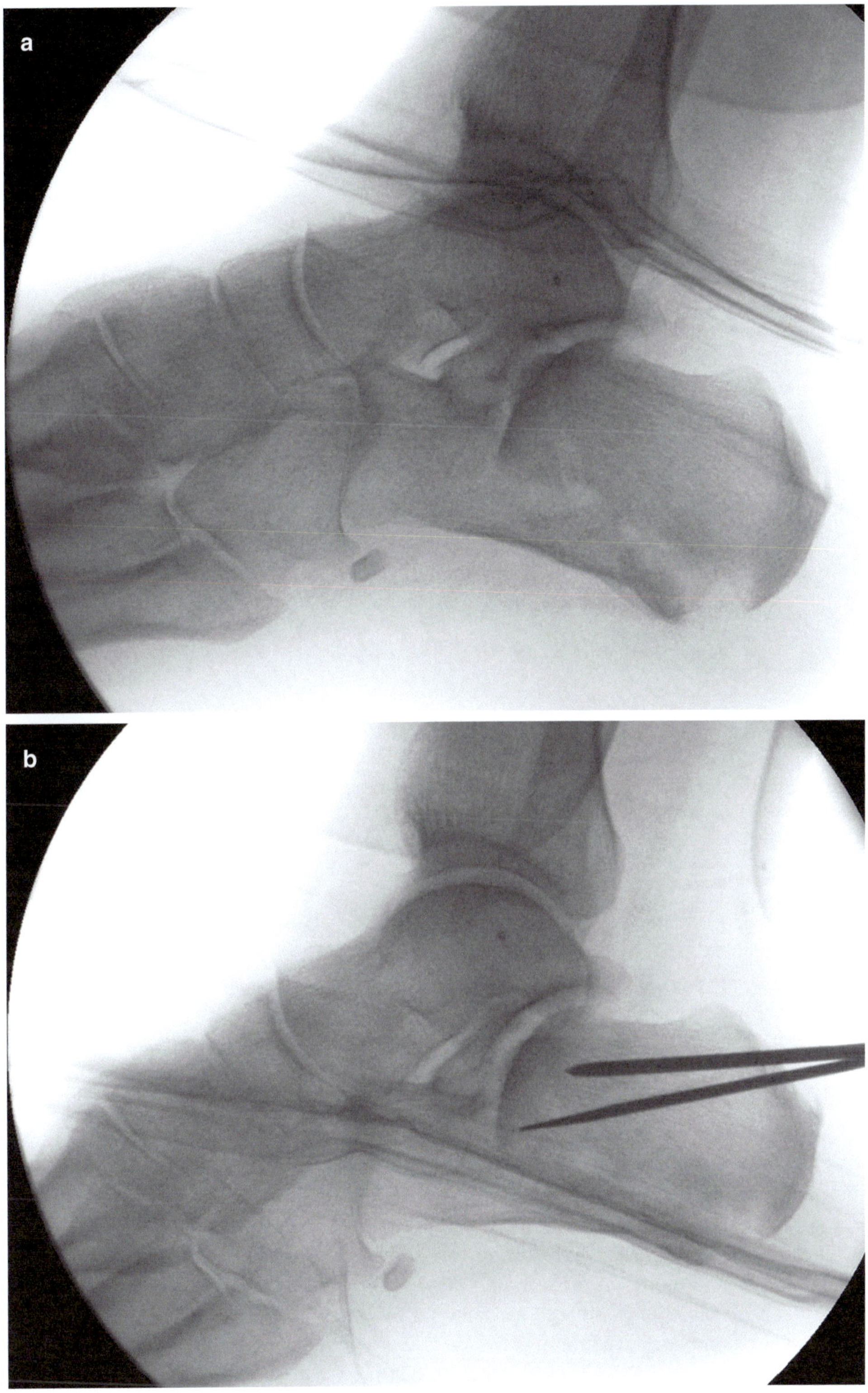

Fig. 5.11 Percutaneous stabilization of a calcaneal fracture: after the posterior tuberosity is identified through fluoroscopy imaging, which is sunken and shifted plantarly (**a**), the tuberosity is hold with two Steinman pins put until the subchondral area of the subtalar joint (**b**)

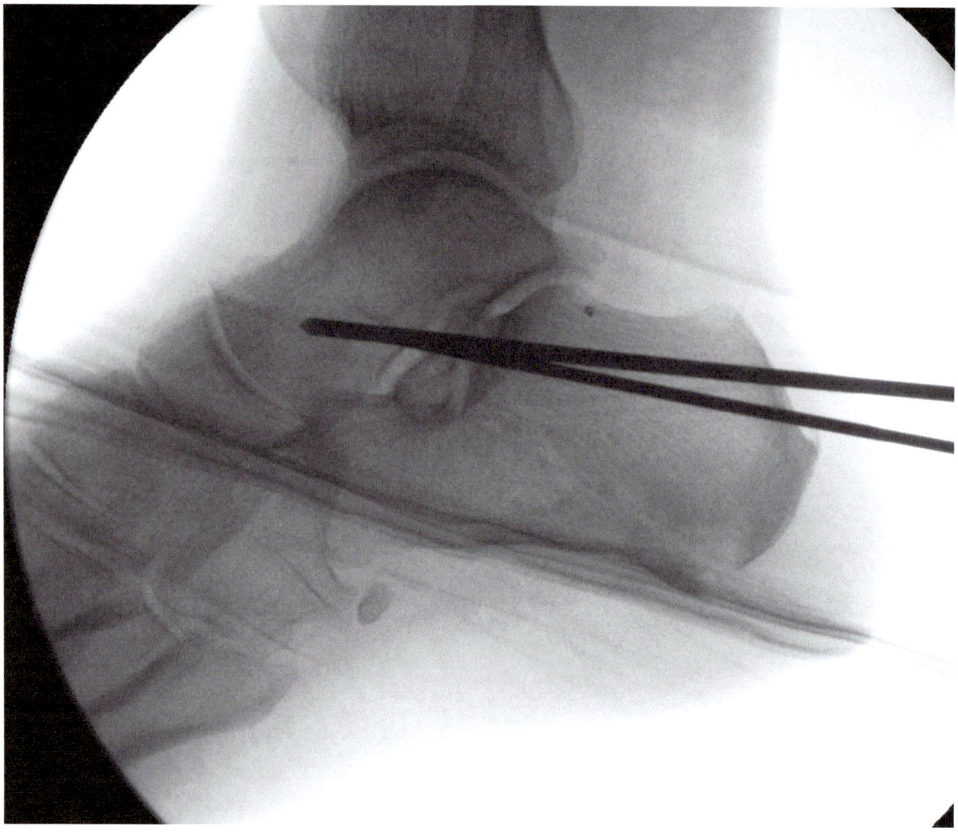

Fig. 5.12 Percutaneous fixation of the calcaneus fracture: after the fracture is reduced, using the pins as levers, the achieved reduction is stabilized through the progression of the same pins into the talar bone, used as a fixed point to gain fixation

The frame that is going to be later built must connect these pins, granting a triangular conformation able to keep length and height previously restored.

Theoretically, any external fixator for little fragments could be used to achieve such geometry. However on the market, it is possible to find specific models of external fixators dedicated to the calcaneal fractures, such as the one developed by Orthofix®, which offers as an advantage to gather in a sterile single use kit all the necessary to build the frame, and it is specifically developed to treat these fractures.

With this device, the fixation elements provided are screws of 3 mm diameter, self-tapping and self-drilling to grant an easy positioning; furthermore, once the frame is connected to the fixation elements, it is possible to partially modify the geometry of the frame, achieved through a system of slays and micrometric screws, producing a mechanic tension between the clamps that increases remarkably the stability of the assembly and consequently between the bone fragments that have been reduced (see Fig. 5.16).

Postoperative Care

The affected limb is positioned in an open plaster cast until the stiches are removed, and then it is possible to allow active movement of the ankle and foot joints without weight bearing.

The pins of the external fixator must be medicated twice per week to prevent any bone infection through the skin incisions; after 40 days, an X-ray is done, and eventually some of the Kirschner wires or Steinmann pins, left percutaneous to increase the stability of the frame, are removed; after 3 months from surgery, subject to X-rays, the external fixator is removed, and a progressive recovery of the weight bearing is allowed, at the beginning eased by the use of crutches.

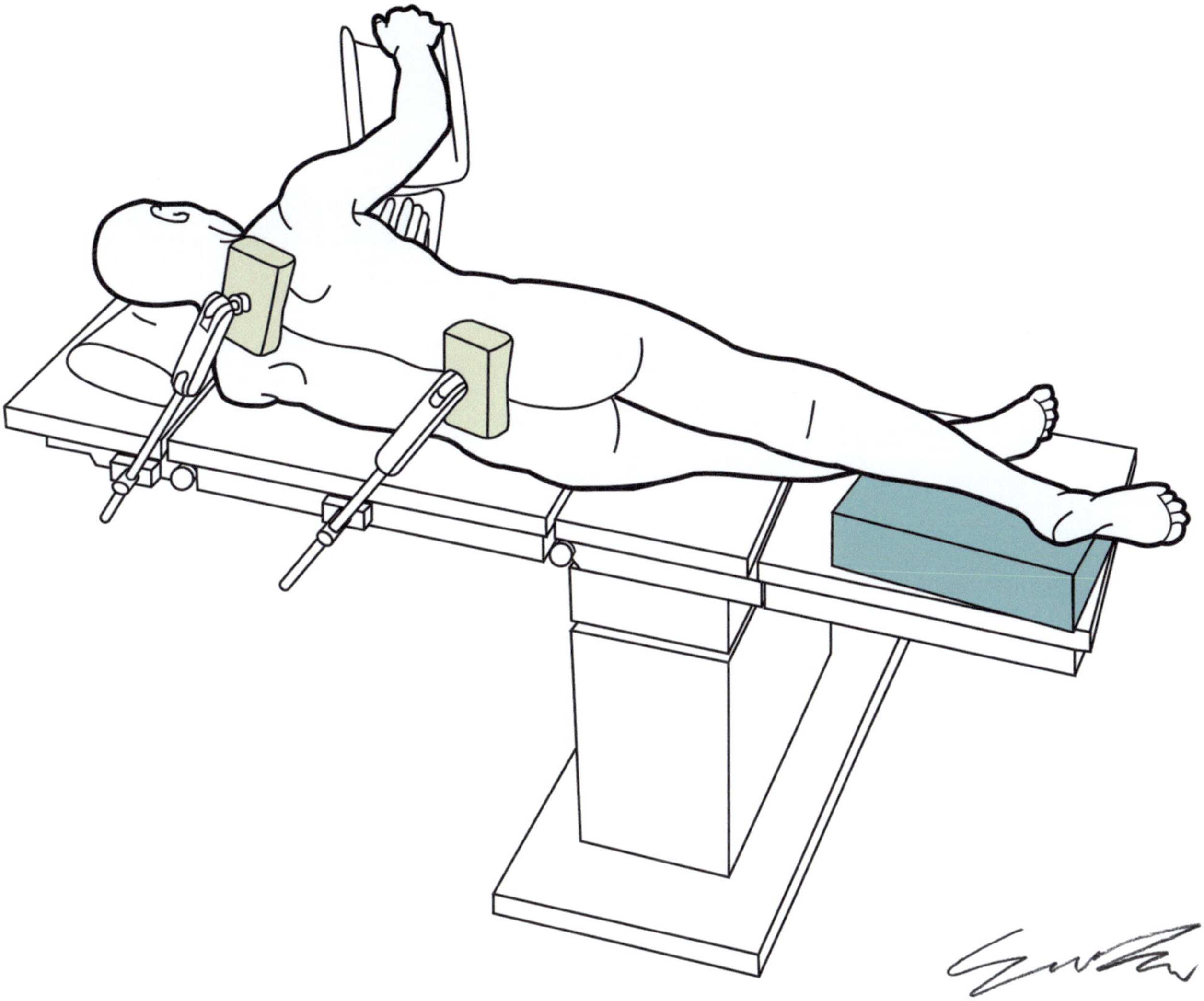

Fig. 5.13 Mini-invasive reduction and stabilization with an external fixator of a calcaneal fracture. Preoperative positioning: the lateral decubitus allows to evaluate the correct restoration of the axis; the cushion under the affected leg grants to have the calcaneus on a different level regarding the other structures, helping to achieve the intraoperative X-ray images

5.1.5 Open Reduction and Internal Fixation (ORIF)

5.1.5.1 Goals

The clinical goal that the surgeon must aim at with this technique is challenging, pursuing the best functional recovery possible, in a pain-free condition. This inevitably passes through the achievement not only of the height and length of the bone and consequently of the spatial volumes of the latter but even through the anatomical reduction of the joint lines, which is directly bound to the best clinical results in the future [1, 14].

5.1.5.2 Surgical Technique

Positioning

The best positioning of the patient to allow the reduction and synthesis with a plate is to be tilted 45° on the healthy side; a radio-transparent table that grants the necessary intraopera-

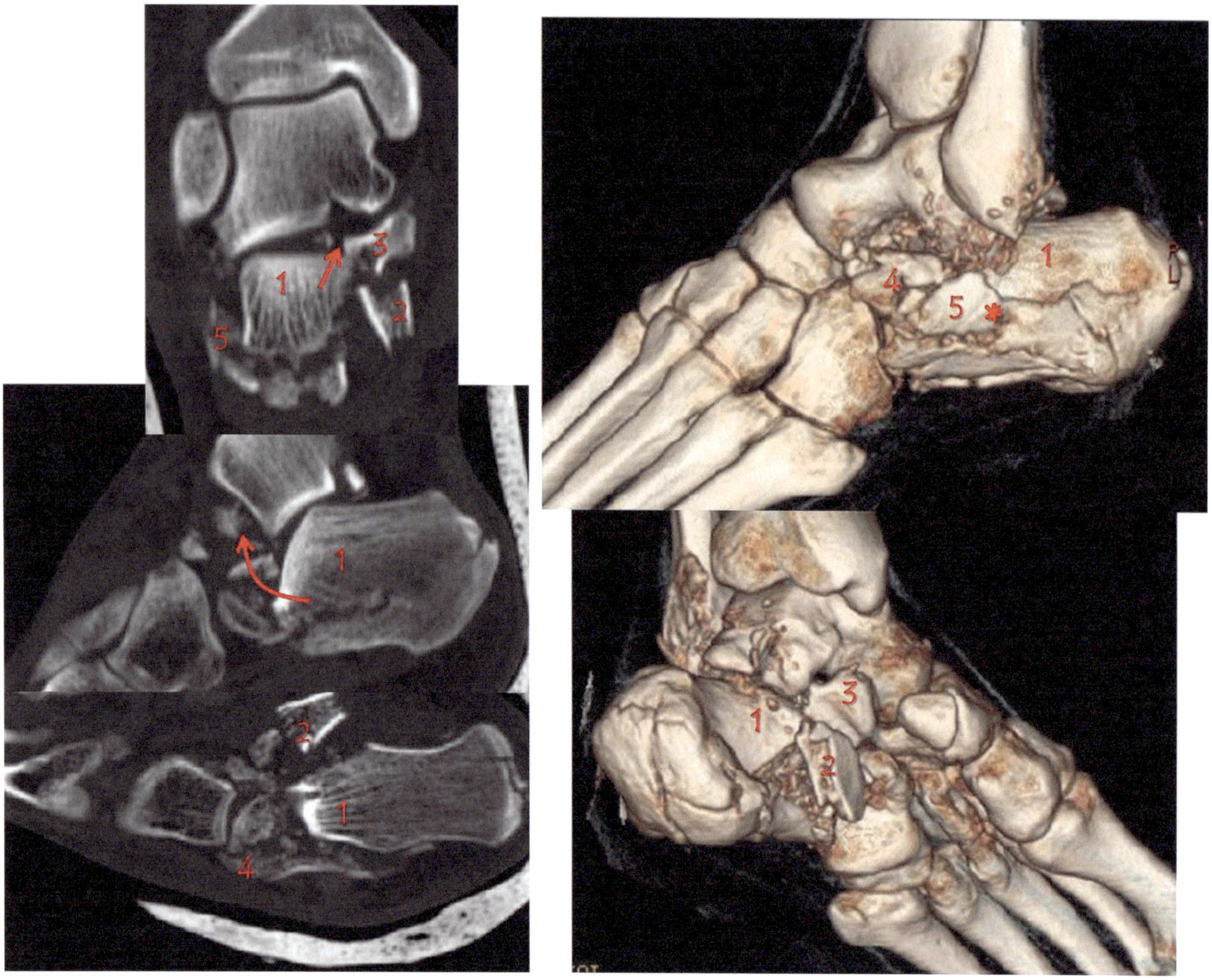

Fig. 5.14 Mini-invasive reduction and stabilization with an external fixator of a calcaneal fracture. The preoperative planning considers the positioning of the fragments and the direction of the forces that are applied through the use of levers to achieve the reduction, spotting the best place to insert the instrumentation (in this case indicated with asterisk)

tive views is necessary, and the tourniquet must be positioned on the thigh of the affected limb.

The positioning is easily kept by a roll positioned under the back and by support devices that will keep the position fixed during surgery; a cushion is inserted between the lower limbs as a support and to avoid the intra-rotation of the lower limb that needs to be treated (see Fig. 5.17).

The lateral and eventually axial views of the calcaneus achieved through fluoroscopy are very difficult to achieve in this position, but it is the only way, without CT or navigation system, to evaluate indirectly the effect of the reduction manoeuvres, and consequently it is essential.

During this phase, it is possible to position the C-arm and the lower limb, before the surgical field is prepared, to achieve the best and reproducible X-ray views (see Figs. 5.18 and 5.19).

Surgical Access

The classic surgical access to the calcaneus fracture is through a lateral incision, which is extensible and allows the exposure of the posterior subtalar and the calcaneocuboid joints, granting also the reduction of the medial wall through indirect manoeuvres.

The so-called "no touch" surgical technique, developed and illustrated by Sanders [8], is the safest way to perform such surgical access, restricting at most the onset of soft tissue complications. Such procedure requires a "hockey-stick"-shaped incision, with a slightly obtuse angle, of which the horizontal arm must be placed over the line between the dorsal and plantar skin of the foot, extending to the calcaneocuboid joint line; the vertical arm must be placed halfway between the posterior border of the fibula

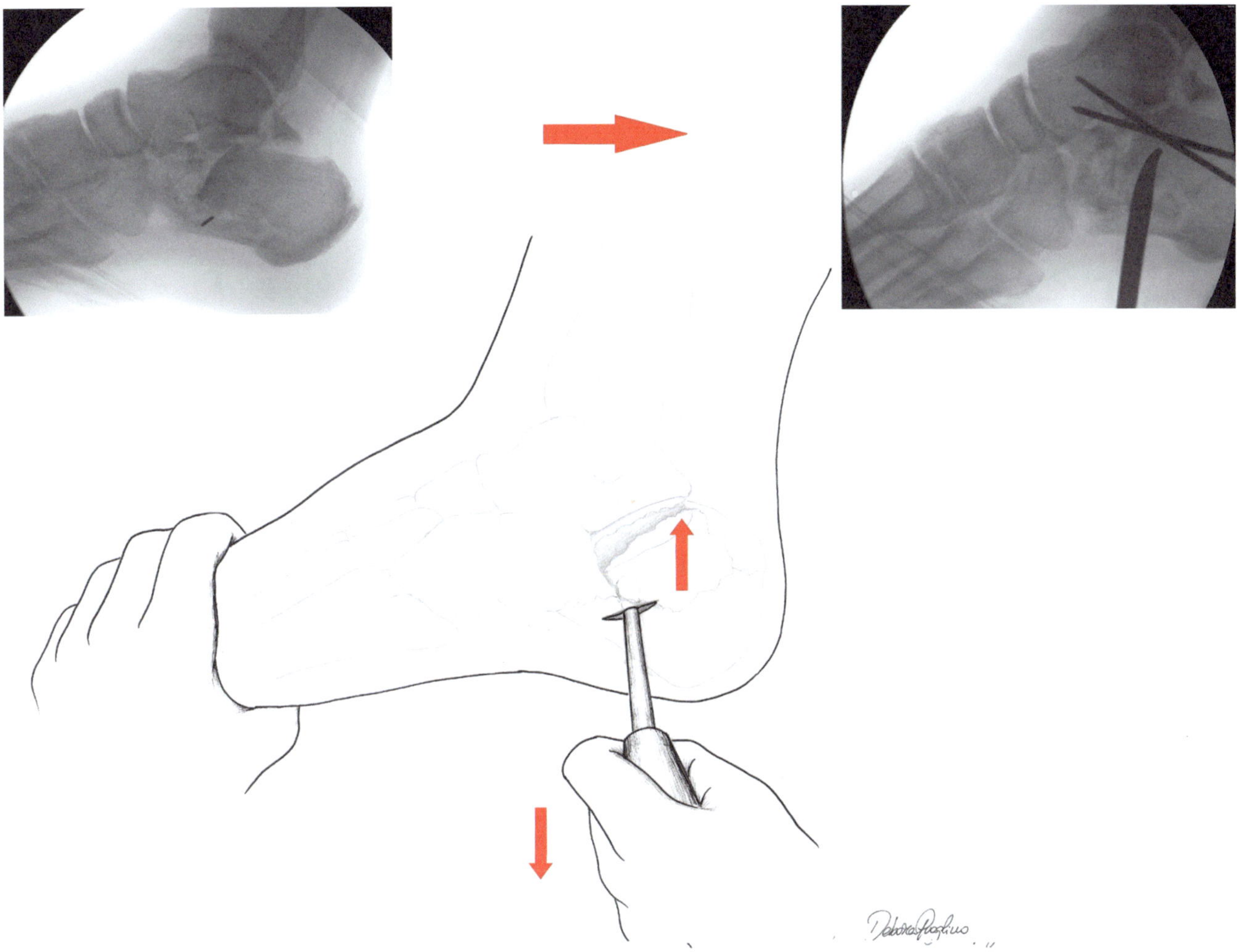

Fig. 5.15 Mini-invasive reduction and stabilization with an external fixator of a calcaneal fracture. The main fragment reduction manoeuvre is performed through a lever introduced by a mini-invasive incision; on the left, the initial radiographic image and, on the right, a picture taken after the reduction, with the lever still inserted, temporarily stabilized by two Steinmann pins

and the lateral border of the Achilles tendon, extending proximally for about four transverse fingers from the apex of the lateral malleolus. During the drawing of the surgical incision, the sural nerve must be signed that it could cross the line of the incision proximally and distally (see Fig. 5.20).

The surgery is performed with the affected limb ischemic, through inflating of the tourniquet to a pressure of 350 mmHg, proceeding with the incision perpendicular to the skin and deepening it to the bone in the same manner, with one single full-thickness cut, avoiding proximally and distally the sural nerve, where the dissection must be careful to enlighten the latter. Once the neurovascular bundle is identified, it is protected by a lace, avoiding any iatrogenic injuries, which could lead to a suffering of the skin flap or to a nervous injury that could be very painful after the surgery. Progressively the skin flap is elevated, through the use of the scalpel, detaching all the soft tissues from the bone and including the peroneal tendons, of which it should be advisable to not open the sheath, sectioning under the periosteum the calcaneal pulley.

During all these steps, it is very important not to mechanically stress the delicate skin of this area, which needs to be elevated through the use of silk wires, avoiding carefully not to use any retractors that can lead to soft tissue suffering [1, 8]. To avoid extended traction, the skin flap is elevated through the use of Kirschner wires, inserted sequentially through the fibula, the talar neck and the cuboid (see Fig. 5.21). The positioning of a Schanz screw or a Steinmann wire in the posterior tuberosity, used as a lever to ease the reduction of the fracture or as a grasp to supinate the posterior subtalar joint, to better see the injury, completes the surgical access phase.

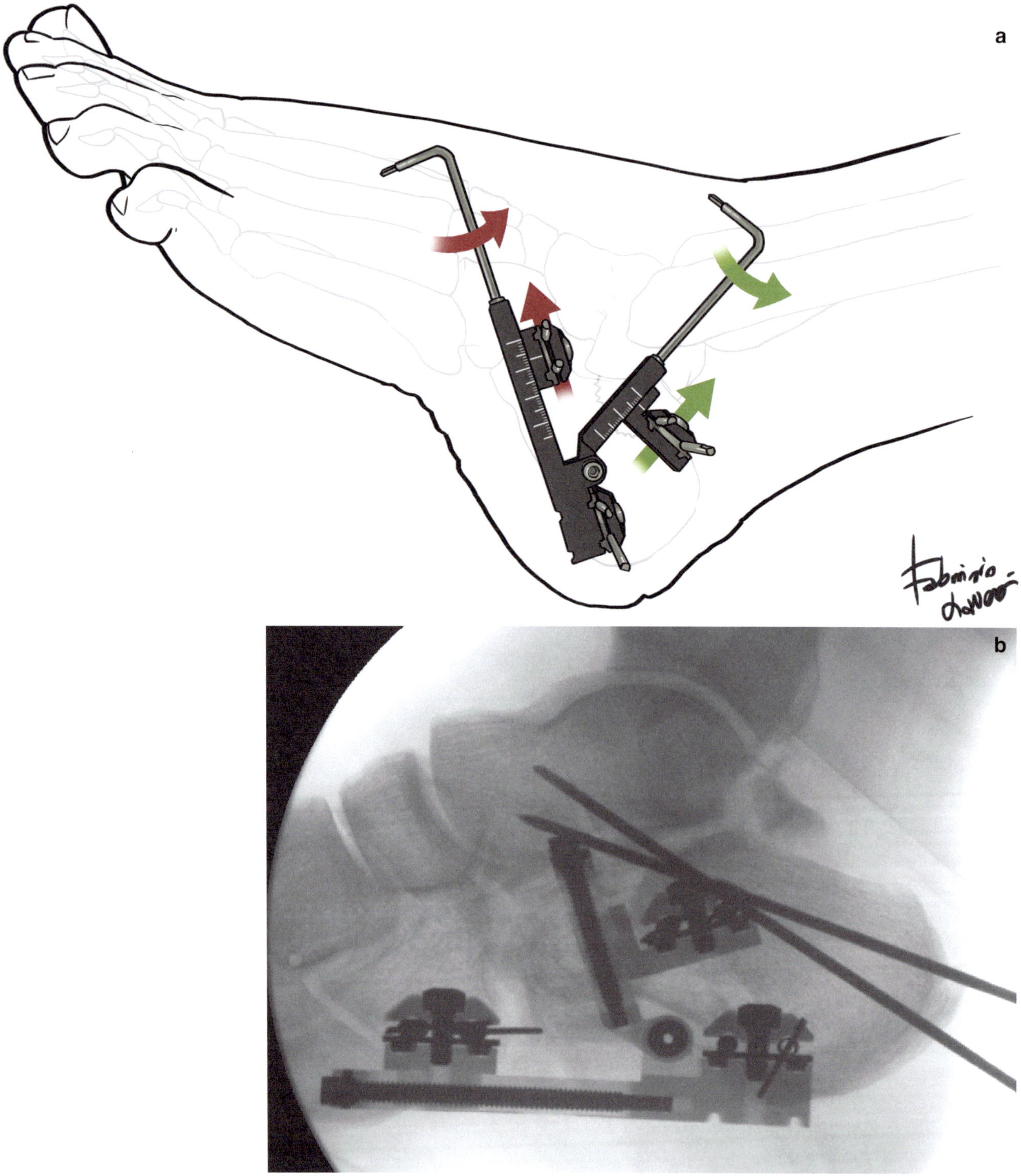

Fig. 5.16 Mini-invasive reduction and stabilization with an external fixator of a calcaneal fracture. After the positioning of the Orthofix external fixator, it is possible to tension the fixation elements through a slay, which increases notably the stability of the frame. In the lower pictures, the radioscopic vision of the external fixator, with the evidence of a good maintenance of the subtalar joint reduction, was further stabilized with Steinmann pins. Because of the fragmentation of the anterior tuberosity, the anterior fixator pin is inserted through the cuboid

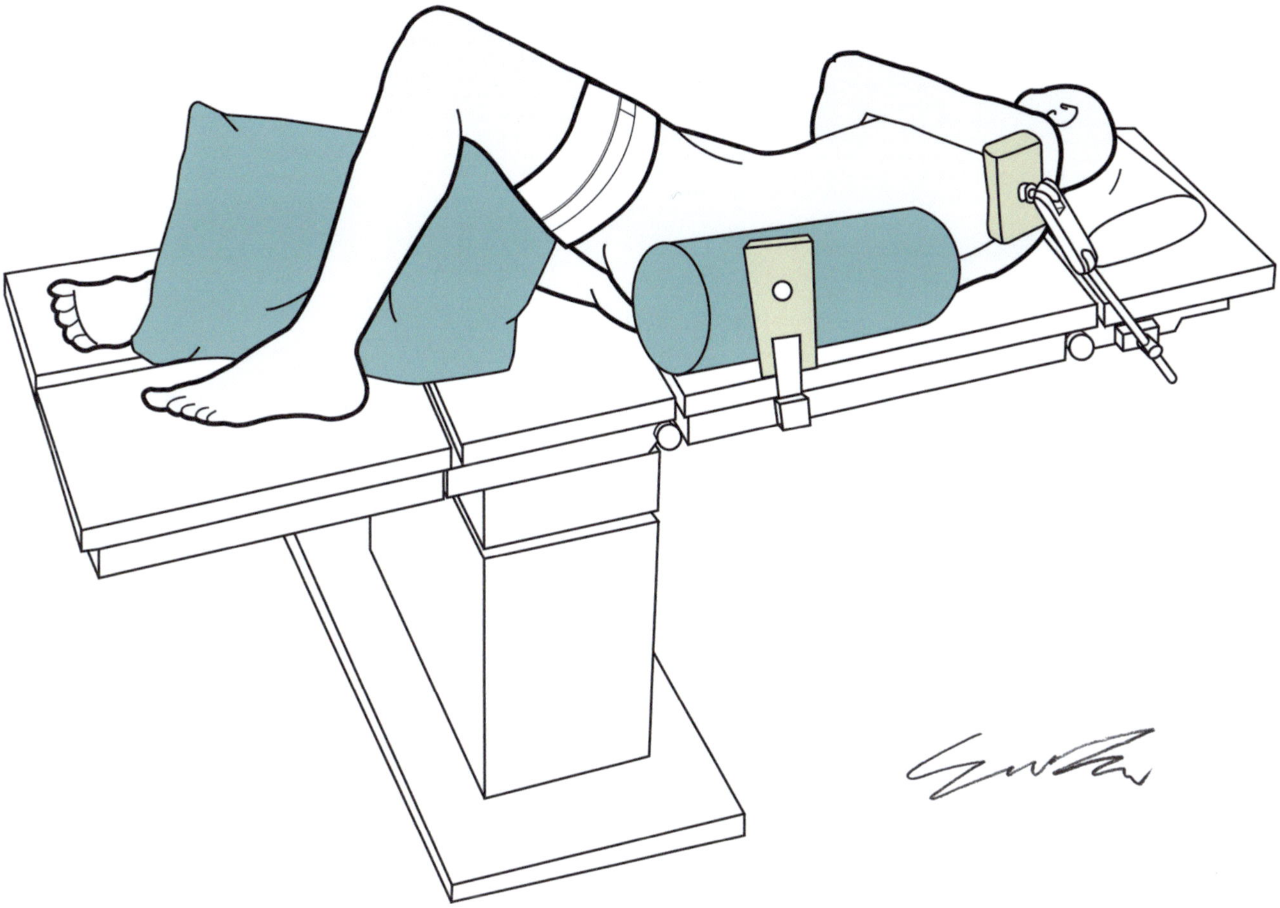

Fig. 5.17 ORIF of a calcaneal fracture: positioning of the patient on a 45° inclined decubitus on the unharmed side and tourniquet at the thigh

Reduction Manoeuvres and Synthesis

To achieve the reduction, the keystone is the surgical anatomy of the sustentaculum tali, which usually keeps its original link with the talus, thanks to the action of the strong interosseous talo-calcaneal ligament; this bone segment becomes the fixed point that drives the progressive reconstruction of the joint anatomy and later will represent a safe target to aim the screws to achieve a solid fixation.

The procedure begins with the mobilization of the sunken osteochondral fragments to gain access to the medial wall of the calcaneus (see Fig. 5.22); if the fracture has two articular fragments, it can be enough to rotate the sunken part of the subtalar joint after having it separated from the surrounding bone fragments, while in case of a Sanders III fracture, it is usually necessary to remove both of the displaced fragments, central and lateral, proceeding to anatomically restore them on the surgical table, stabilizing them with absorbable poly-L-lactic acid (PLLA) pins (see Fig. 5.23).

If there is a dislocation of the medial wall, at this point, the interpenetrated fragments in this area are freed, using a lever inserted at the apex of the deformity (see Fig. 5.24), previously spotted during preoperative planning and eventually later using a laminar spreader to increase gradually the distraction force applied. Considering the landmarks of the deformity deducted from the preoperative planning, once freed from the impaction of the medial wall due to the impact of the posterior tuberosity, the latter is rotated and shifted opposite to the varus-valgus and procurvatum-recurvatum generated by the trauma, repositioning it along the original axis and temporarily stabilizing it, with 2 mm Kirschner wires, from the posterior tuberosity to the sustentaculum tali (see Fig. 5.25) and eventually further onto the talus to gain a better temporary stability.

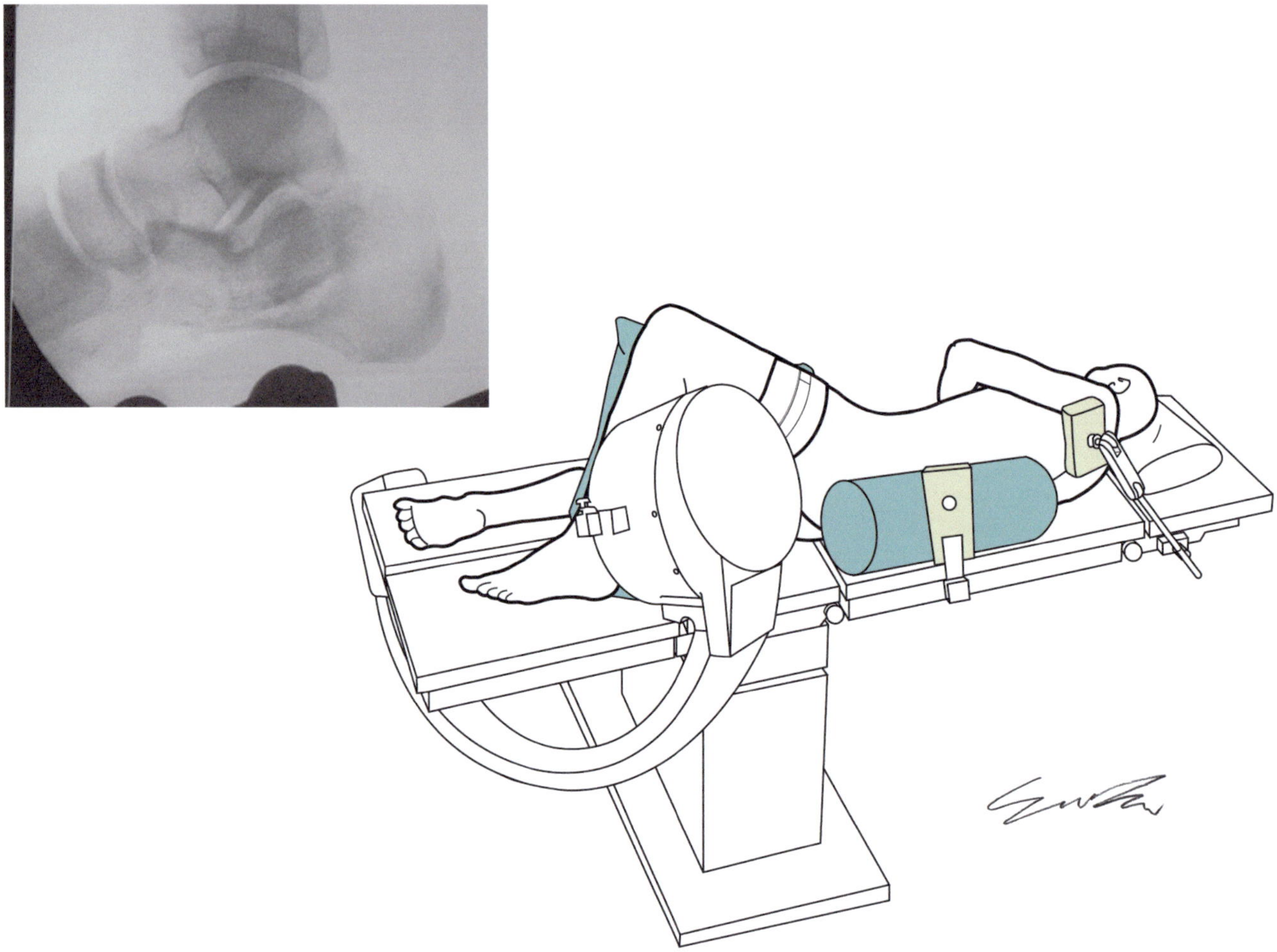

Fig. 5.18 ORIF of a calcaneal fracture: with the patient positioned, the lateral projection is performed rotating laterally the C-arm to bring the beam perpendicular to the hindfoot. In the square, the image that is generated with the projection is correctly performed

Once the medial side is reduced, it is possible to proceed to the reduction of the lateral fragment, single or reconstructed, of the subtalar joint; if the reduction obtained is good, the latter finds its spatial collocation easily, and it fits in its area with a click, restoring the Gissane angle; even this reduction is temporarily stabilized with at least two 1.6 mm Kirschner wires (see Fig. 5.26), and it is checked under fluoroscopy.

If everything is okay, the subtalar joint is fixed through two free-handed compression screws, carefully orientating the latter from posterior to anterior and proximal to distal, to achieve a good grip on the sustentaculum tali strong bone and to mainly avoid the accidental interpenetration of the screws in the joint [15], considering the obliquity of the subtalar joint line (see Fig. 5.27); otherwise and in a more difficult manner, even if less time-consuming, the screws that fix the subtalar joint can be inserted directly on the plate, keeping the insertion point a little lower, mostly for the locking screws, which have a fixed direction.

The osteosynthesis must be performed through the use of the thinnest plate possible to minimize the impact on the soft tissues, but, keeping in mind this attribute, it is more advisable to use a rigid plate not bendable, such as the LCP Synthes®. Even if they require a more precise surgical technique for the positioning, it is important to use titanium devices, because they seem to be less attractive for bacteria and more suitable to reduce problems if there is an infection [16]. This plate is anatomical for the side, in the classic version it needs to be mod-

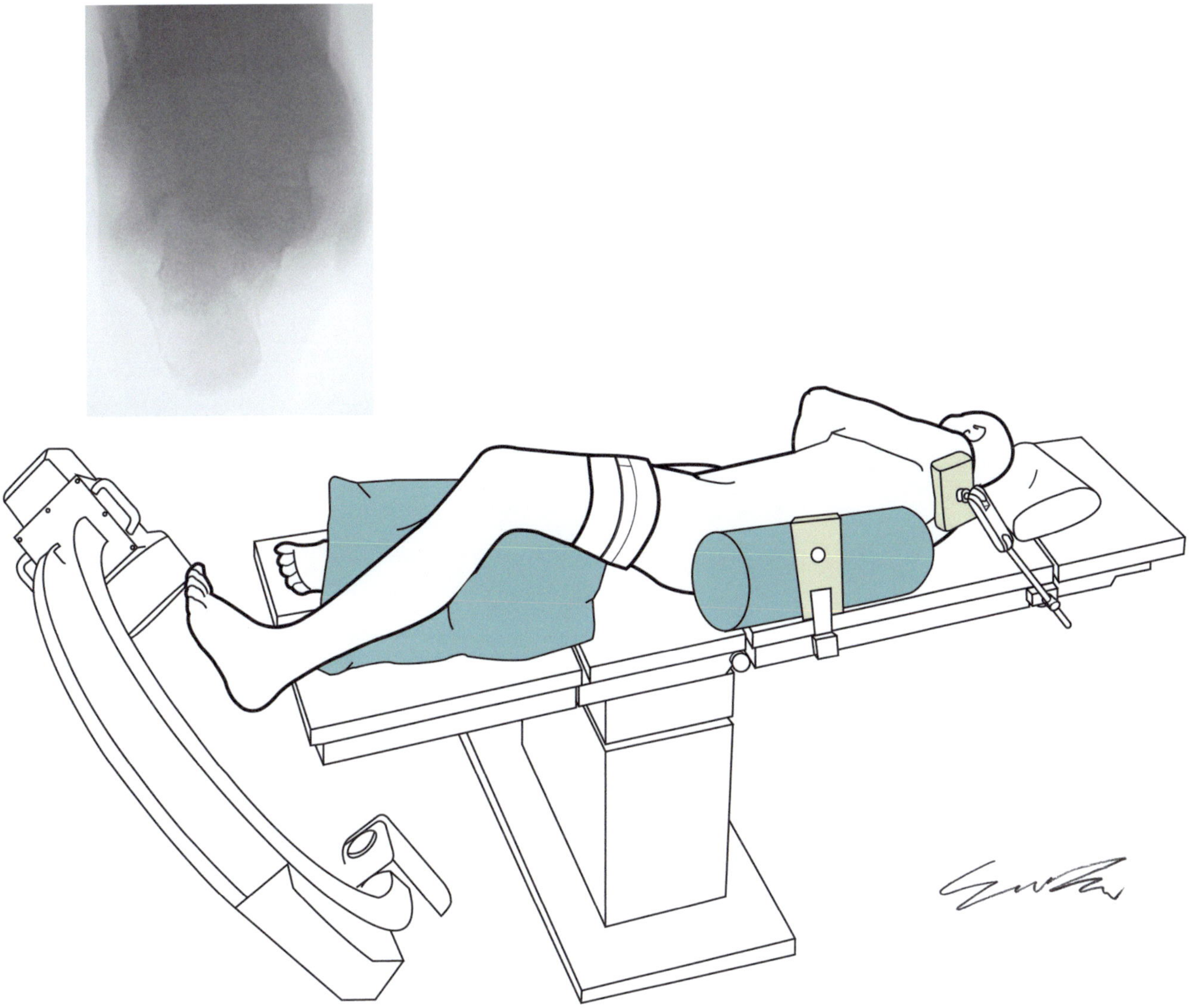

Fig. 5.19 ORIF of a calcaneal fracture: with the patient already positioned, the axial X-ray projection is difficult to do; it is performed through an external rotation of the lower affected limb and resting it on the C-arm, to have the beam passing through the calcaneus. In the square, it is possible to see the correctly obtained image

elled, cutting of eventual holes not needed, adapting it to the bone anatomy, thanks to a plastic phantom, that is used as guide (see Fig. 5.28). The plate holes accept both conventional and locking screws, the latter increasing notably the stability of the synthesis [17, 18]. The screws, diameters 2.7 and 3.5 mm, must be positioned in the areas where there is the best bone grasp, which are the anterior and posterior tuberosity and the subtalar joint. If a combination of locking and conventional screws is used, the normal screws must be placed before the locking ones, to avoid any accidental loosening of the latter. It is advisable to insert in every of the three valid grasp points one conventional screw, to adapt the plate to the bone in all its parts, reducing the mass effect of the device; further on, the synthesis is completed through the insertion of at least three locking screws, always one per segment, increasing the overall stability (see Fig. 5.29). As a rule, to avoid loss of reduction, it is essential to position the screws bi-cortically, gaining grasp on the medial wall, achieving strength and mechanical validity [17]. The main advantage of using a rigid and anatomic plate is that, if it adapts flush to the lateral wall of the reconstructed calca-

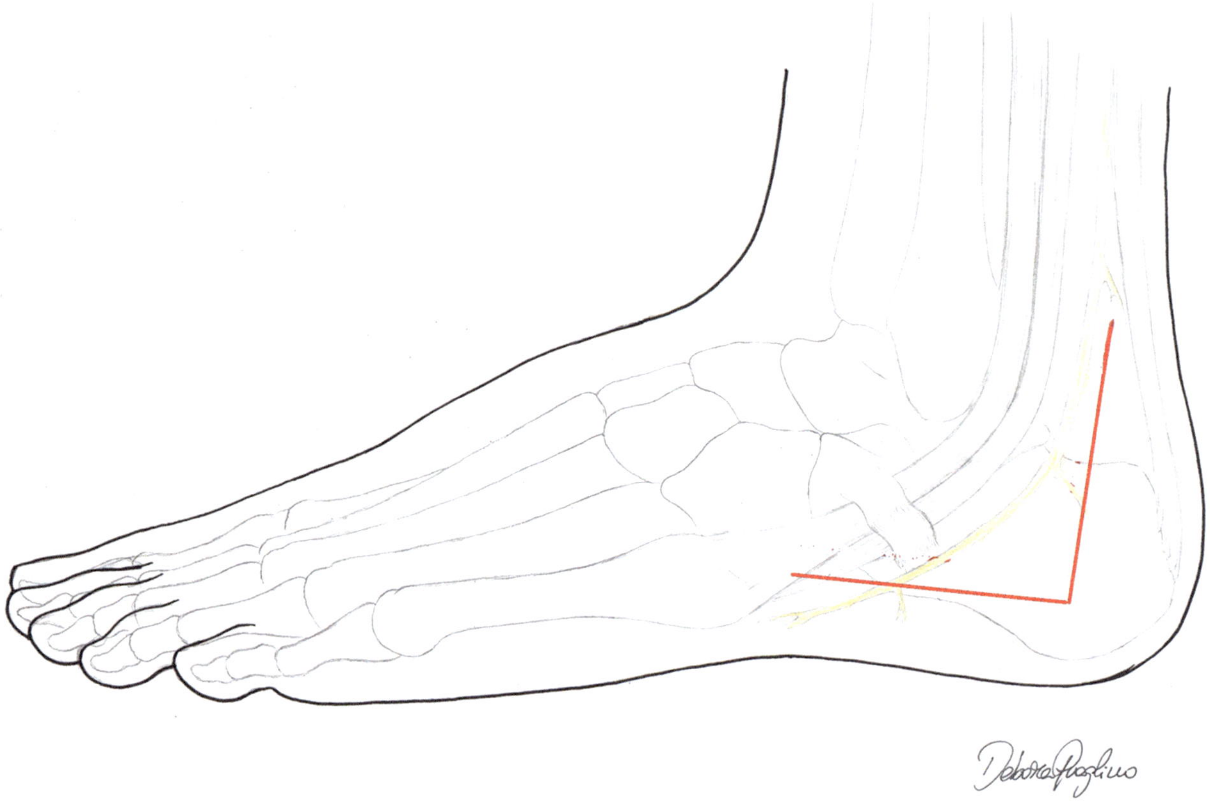

Fig. 5.20 ORIF of a calcaneal fracture: hockey-stick incision with the horizontal part that lays between the dorsal and the plantar skin and the vertical portion lays halfway between the Achilles tendon and the posterior edge of the fibula. With this access, attention must be paid to the sural nerve, which is near and crossing the incision line either proximally or distally

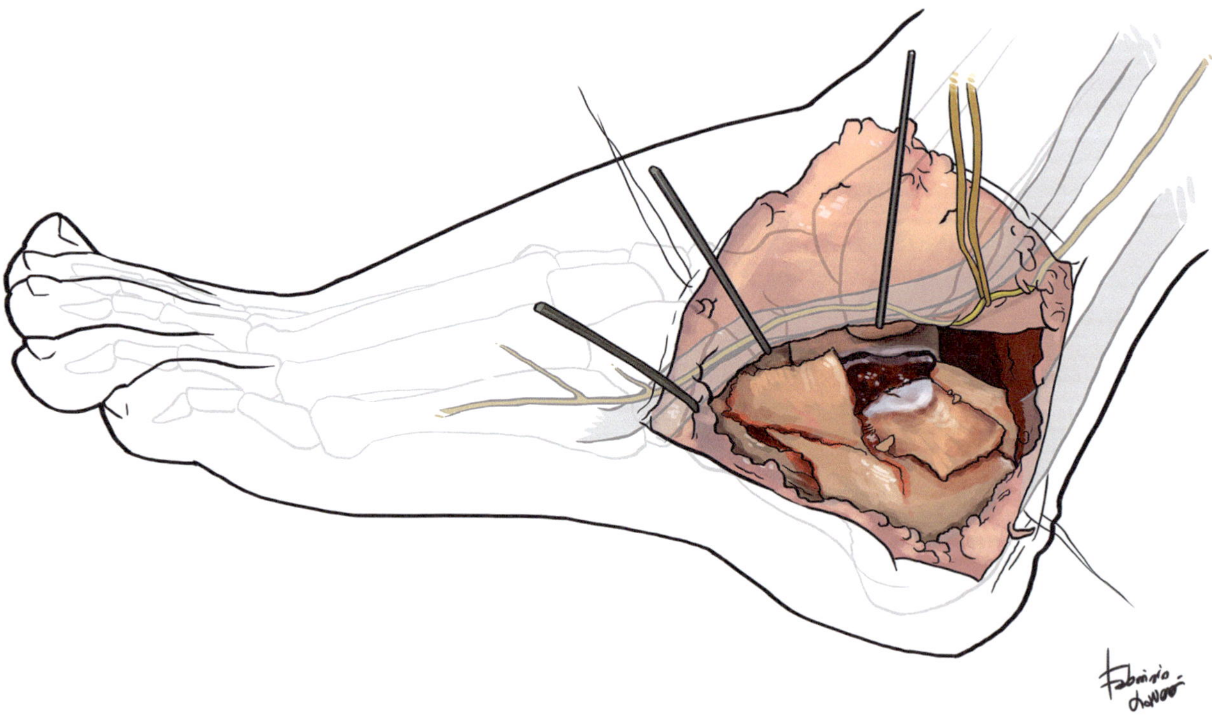

Fig. 5.21 ORIF of a calcaneal fracture: lateral access—the skin flap is performed using silk wires, avoiding any tractions with retractors, keeping it elevated through the use of three Kirschner wires, one on the fibula, one on the neck of the talus and one on the cuboid. Proximally the anatomical dissection has enlightened the sural nerve and its vascular complex, isolated and protected with a silicone lace

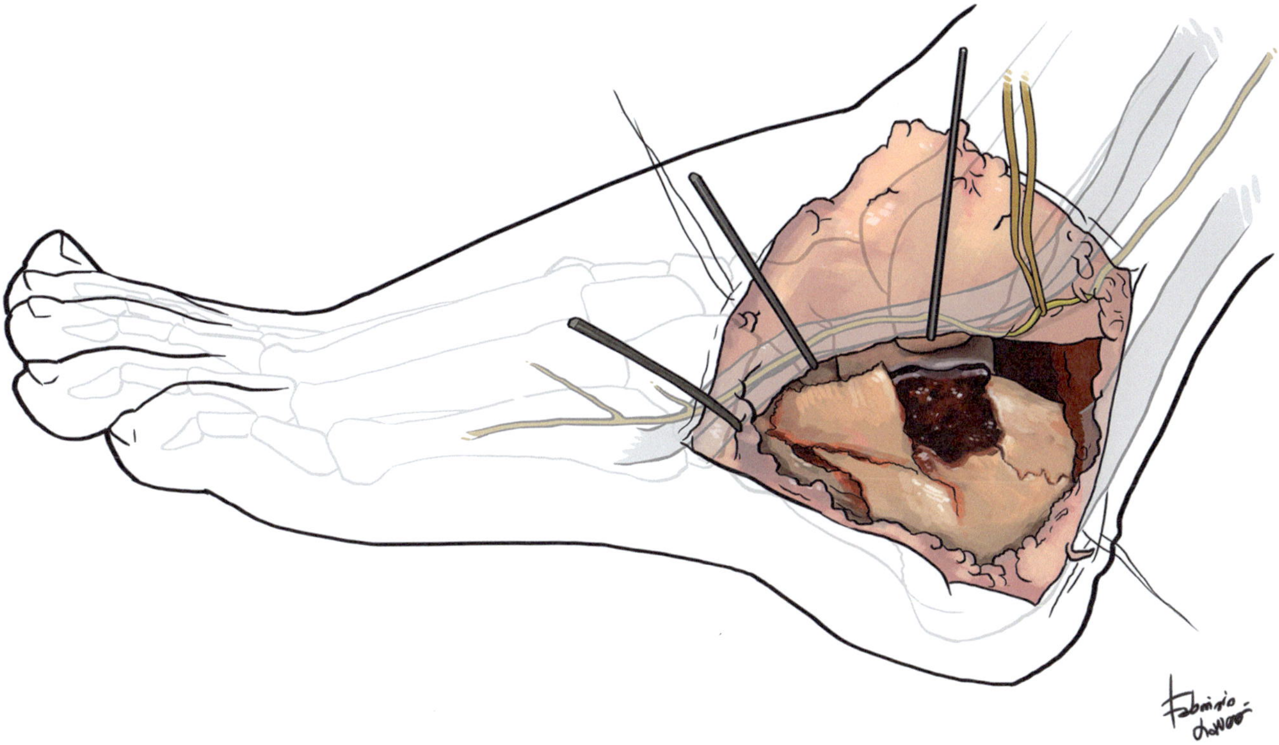

Fig. 5.22 ORIF of a calcaneal fracture: once the lateral wall and the lateral and central subtalar joint fragments have been removed, it is possible to gain access to the medial wall, and it is possible to achieve a reduction

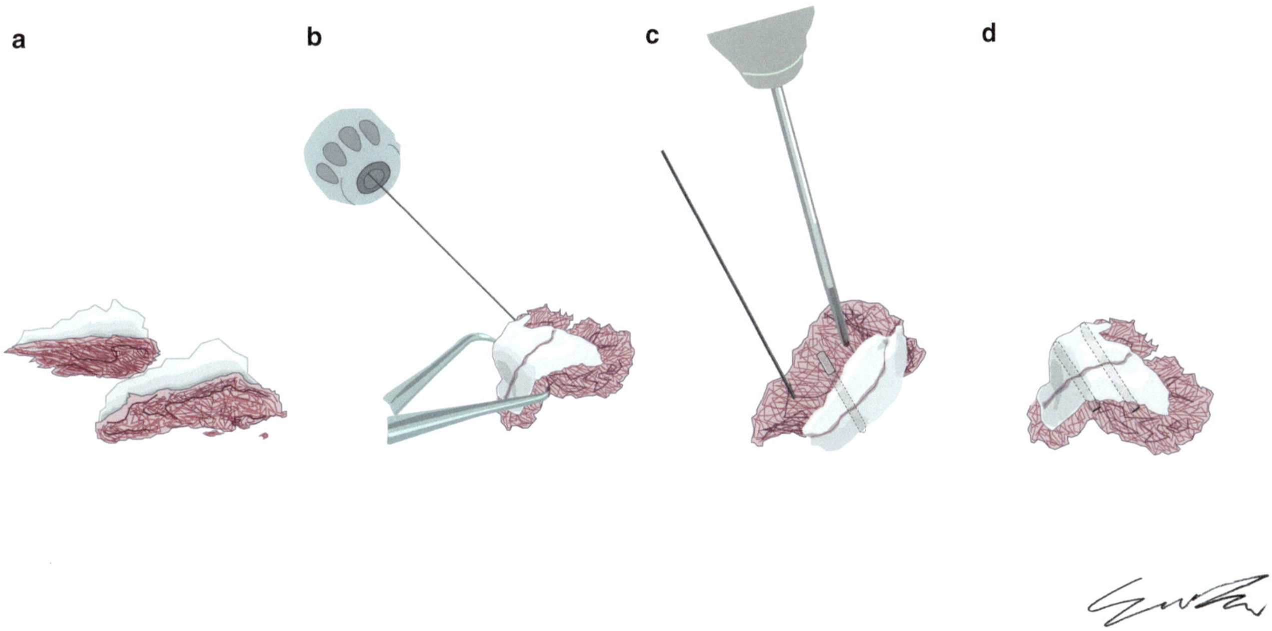

Fig. 5.23 ORIF of a calcaneal fracture: in case of three articular fragment fractures, the lateral fragment and the central one are more conveniently controlled by removing them and providing an anatomical reduction on the serving table (**a**). Once a temporary fixation is achieved with Kirschner wires (**b**), some PLLA pins are inserted to unite the fragments, previously drilled with a dedicate drill bit (**c**) and at the end cut flush to the bone (**d**)

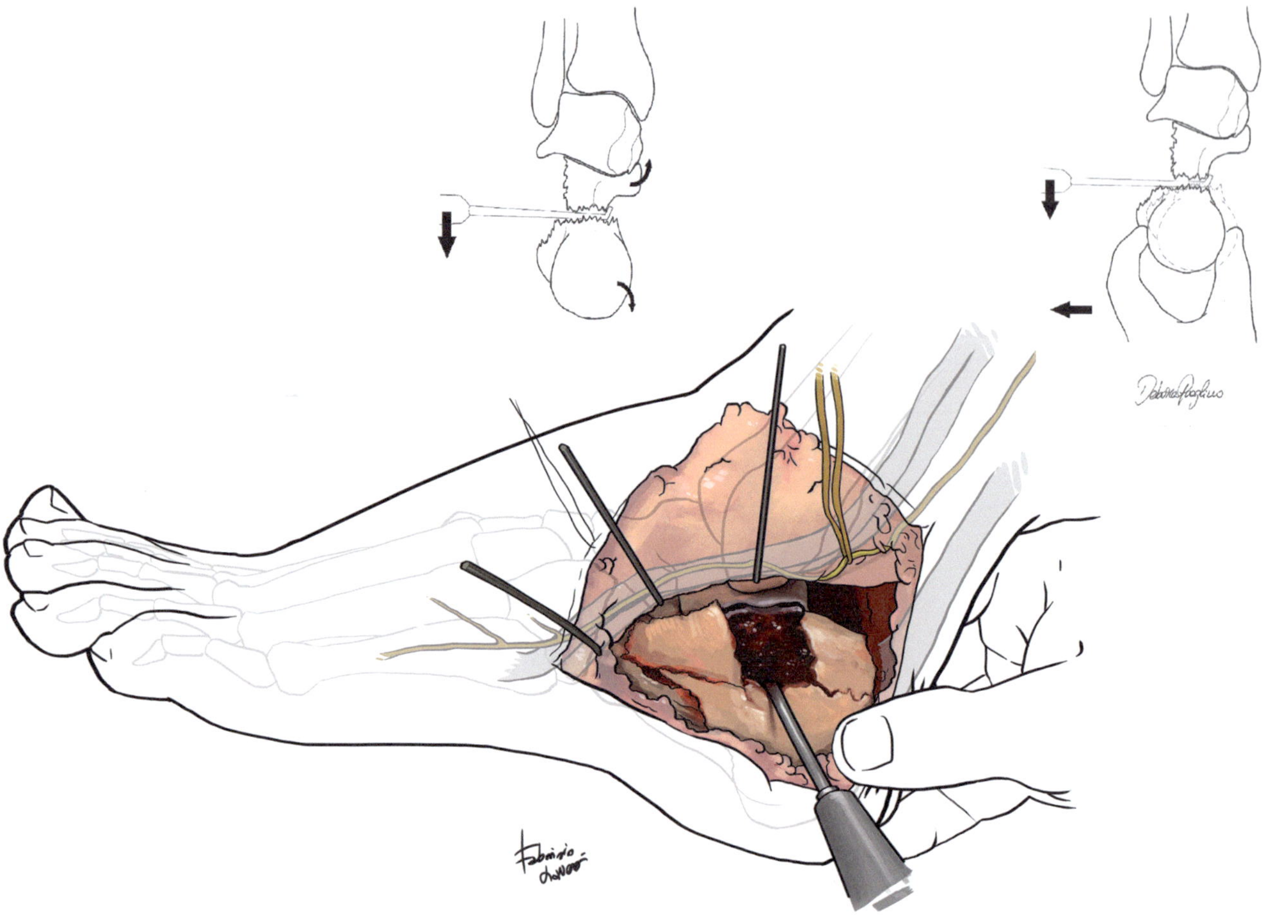

Fig. 5.24 ORIF of a calcaneal fracture: reduction of the medial wall—with the use of a lever, the impacted fragments are freed, and consequently a specific lateral/medial translation combined with a varus-valgus solicitation is applied to restore the correct position of the posterior tuberosity in line with the bony segment and realign the medial profile of the calcaneus

neus, mainly straight, without the need of any bending on its main side, it represents an indirect index of the good realignment of the medial wall, allowing to avoid the axial view of the calcaneus during the fluoroscopy check, earning time and avoiding excessive dorsiflexion solicitations to the foot. The bone synthesis achieved through locking plates makes unnecessary the use of bone graft to fill the defects, allowing to spare more surgical time, to avoid the need of further surgical accesses to obtain any bone graft [8, 19] and to reduce the risk related to the positioning of further foreign materials that it would be inevitable if synthetic bone graft is used.

The surgery is completed through the closure of the wound through single stiches of the deep soft tissues with an absorbable 3.0 suture and a continuous single thread 3.0 or 4.0 skin suture. This continuous suture will tension by itself once the tourniquet is released, avoiding mechanical stresses in single spots. With the growing experience of the surgeon and the use of optimized instrumentation, it is possible to constantly keep the tourniquet time under the 2½ h, preventing the removal of the tourniquet before the ending of the surgery. This is essential because releasing the tourniquet once the suture is ended, an elastic dressing is completed and an open plaster cast is positioned avoids to develop any tensioning on the incision and to contemporarily perform effective haemostasis, reducing at minimum any sufferance of the soft tissues [1].

Postoperative Care

Once the drainage is removed, a closed plaster cast is performed, putting the foot in a functional position preventing to have any equinus contracture tendency; such plaster cast must be kept for 3 weeks as a protection of the wound, taking care of observing the absolute and correct elevation of the foot.

After 20 days, the plaster cast and the stiches are removed, and active mobilization of the ankle without weight bearing is started; after 40 and 90 days from surgery, a clinical and radiological check is performed; after 3 months, the weight bearing is gradually and progressively recovered, starting as soon as possible hydrokinesitherapy to recover muscular strength and to complete the rehabilitation process.

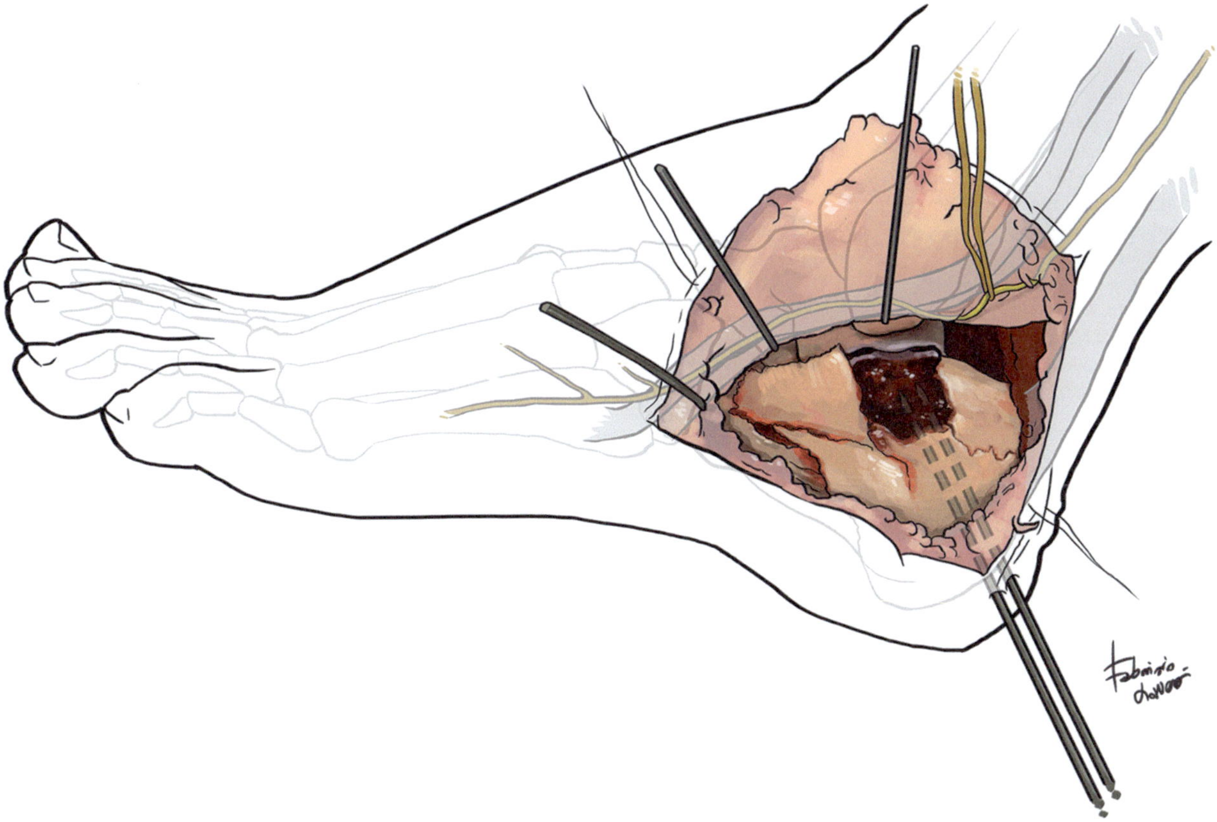

Fig. 5.25 ORIF of a calcaneal fracture: once the medial wall of the calcaneus is reduced, a temporary stabilization with 2 mm Kirschner wires is performed

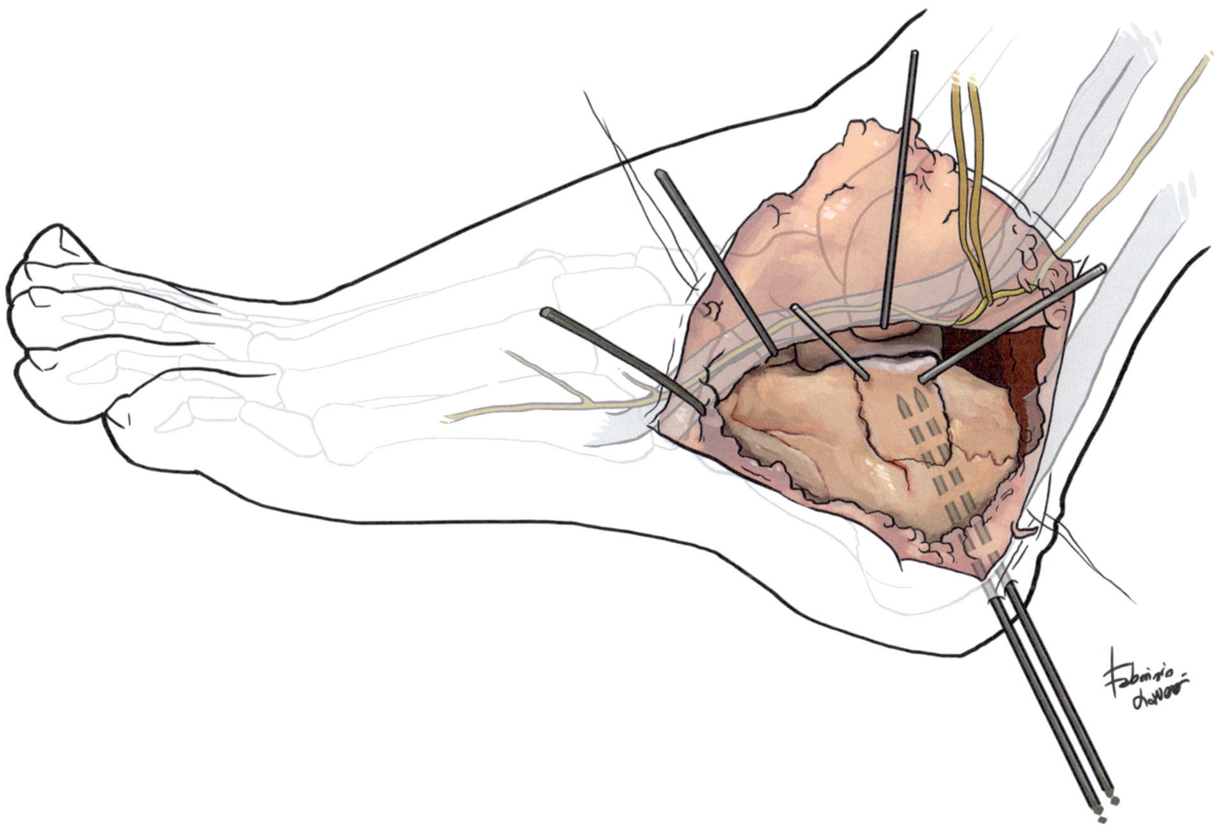

Fig. 5.26 ORIF of a calcaneal fracture: once the medial wall is restored, the residual space is enough to reposition the osteochondral fragment previously rebuilt, which is going to be inserted and temporarily stabilized with 1.6 mm Kirschner wires (at least two)

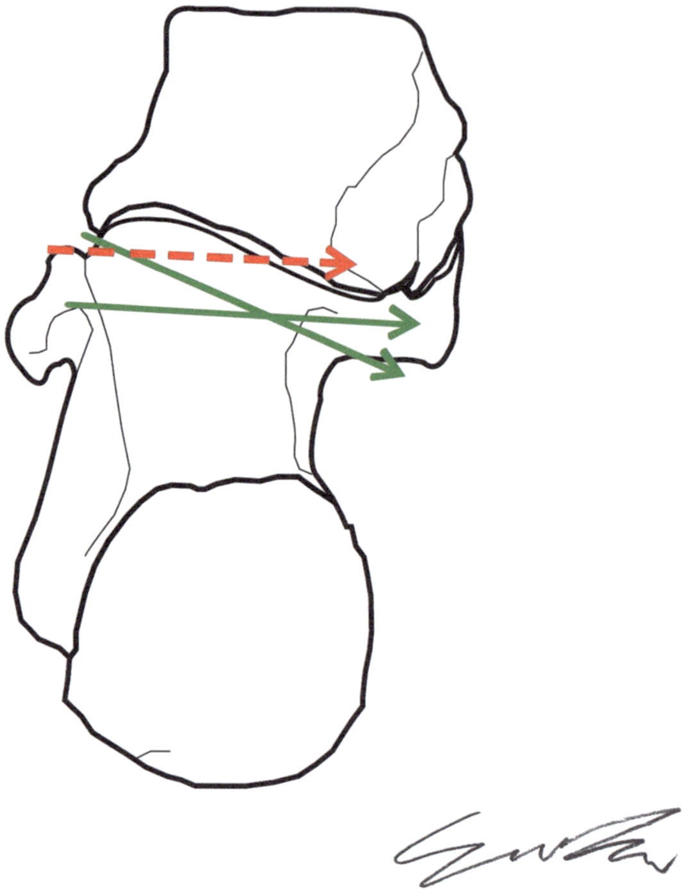

Fig. 5.27 ORIF of a calcaneal fracture: when the screws are inserted in proximity of the subtalar joint line, which are going to be inserted with an anterior direction aiming to the sustentaculum tali, it must be considered the lateral-to-medial obliquity of the subtalar joint, aiming the holes oblique or starting lower as inserting point (green arrows), to avoid accidental intra-articular penetration (red arrow)

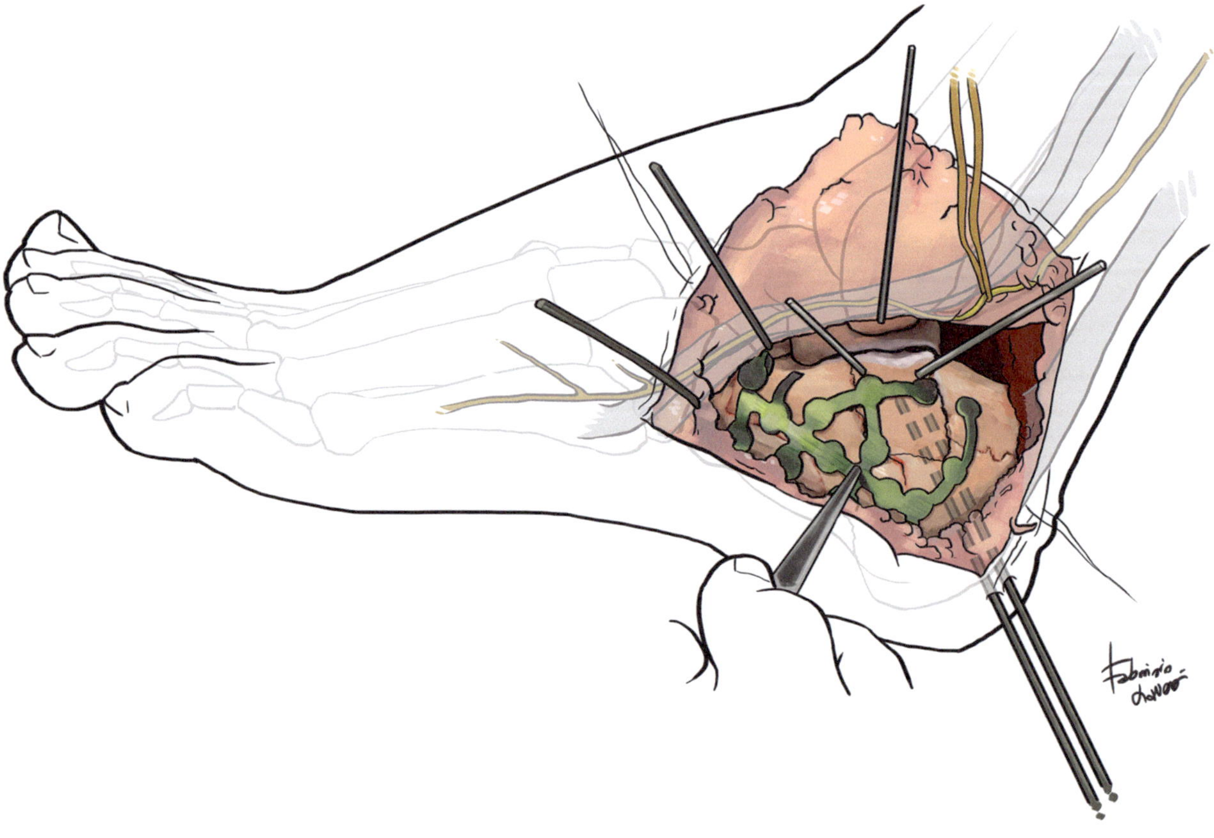

Fig. 5.28 ORIF of a calcaneal fracture: the soft mask is adapted to the lateral wall of the calcaneus after the temporary fixation is achieved; it will serve as a guide to achieve the best modelling of the definitive plate

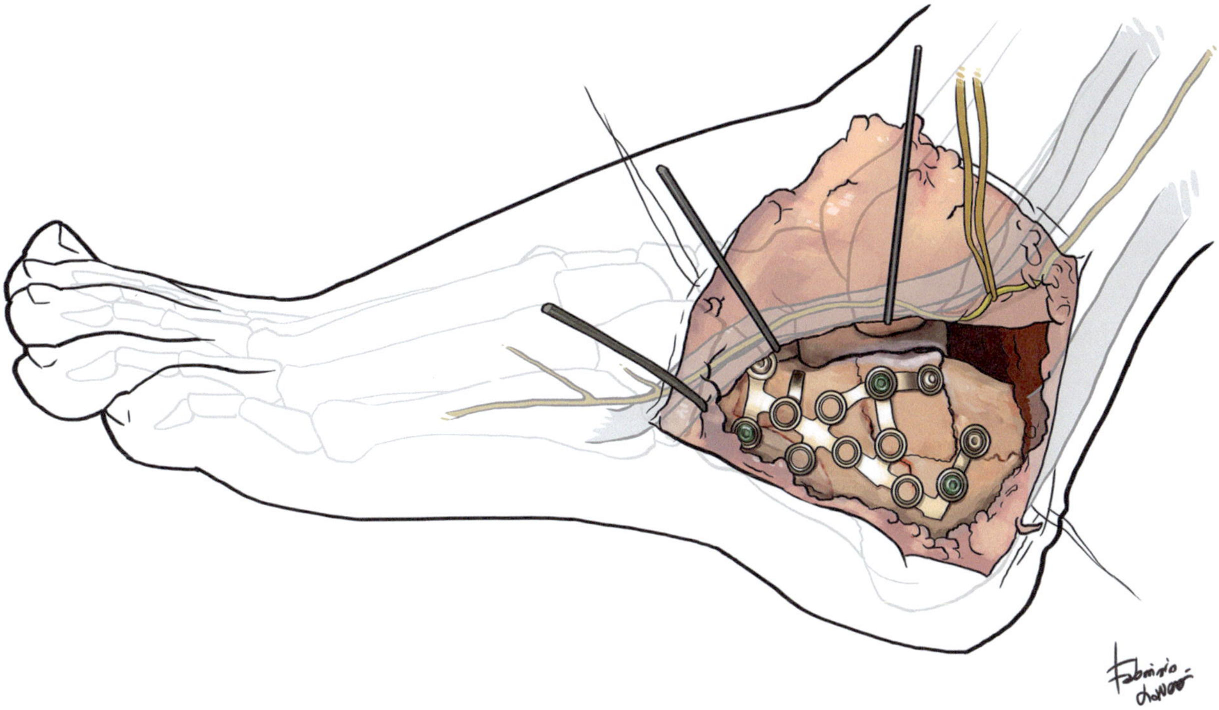

Fig. 5.29 ORIF of a calcaneal fracture: after the Synthes LCP plate is modelled, the osteosynthesis is perfected, inserting at least two screws for every good-quality bone zone, which are represented by the posterior subtalar joint and the anterior and posterior tuberosity

References

1. Sanders RW, Clare MP (2007) Fractures of the calcaneus. In: Coughlin MJ, Mann RA, Saltzman CL (eds) Surgery of the foot and ankle, 8th edn. Mosby Elsevier, Philadelphia, pp 2017–2073
2. Tscherne H, Zwipp H (1993) Calcaneal fractures. In: Tscherne H, Schatzker J (eds) Fractures of the Pilon, talus, and the calcaneus. Current concepts in treatment. Springer, Berlin, pp 153–174
3. Heier KA, Infante AF, Walling AK et al (2003) Open fractures of the calcaneus: soft-tissue injury determines outcome. J Bone Joint Surg Am 85-A(12):2276–2282
4. Csizy M, Buckley R, Tough S et al (2004) Displaced intra-articular calcaneal fractures: variables predicting late subtalar fusion. J Orthop Trauma 17(2):106–112
5. Schepers T, van Lieshout EM, van Ginhoven TM et al (2008) Current concepts in the treatment of intra-articular calcaneal fractures; results of a nationwide survey. Int Orthop 32:711–715
6. Brauer CA, Manns BJ, Ko M et al (2005) An economic evaluation of operative compared with nonoperative management of displaced intra-articular calcaneal fractures. J Bone Joint Surg Am 87:2741–2749
7. Gilmer PW, Herzenberg J, Frank JL et al (1986) Computerized tomographic analysis of acute calcaneal fractures. Foot Ankle 6(4):184–193
8. Sanders R, Fortin P, Di Pasquale T et al (1993) Operative treatment in 120 displaced intraarticular calcaneal fractures. Results using a prognostic computed tomography scan classification. Clin Orthop Relat Res (290):87–95
9. Schepers T, Den Hartog D, Vogels LMM et al (2013) Extended lateral approach for intra-articular calcaneal fractures: an inverse relationship between surgeon experience and wound complications. JFAS 52:167–171
10. Buch BD, Myerson MS, Miller SD (1996) Primary subtalar arthrodesis for the treatment of comminuted calcaneal fractures. Foot Ankle Int 17(2):61–70
11. Buckley R, Leighton R, Sanders D et al (2014) Open reduction and internal fixation compared with ORIF and primary subtalar arthrodesis for treatment of Sanders type IV calcaneal fractures: a randomized multicenter trial. J Orthop Trauma 28(10):577–583
12. Essex-Lopresti P (1952) The mechanism, reduction technique and results in fractures of the os calcis. J Bone Joint Surg Br 39:395
13. Magnan B, Bortolazzi R, Marangon A et al (2006) External fixation for displaced intra-articular fractures of the calcaneum. J Bone Joint Surg Br 88(11):1474–1479
14. Barei DP, Bellabarba C, Sangeorzan BJ et al (2002) Fractures of the calcaneus. Orthop Clin North Am 33(1):263–285
15. Phisitkul P, Sullivan JP, Goetz JE et al (2013) Maximizing safety in screw placement for posterior facet fixation in calcaneus fractures: a cadaveric radio-anatomical study. Foot Ankle Int 34(9):1279–1285
16. Arens S, Schlegel U, Printzen G et al (1996) Influence of materials for fixation implants on local infection. An experimental study of steel versus titanium DCP in rabbits. J Bone Joint Surg Br 78(4):647–651
17. Ackermann O, Mauk PJ, Beuke T et al (2015) Comparison of stability of plate fixateurs with parallel and oblique screw directions. Z Orthop Unfall 153(2):160–164. https://doi.org/10.1055/s-0034-1396187
18. Lenz M, Wahl D, Gueorguiev B et al (2015) Concept of variable angle locking—evolution and mechanical evaluation of a recent technology. J Orthop Res 33(7):988–992
19. Tufescu TV, Buckley R (2001) Age gender, work capability, and worker's compensation in patients with displaced intraarticular calcaneal fractures. J Orthop Trauma 15(4):275–279

Surgical Treatment of Midfoot Traumatic Injuries

6

Contents

6.1 Traumatic Injuries of the Midfoot

The injuries of the midfoot are extremely infrequent and insidious: they present an incidence of 1.5–3.6 cases/100,000 people/year [1]; because of the scarce familiarity of the surgeons with such rare injuries, united with the complex regional anatomy, it can be difficult to do a correct diagnosis, with a very high risk of being unidentified [2].

6.1.1 Diagnostic Help Orientated to Surgery

The classical radiologic sensibility is reduced in these types of injuries because of the overlapping of all the bony components [2]. If there is a suspected Lisfranc injury, it is useful to perform a comparative X-ray, in a cranial-caudal projection, which will allow to compare all the articular relationships of the tarso-metatarsal bones with the unaffected side, frequently resulting in helping to achieve the diagnosis or to solve any doubts in the more tricky injuries (see Fig. 6.1).

In all the cases, for any midfoot segment, it is fundamental to complete the classic X-ray images with an oblique projection and, if any doubt remains, to perform a CT.

When performing a CT study of this anatomic area, it is very important to obtain images that can show all the connections between the tarsal bones and between the tarsal and metatarsal bones, to grant the vision of any joint dislocations. Considering the plantar arch inclination, to obtain such images, it is mandatory to perform the axial reconstructions not parallel to the foot, like is usually done, but along the metatarsal bones (see Fig. 6.2).

W. Daghino et al., *Foot and Ankle Trauma Injuries*, https://doi.org/10.1007/978-3-319-69617-1_6

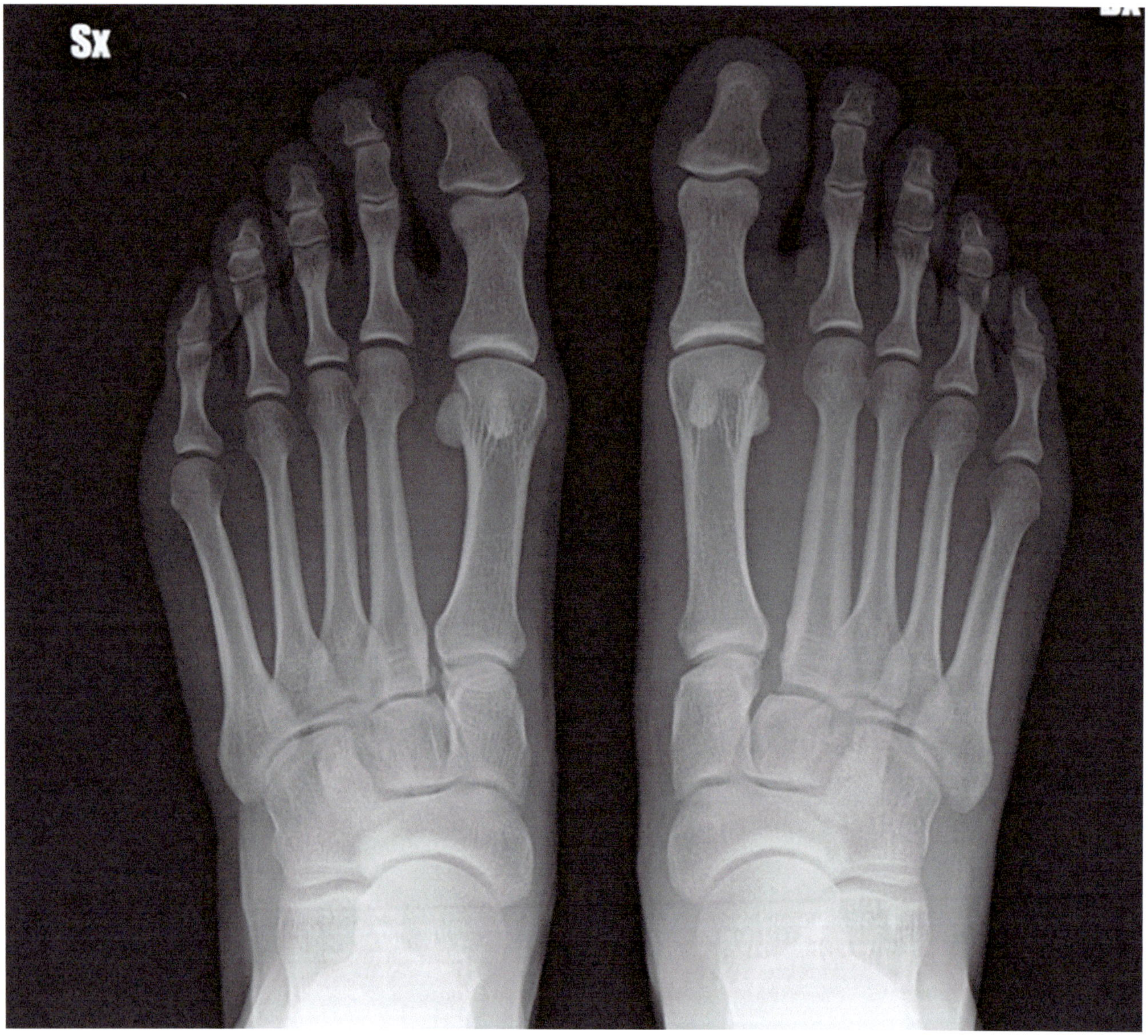

Fig. 6.1 A comparative projection can be useful to recognize a Lisfranc injury: in this case on the right, the increase in the space between the base of the second and first metatarsals is evident

6.1.2 Preoperative Planning and Instrumentation

The CT study becomes fundamental and undeniable in those cases in which surgery is needed, because it is the basis of the preoperative planning that allows to identify the number of fragments and segments involved, it is possible to obtain the pathologic anatomy of the injury and to spot the translations of fragments, it is possible to programme the timing and the necessary reduction manoeuvres, and it is possible to determine the instrumentation needed (see Fig. 6.3).

The availability of dedicated instrumentation especially in this area is crucial, and, together with the experience and formation of the surgeon and his team that will perform the surgery, they are critical to achieve good results even in the more serious cases [3]. Such specific instrumentation needs to be ordered and prepared before the surgery, and it must include, besides the classic Kirschner wires of different diameters between 0.8 and 3 mm, a little segment distractor, useful to grant the sight of the joint surface fragments that need to be restored and temporarily stabilized; double-threaded cannulated screws of little diameter, less than 3 mm; pins and screws made of absorbable materials; syn-

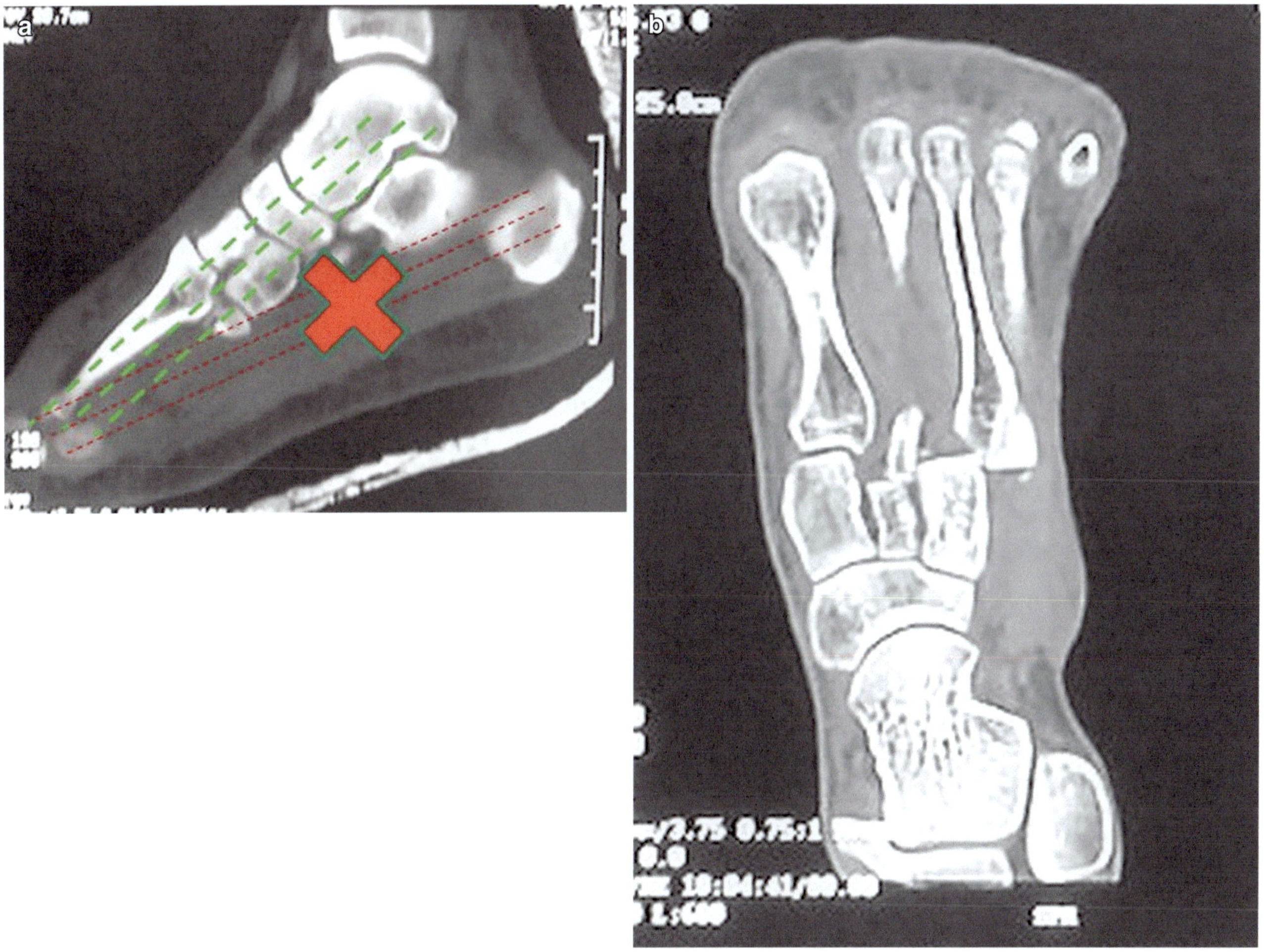

Fig. 6.2 (**a**) The axial reconstructions that need to be acquired and evaluated in the study of the midfoot are not the classic ones, parallel to the foot (red line), but the ones that result to be parallel to the metatarsal bones (green lines); in this way, it is possible to achieve images that enlighten contemporarily the bones of the metatarsus and the tarsus (**b**), allowing to see correctly the joint relationships

thetic bone graft; plates and locking screws, generic or specifically designed for the segments; and mini-external fixators with a gliding system. Any of these systems, even if not daily used, can result irreplaceable to resolve specific technical difficulties tipical of these segments. Therefore, to prevent that the surgeon needs to adapt to alternative less effective solutions, it is advisable to list these instruments during the preparation to the surgery, in course of preoperative planning, so to have time to prepare them correctly. This is crucial to achieve good outcomes.

6.2 Traumatic Injuries of the Chopart

6.2.1 Classification

For this segment, no prognostic classification has been published; for this reason, usually the injuries are defined through merely descriptive and mechanic criteria [4], dividing them into:

Compression injuries: extremely polymorphic, consequent to a direct crush of the tarsal bones; they represent the more serious injuries, because of the important fragmentation and because of the frequent association with bone exposition.

Longitudinal stress injuries: they develop through a nutcracker-type mechanism, in consequence of the opposed actions of kinetic energy and the strength of the ground on which the force lines act along the major axis of the foot (see Fig. 6.4); frequently they are associated with Lisfranc injuries.

Medial or lateral stress injuries: they are so described depending on where the dislocation of the forefoot is present, which is a consequence of solicitations between the latter and the rest of the bone segment, which is held fixed, variably associated with torsional forces (see Fig. 6.5).

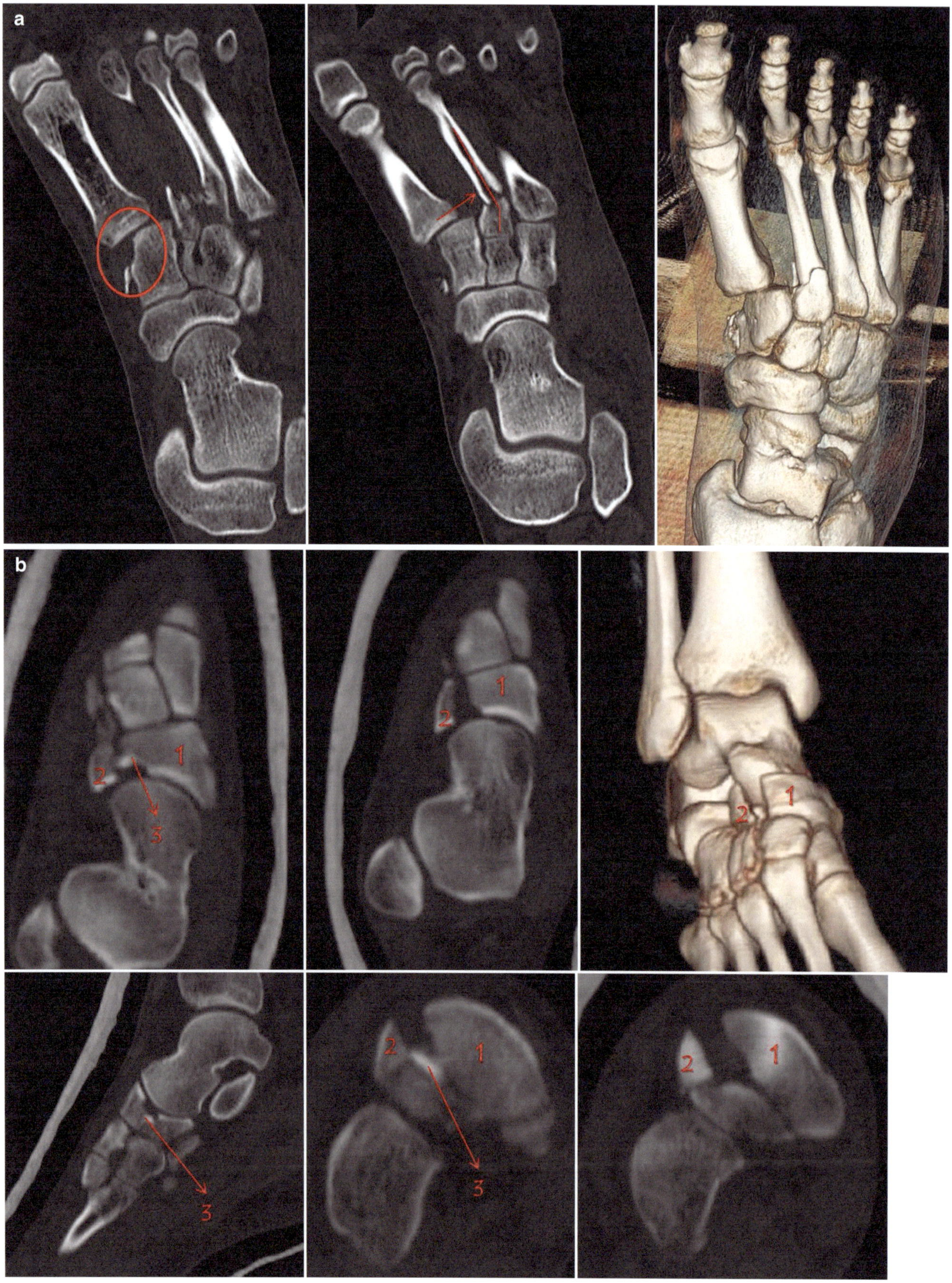

Fig. 6.3 Examples of a preoperative planning: (**a**) Lisfranc injury, where the key problem is in the angulation of the base of the second metatarsal bone and consequently in the subluxation of the first cuneo-metatarsal joint; (**b**) fracture of the navicular bone, where it is evident that the key for a satisfying reduction must be the repositioning of the osteochondral fragment, centrally sunken (shown as nr. 3)

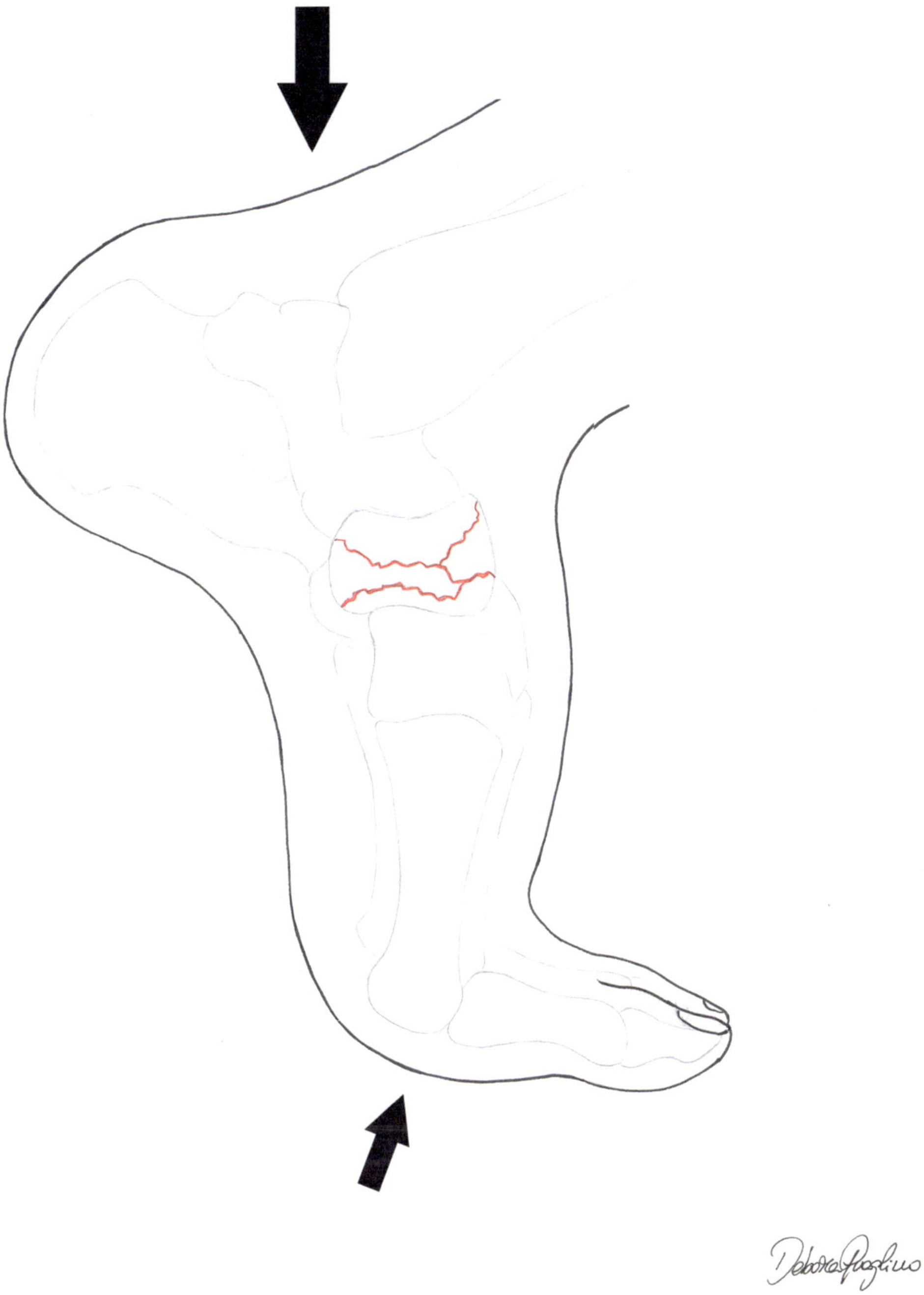

Fig. 6.4 Descriptive classification of the Chopart injuries: the longitudinal stress fractures are induced by a nutcracker mechanism, resulting from the contemporary and opposed action of the kinematic energy and the resistance of the bearing surface, which are acting against the metatarsal bones

Plantar stress injuries: the more rare, with plantar/dorsal dislocation of the tarsal component (see Fig. 6.6).

6.2.2 Indications and Goals

Whichever Chopart segment is involved, the guiding principle to the treatment indication is common, based on the presence of an isolated dislocation, of an isolated fracture or a combination of the two.

Established that a nonsurgical treatment is dedicated to the stable and undisplaced injuries [3], in all the other situations, it is necessary to reduce the joint dislocation and to evaluate the stability of the segment, which can be kept even through a percutaneous positioning of Kirschner wires if not safe. Particular caution must be reserved to the indication of a closed reduction and percutaneous stabilization through Kirschner wires that can be acceptable in the case of a pure dislocation in which a closed reduction allows to achieve an anatomic restoration, which needs to be always checked

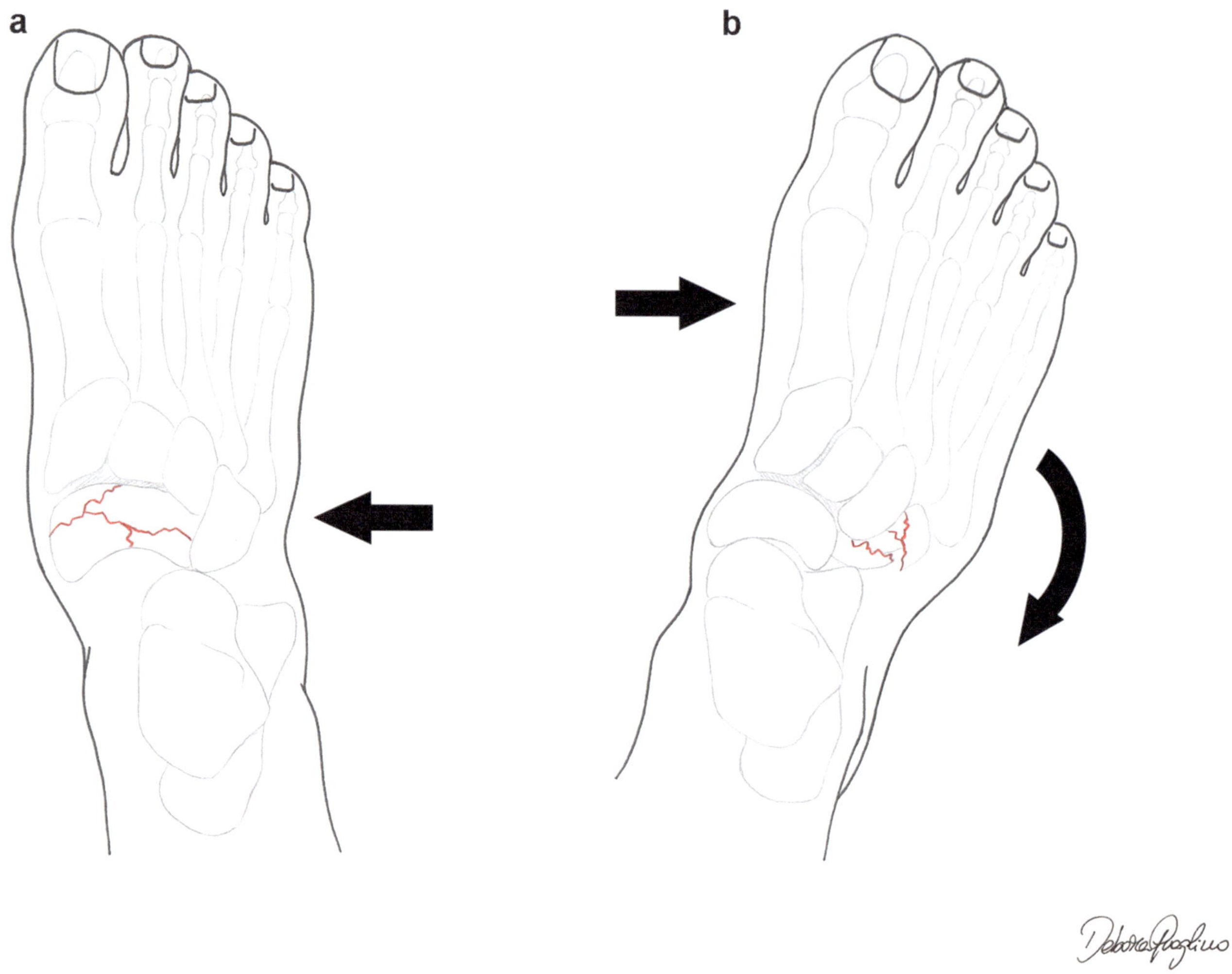

Fig. 6.5 Descriptive classification of the Chopart injuries: the injuries related to a medial stress (**a**) are distinguished from the ones related to a lateral stress (**b**) considering the direction of the forefoot dislocation in comparison with the hindfoot

through imaging. In all the other fracture dislocations or nonanatomic reductions, it is necessary to proceed to an open reduction, which has the aim to restore the anatomy of the joint surfaces and to achieve a stable fixation of the fragments. This aspect may differ depending on the involved segment and the pathologic anatomy of the injury: in the case of an avulsion of fragments from the navicular bone, when these are dorsal, due to the talo-navicular ligament action, the surgery of choice is the reinsertion of the detached ligament through anchors; if the avulsion involves the medial tuberosity of the navicular bone, like the detachment of large osteochondral fragments of any segment of the midtarsal joint, the preferred treatment is the double-threaded screw fixation; finally, the conventional osteosynthesis, eventually associated with bone grafting to increase the stability of the construct, is the best technique for the more complex and extended fractures [5].

If the morphologic restoration is not enough to achieve stability in consequence of the injured ligaments and of the soft tissues, the use of a plaster cast or the positioning of an external fixator that needs to be kept until the scar is able to substitute safely such structures is indicated. The external fixation associated with the Kirschner wire stabilization, from a complementary option, is considered the only option when there is such a fragmentation of the fracture, which leads to an impossibility of a synthesis through the other methods or if there is an important soft tissue suffering: in these cases, the aim of the surgery is only to restore the length of the two foot columns, medial and lateral [5, 6].

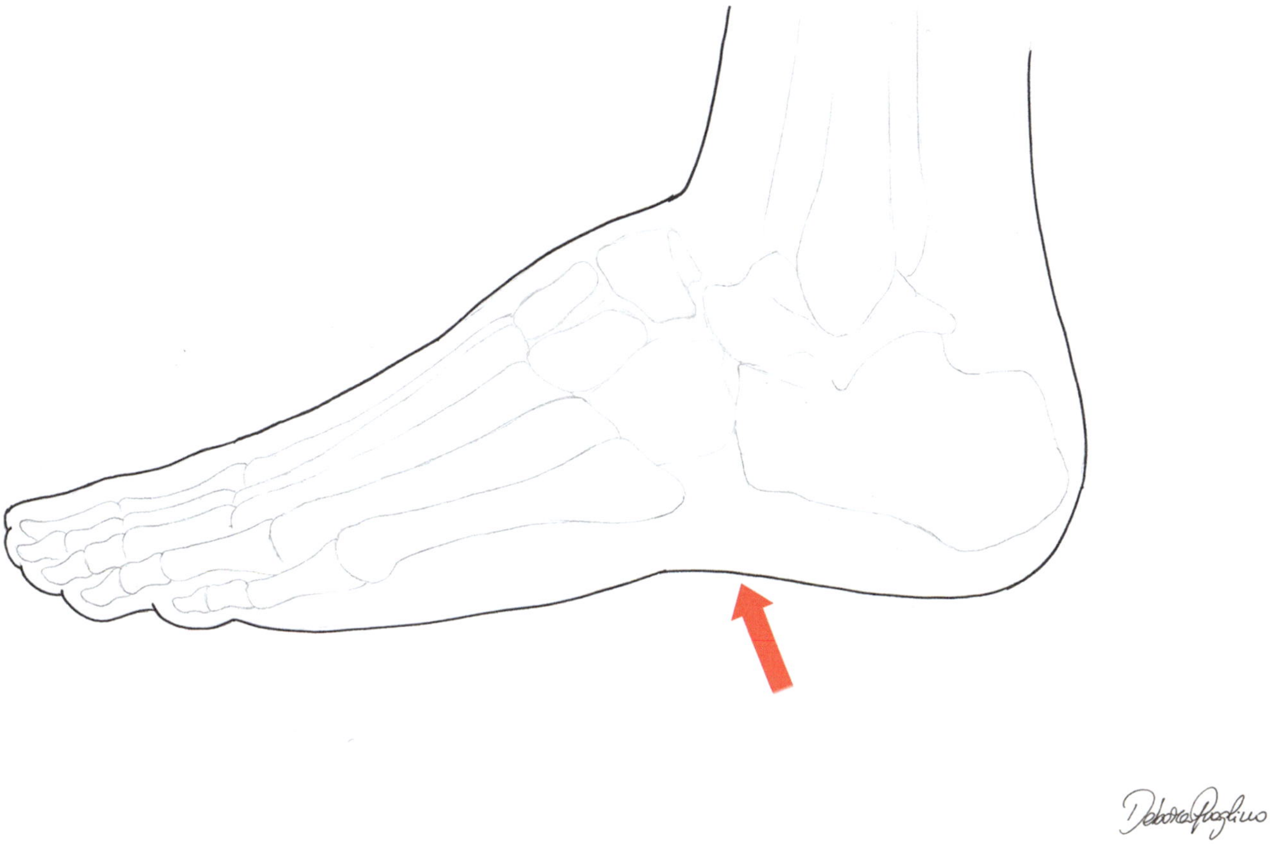

Fig. 6.6 Descriptive classification of the Chopart injuries: in the injury related to a plantar stress, a dorsal or plantar dislocation of the midfoot in relationship to the rear foot is present

6.2.3 Surgical Technique

6.2.3.1 Patient Positioning

The patient is positioned on a radio-transparent table, supine, with a tourniquet on the thigh and a cushion under the gluteus of the affected limb to nullify the natural tendency to extrarotate the leg. The other lower limb is elevated with the knee flexed and positioned on a support, removing or lowering the adjacent part of the table, allowing the access of the surgeon to both sides of the foot and permitting to position the nearest as possible the C-arm to grant the best imaging (see Fig. 6.7).

As in every complex bone injury of the foot and ankle, at this time, an X-ray in the two basic projections is done allowing to check the correct positioning of the patient that grants the best vision of the fracture and to save such images as a starting point useful to be compared to the future images done after the reduction manoeuvres. This part ends the positioning of the patient.

6.2.3.2 Surgical Access

The surgical access used depends on the anatomy of the injury: an incision is performed more or less dorsal, medial or lateral depending on the manoeuvres necessary for the reduction and the type of osteosynthesis decided during the preoperative planning.

Generally for the calcanear foot, direct lateral or dorsolateral access is used, being careful to avoid and protect the peroneal tendons and the branches of the saphenous and superficial peroneus nerve, while for the medial structures, the choice falls on the classic medial accesses, laying between the anterior tibial tendon and the posterior tibial tendon and, on more dorsal accesses, laying between the extensor tendons and the neurovascular bundle (see Fig. 6.8).

6.2.3.3 Reduction Manoeuvres

Before proceeding to the reduction of the fracture, the starting point is always the preoperative planning; on the count of

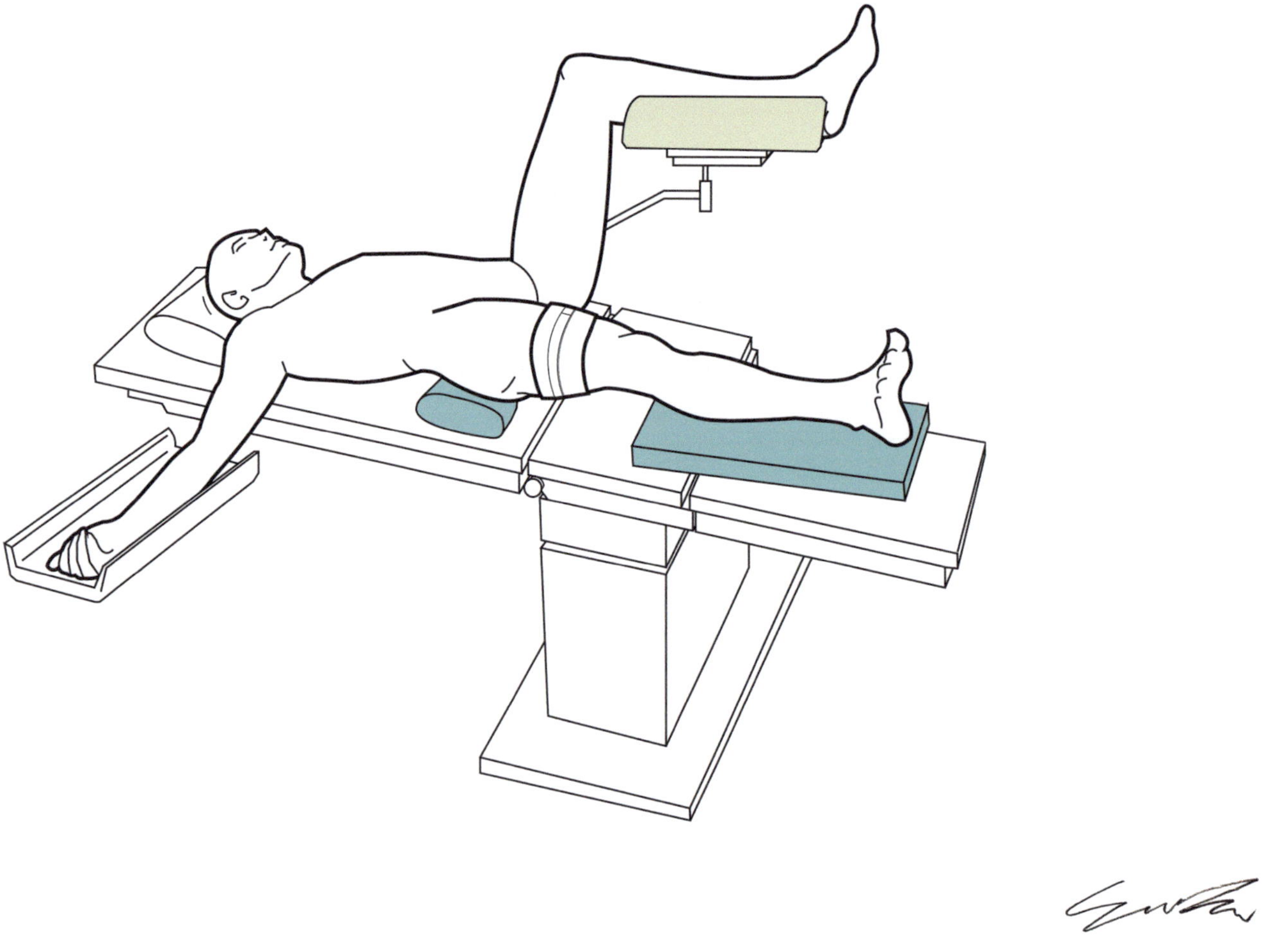

Fig. 6.7 Chopart injury: during the preoperative positioning, the rising of the opposite lower limb will grant the surgeon an access to the medial side of the foot, and it will ease the lateral fluoroscopic imaging

the latter, it is decided where the distractor for the little joints is going to be positioned that is central for the accomplishment of the surgery.

Once the articular distraction is positioned, it is much more easy to identify all the joint fragments that were previously spotted with the CT; in this phase, it is important to respect as much as possible the position of these fragments: this will allow of maintaining the preoperative planning as a guide, reducing the risk of lose the references, that are the more important the more is complex the fracture. Only after having spotted all the components and correctly evaluated the pathological anatomy, it is convenient to begin their mobilization and movement, using thin and delicate elevators to free any impacted fragments (see Fig. 6.9), without altering the anatomical landmarks that will be necessary to the reduction process. In navicular bone injuries, it is possible to find a sunken central osteochondral fragment; in the case in which the bony component is too little to be stabilized through osteosynthesis, once it has been identified, split opened one of the dorsal fragments with a spreader and freed and repositioned in its place, it is possible to keep the correct joint line shouldering it through a bone graft. This graft, synthetic or autologous, must be set near to the osteochondral reduced fragment, with a mechanical function; later the dorsal fragments are reduced and stabilized through the use of temporary Kirschner wires (see Figs. 6.10 and 6.11).

6.2.3.4 Stabilization/Osteosynthesis

If the fragments are sufficiently big to allow it, it is preferable to synthetize the fractures with free mini screws, conventional or double threaded; if the comminution is extensive or the bone quality is compromised, it can be useful to use dedicated anatomical plates with locking screws, which increase the grip and the solidity of the construct. Only in limited cases or in severe soft tissues suffering that are in conflict with an internal fixation, the stabilization is achieved through Kirschner wires or Steinmann pins, neutralizing the displacing forces through the use of an external fixator that bridges the fracture, which will allow to keep the correct length of the affected column (see Fig. 6.12).

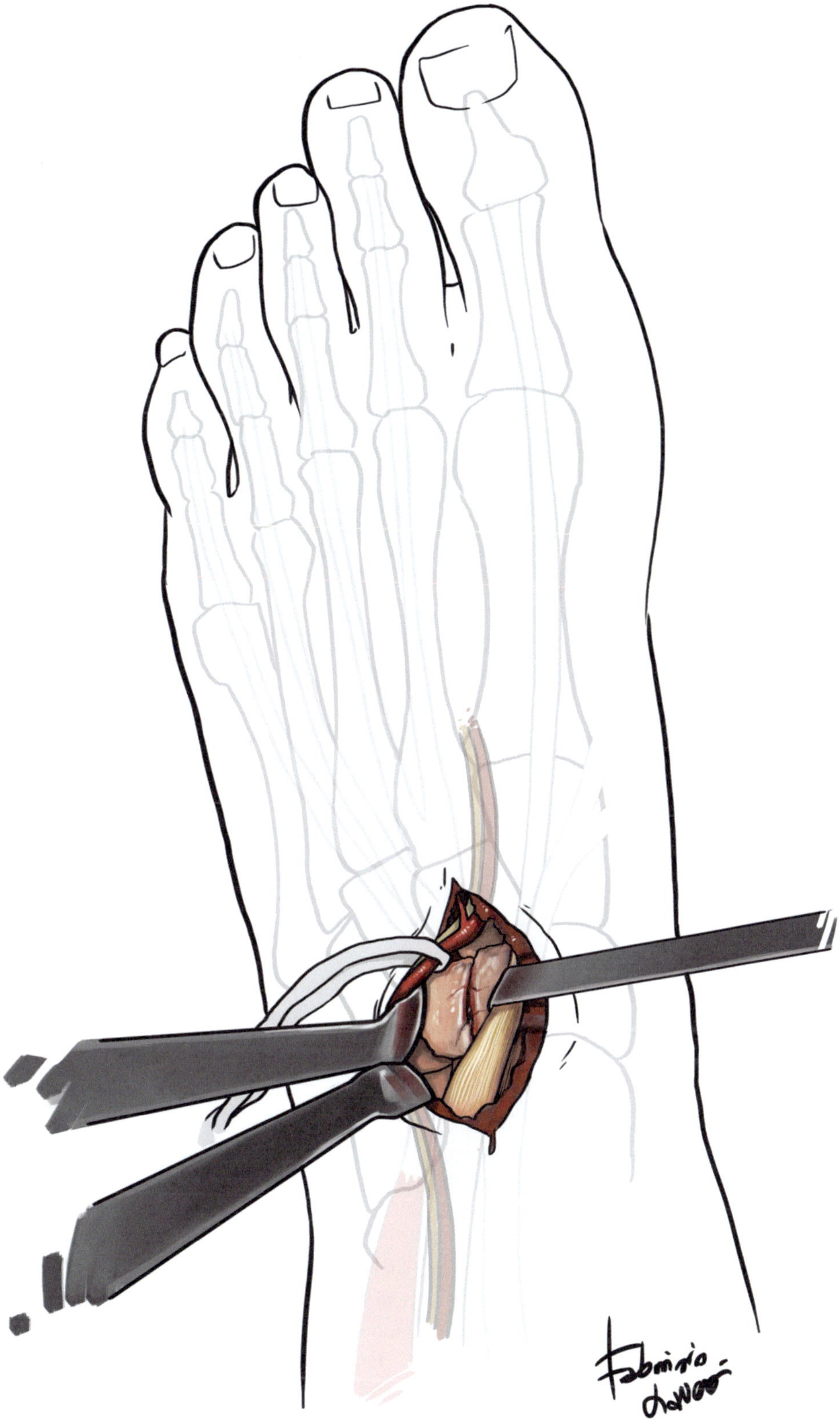

Fig. 6.8 Surgical access to the navicular bone of the tarsus: the incision is done following the preoperative planning; in this case (see Fig. 6.3b) to land on the fractured fragments, a pure dorsal incision was indicated, which has been done passing between the tibialis anterior and extensor hallucis tendons, which are medially retracted, and the extensor digitorum longus tendon, which is retracted laterally together with the neurovascular bundle

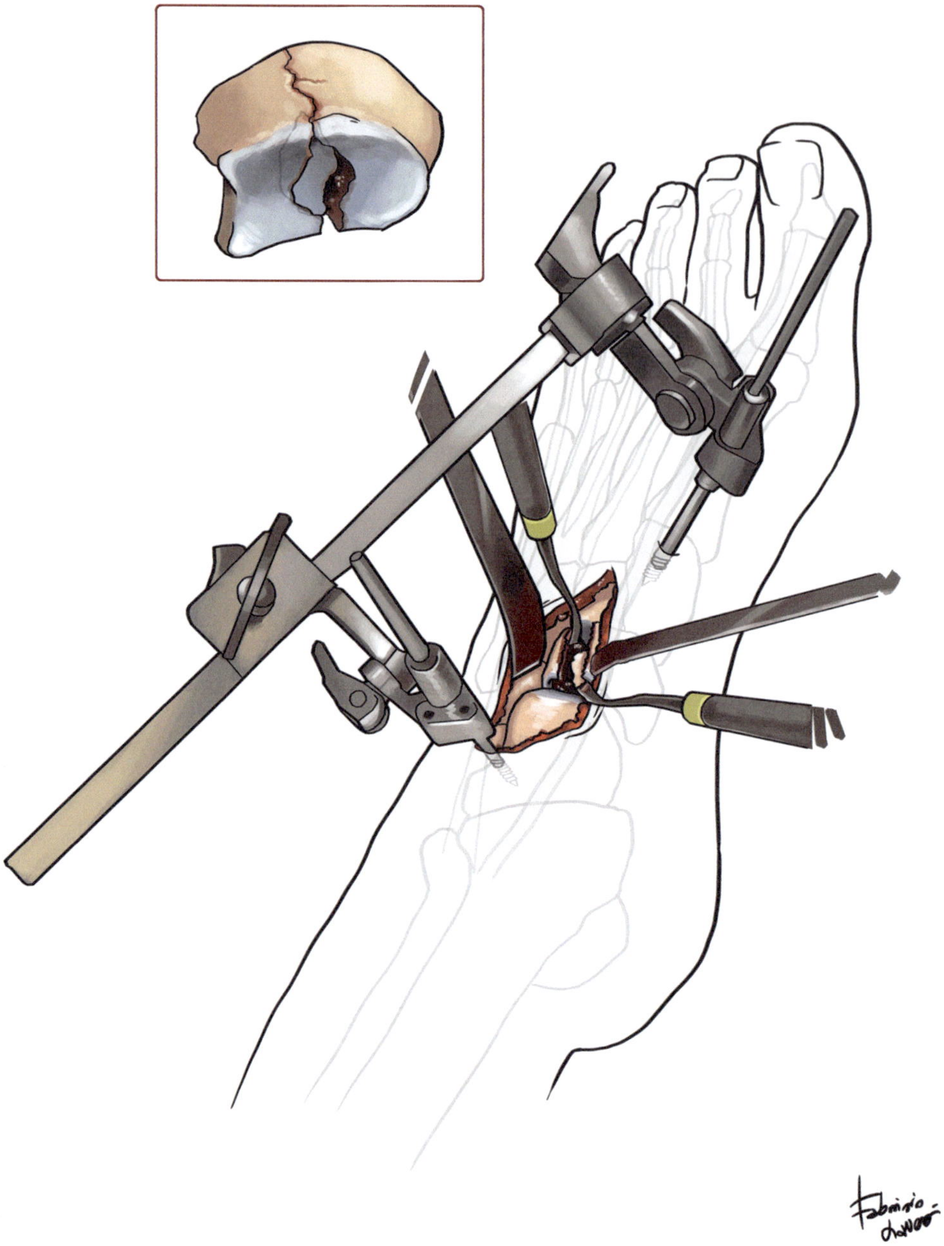

Fig. 6.9 Injury of the navicular tarsal bone: after the type of injury and the presence of impacted fragments (in the square) are correctly identified, it is possible to mobilize all the stuck fragments through the use of specific instrumentations

In the cases in which at the end of the surgery there is a remaining instability, it is necessary to strengthen the construct with trans-articular Kirschner wires and Steinmann pins or, as an alternative, use absorbable pins, which do not have all the disadvantages of the percutaneous devices, equally granting the temporary fixation of the joint and losing their mechanical stability in a few months [7].

6.2.3.5 Postoperative Care

The stiches are removed after 2 weeks from surgery; if any percutaneous Kirschner wires are present, these usually are removed after 6 weeks, together with the removal of any immobilization achieved with plaster casts or braces that limit the range of motion in all those cases in which the synthesis is unstable.

Especially for the navicular fractures, where the unstable terminal vascularization can impede the healing process, increasing contemporarily the risk of an avascular necrosis, but more in general in all the situations in which the synthesis includes an articular segment, because the principle of bony restoration is achieved through a cortical fusion, it is necessary to wait for the bone healing before allowing the weight bearing, which should be postponed for at least 12 weeks [8].

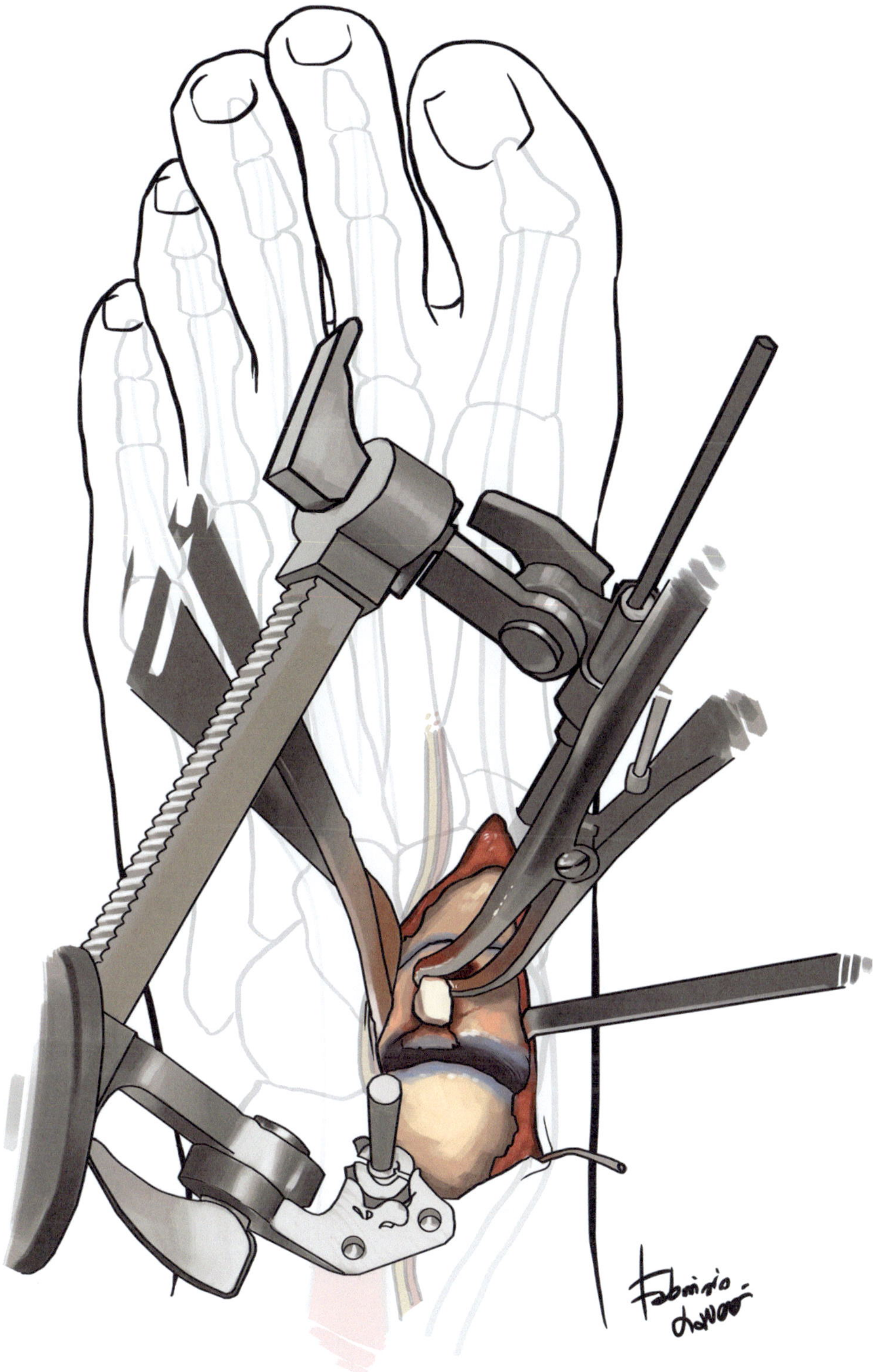

Fig. 6.10 Once all the osteochondral fragments have been reduced at the correct height, but they are not sufficiently large to be synthetized, it is possible to keep them in the right spot positioning a bone graft that will function as mechanical support

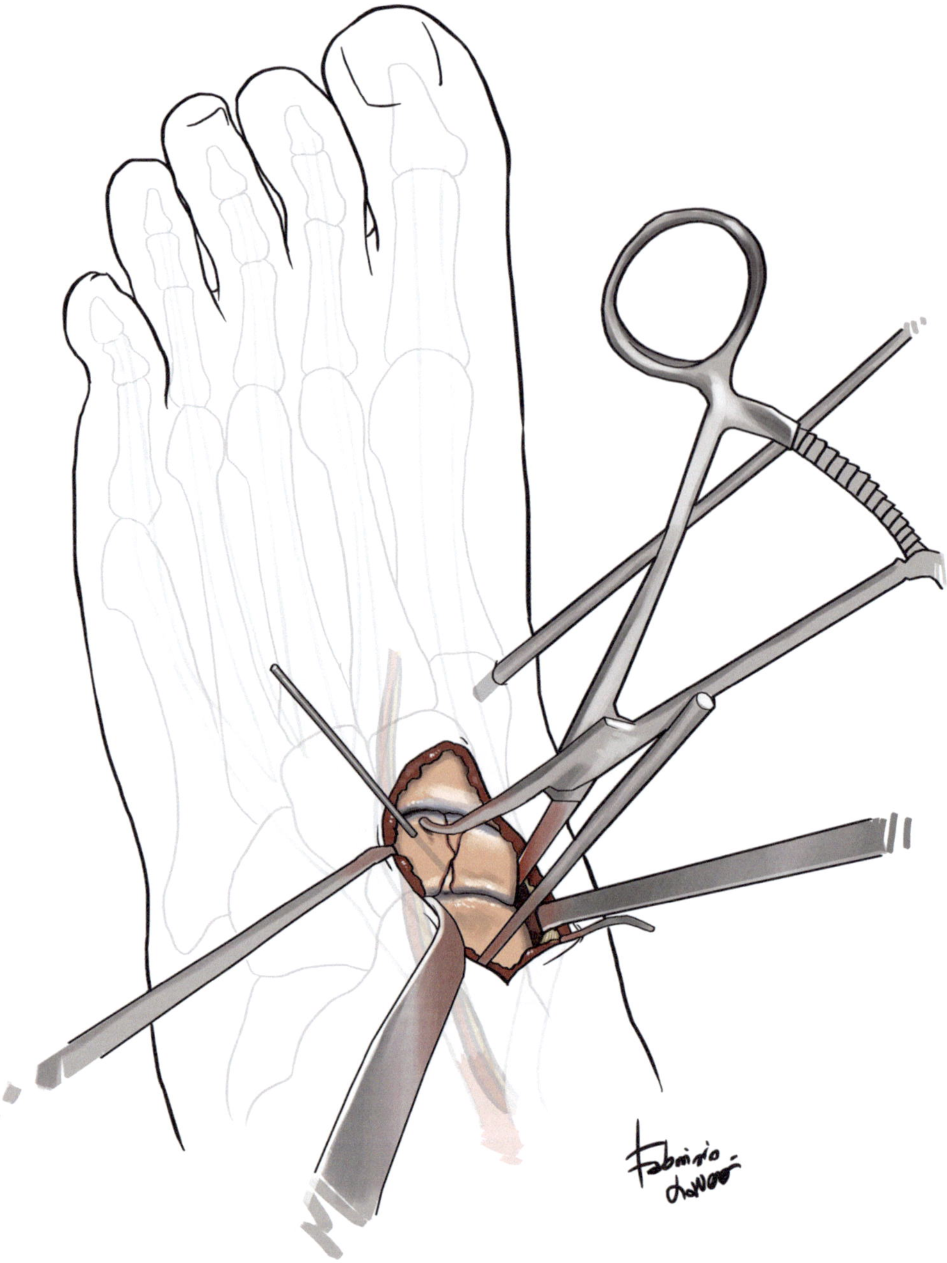

Fig. 6.11 Once closed the superior fragment, previously opened as a book to grant the joint reconstruction, it is possible to proceed to the stabilization with thin Kirschner wires. The distraction is then removed, checking that all the articular relationships are corrected

6.3 Traumatic Injuries of the Lisfranc Joint

6.3.1 Classification

As the Chopart injuries are extremely rare, there is no classification with a prognostic factor but only descriptive classifications. The more used system is the one proposed by Quenu and Kuss, introduced during the first years of the past century, and modified by Mayerson in 1986 (see Fig. 6.13), which distinguishes between the cases in which the injury includes all the metatarsal tongue, which remains integral (type A), from the ones where there is a partial incongruity, including only the first ray in isolation or all the lateral metatarsal bones (types B1 and B2, respectively), and the injuries where there is a complete incongruity with a divergence between the first ray and the lateral rays (type C) [9].

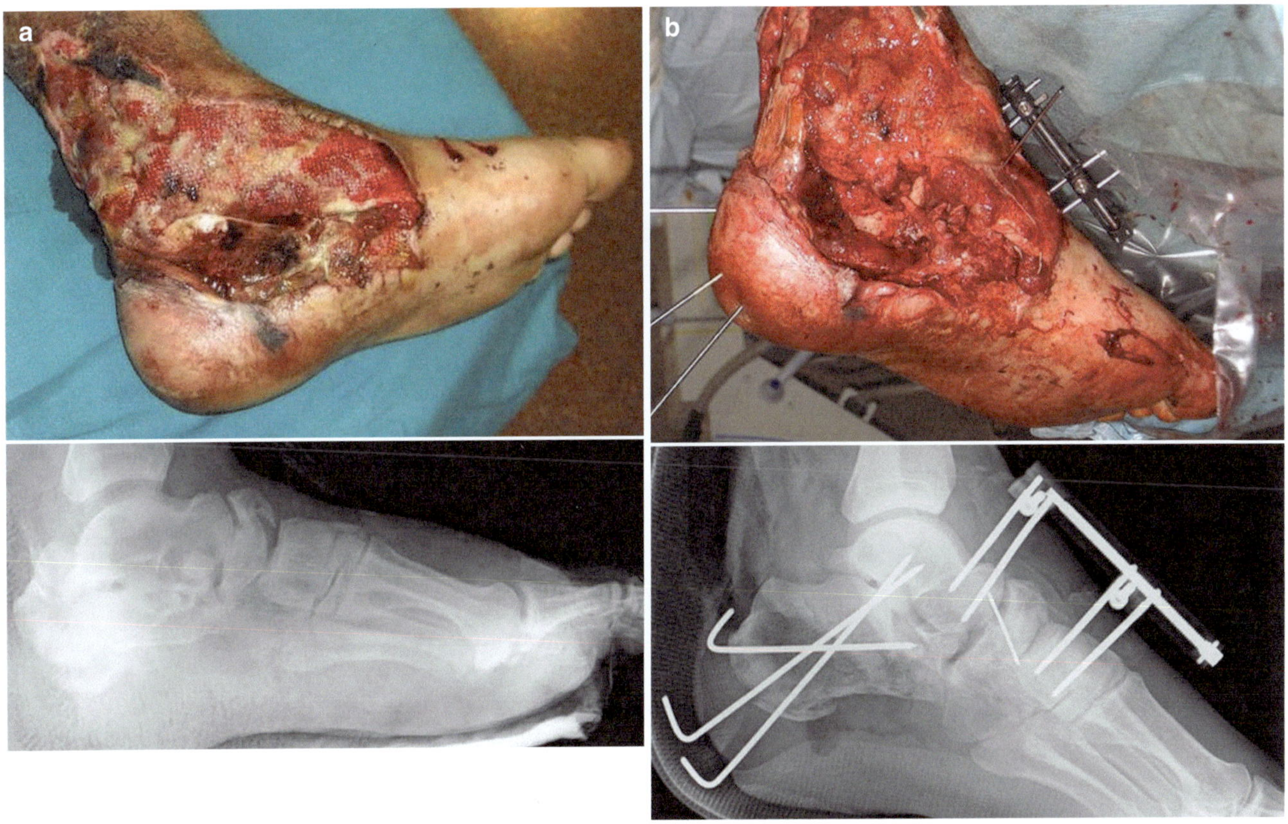

Fig. 6.12 When it is impossible to proceed to an internal fixation because of the severe comminution or of the presence of concomitant injuries of the soft tissues (**a**), after a Kirschner wire stabilization is achieved, it is possible to neutralize the tendency to dislocation and to lose length of the column through the use of a bridging external fixator (**b**). In this case, the severity of the soft tissue injury allowed only to achieve a minimal synthesis even because of the calcaneal fracture

6.3.2 Indications and Goals

Because they are injuries that frequently hesitate in a symptomatic rigid and degenerative joint and since it is acknowledged that the adverse evolution is proportional to the anatomical alteration, in these cases, the behaviour must be extremely aggressive, considering unacceptable even displacements of 1–2 mm that are spotted during the imaging, above all in the young patients. The goal to pursue is to achieve a pain-free foot, stable and plantigrade, and this is obtained only through an anatomical reduction [5]. And for this reason, any percutaneous synthesis must be considered extremely dangerous and an option only if the surgeon is certain that the reduction achieved through external manoeuvres is perfect, which is mostly infrequent. For these reasons, this kind of injury is mainly treated through open reduction and stabilization [5, 9–12].

Regarding the surgical timing, considering that in these lesions it is always theoretically possible to develop a compartment syndrome, the neurologic evaluation is discerning: if a neurological loss is uprising, the treatment becomes an urgency, and the swelling is not any more pivotal even if massive, because the surgical access is by itself able to reduce the tissue tension [5, 13]. In all the other situations, in the absence of a compartment syndrome, it is best to immobilize the injury with a posterior half cast, checking periodically the neurological and vascular parameters, keeping the lower limb elevated and performing surgery only if there is a specifically trained surgeon with all the necessary instrumentation and with a complete diagnostics that allow to have an accurate preoperative planning and in any case proceeding to surgery at the most 3 weeks after the trauma [3].

6.3.2.1 Surgical Technique

6.3.2.2 Patient Positioning

The patient is positioned supine on the radiolucent surgical table, with a tourniquet at the thigh and a cushion under the gluteus of the affected side to nullify the tendency to extrarotate the lower limb, checking that a three-projection radioscopic imaging is obtainable; the limb that is going to be treated must be elevated by a cushion (see Fig. 6.14), or

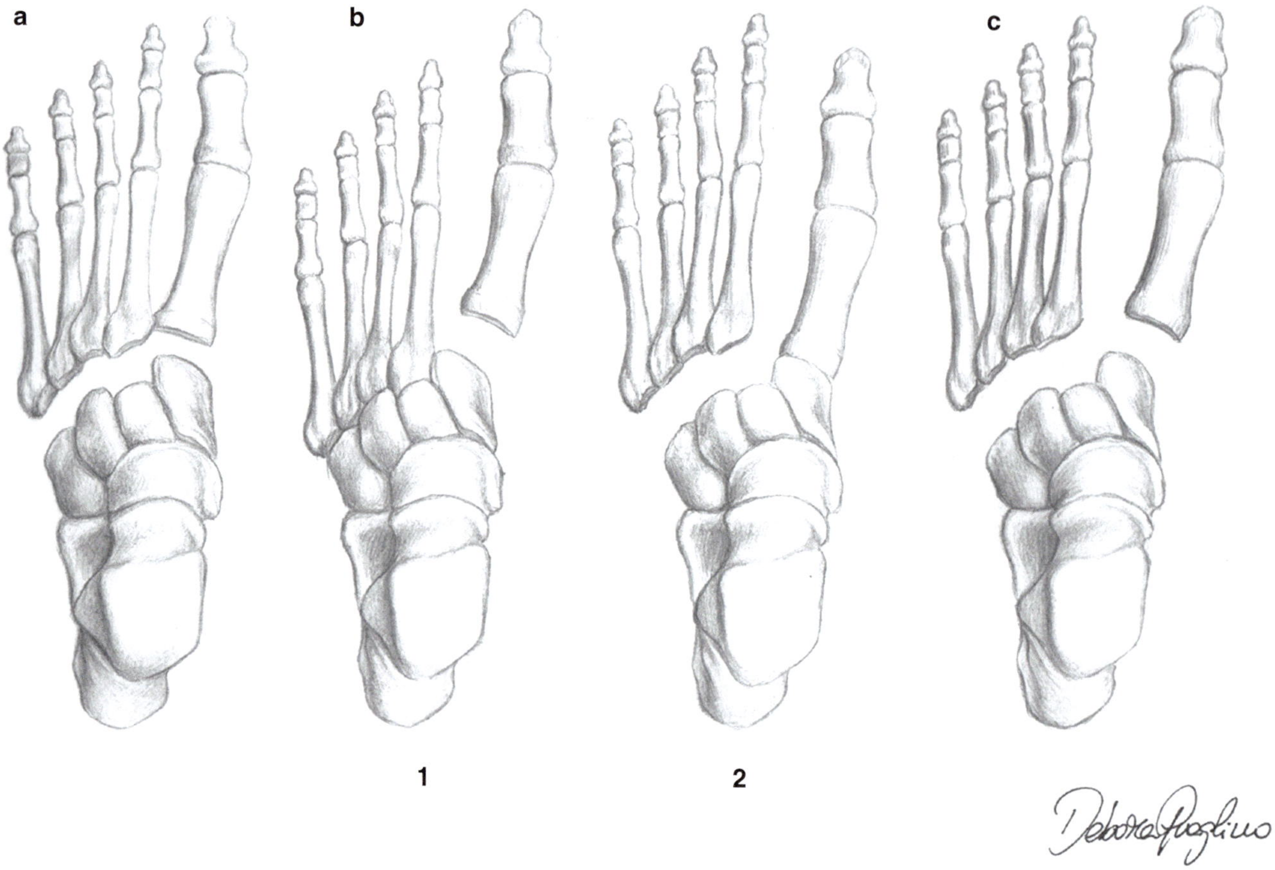

Fig. 6.13 Lisfranc injury classification: the type A relates to a complete dislocation of the entire metatarsal tongue; the type B includes the injuries of the first ray (B1) or only of the lateral rays (B2); the type C includes all the divergent injuries

alternatively the opposite limb must be elevated, flexed, abducted and extrarotated on a support. A final check before the surgical field is prepared grants to confirm the correct imaging and to have a starting point as a paragon for the following reduction manoeuvres. This final step completes the preoperative positioning of the patient.

6.3.2.3 Surgical Access

The classic access considers dorsal longitudinal incisions, the first near the 2° ray on the 1° intermetatarsal space, which is always necessary; a second optional incision along the fourth ray must be performed if the lateral portion of the tarso-metatarsal joint is not reducible (see Fig. 6.15).

After having moved aside the two margins of the wound through silk wires, to avoid any tractions with retractors on this extremely delicate skin, the dissection is completed, loading and protecting with laces the branches of the superficial peroneal nerve, which cross the incision line, and the dorsalis pedis neurovascular bundle, which passes deeply underneath, under the retinacula of the extensors, inferiorly to the extensor hallucis longus tendon and medially to the extensor hallucis brevis tendon (see Fig. 6.16).

The journey of the bundle must be followed during the dissection, so to have it mobilized and to be able to move it freely in the best position in relation with the manoeuvres needed; following the neurovascular bundle, just before it deepens into the first intermetatarsal space, it is possible to arrive in the proximity of the base of the second metatarsal bone and into the key area of the injury, completing the surgical access (see Fig. 6.17).

6.3.2.4 Reduction Manoeuvres

Even in this type of injuries, the best starting point to achieve a good reduction is a rigorous preoperative planning: starting from the latter, it is possible to foresee the dislocations and translations generated by the trauma and to identify all the various fragments if any fracture lesions coexist. Once the pathologic anatomy study and the surgical landmarks coupling with the ones shown by the CT are achieved, the reduction is completed following the planned order.

Usually the first structure that is reduced, because it represents the keystone to achieve a good anatomical reduction of the entire tarso-metatarsal joint, is the base of the second metatarsal bone, which must be wedged between the three

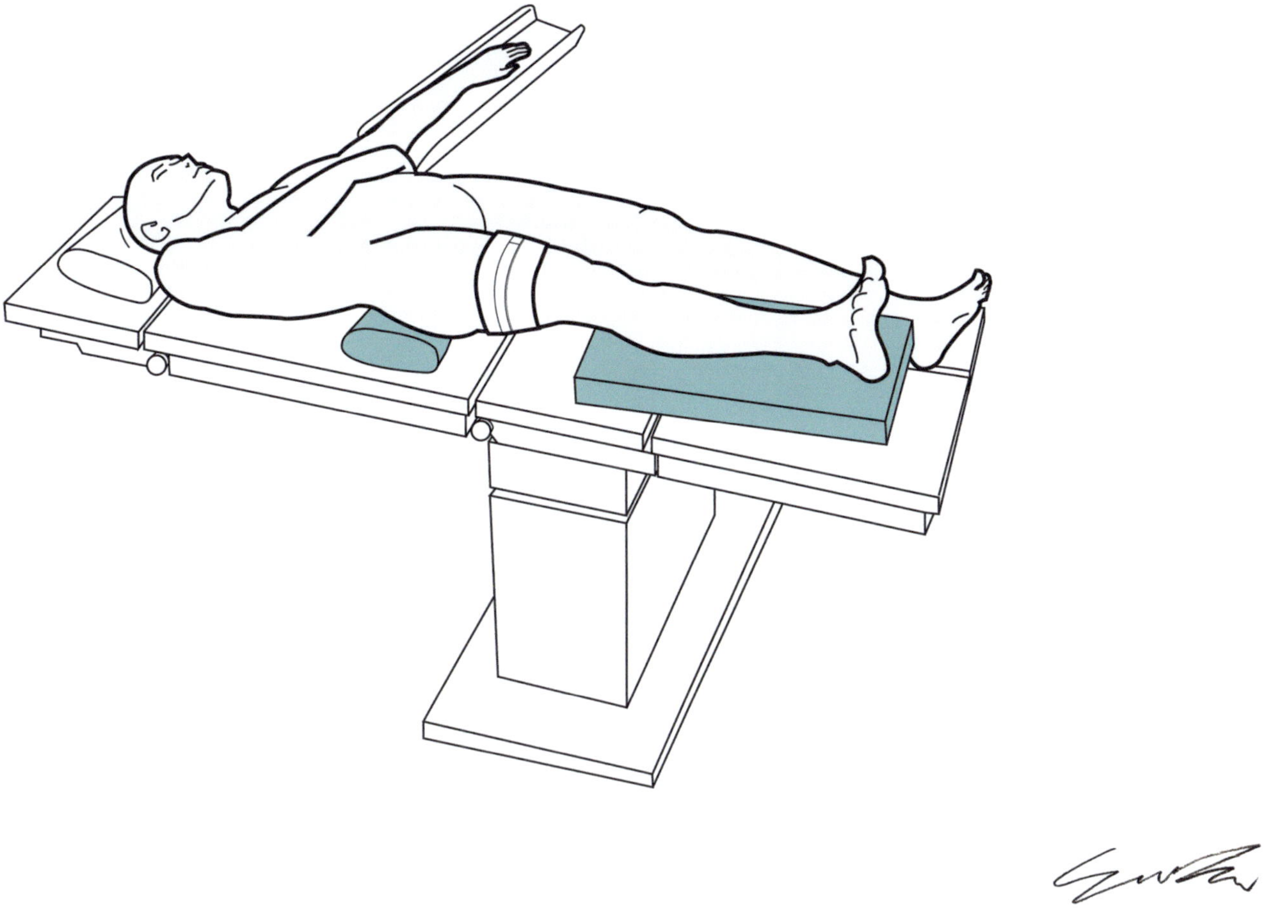

Fig. 6.14 Lisfranc injury surgical treatment: preoperative positioning—a cushion under the gluteus will nullify the tendency to extrarotate the lower limb; one under the foot will allow to have the foot on a different level regarding the opposite unharmed side, granting the execution of the fluoroscopic intraoperative imaging

cuneiforms, restoring the relationship between the cuneometatarsal joint and base of the first metatarsal bone (see Fig. 6.18).

Once the normal regional anatomy is restored, a temporary Kirschner wire stabilization is performed to allow checking with the C-arm the quality of the reduction that must be imperative, proceeding with further manoeuvres, solicitations and further X-ray imaging until the planned result is achieved.

During this phase, it is essential to obtain the radiological images with the same angles to the ones done prior to surgery, so to nullify the confounding effect results from images with different obliquities, granting the possibility to evaluate precisely the result of the manoeuvres performed and the restoration of the bony anatomy.

After the reduction of the second metatarsal bone base, if there was a coexistent dislocation of the lateral metatarsal bone bases, the correct reduction of the latter is checked under fluoroscopy. Usually the reduction is achieved through the action of the ligamentous apparatus if unharmed, proceeding afterwards with a Kirschner wire stabilization. If the reduction of the lateral components is not achieved, it is necessary to perform the accessory lateral incision on the fourth metatarsal bone to complete the open reduction of the Lisfranc joint.

6.3.2.5 Stabilization/Osteosynthesis

If there is a fracture of the metatarsal base, a synthesis with titanium-free screws of a diameter between 2.0 and 2.7 mm is necessary; the use of preformed L or T plates of adequate dimension is possible in these segments, but because the soft tissue covering is thin, it must be considered the necessity of removal. For these reasons, such type of synthesis is reserved only in case of highly comminuted injuries, where it has the advantage of keeping the segment length and the possibility of performing a minimally invasive technique, or, if it is not possible to achieve an anatomic reduction, it allows to bridge the comminuted area performing an arthrodesis of an area that is irreparable. Considering the stabilization of the articular segments, two different philosophies are codified: one

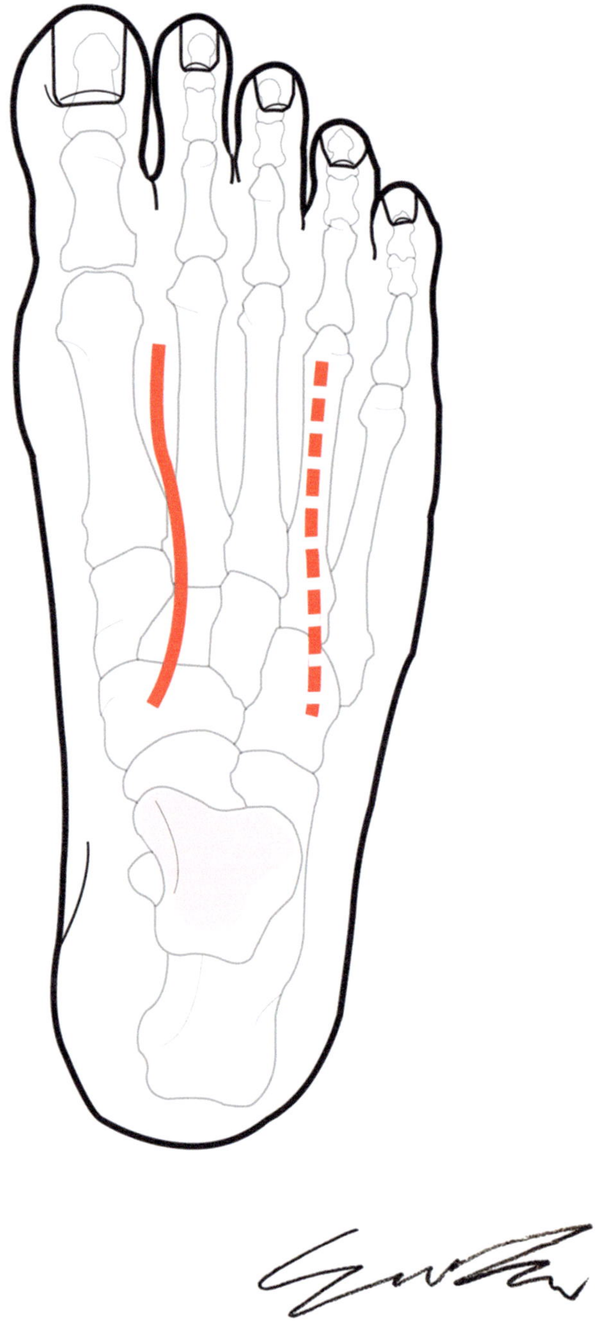

Fig. 6.15 Stabilization of the Lisfranc: the classic surgical access is dorso-longitudinal, and it lays over the first intermetatarsal space, staying on the side of the second ray; if necessary, it is possible to perform a secondary access, with an incision aimed on the fourth metatarsal bone

foresees the use of percutaneous Kirschner wires, which have the advantage of being removable in clinic and to create little holes into the cartilage [5], but they can lead to a certain loss of reduction once they are removed [10]. The second option is to use 3.5 mm diameter metal screws, positioned bridging the tarso-metatarsal joints, granting a reliable and efficient conservation of the achieved reduction, but, on the other side, they leave bigger holes into the joint cartilage, and, above all, being trans-articular, they necessarily need to be removed after a few months, to avoid any rupture with the consequent issue of having intra-articular materials or to create de facto an arthrodesis [5, 13].

A brilliant solution to this debate is the use of absorbable poly-L-lactic acid (PLLA) devices to temporarily have a trans-articular stabilization: besides the common bars, of diameter 1 to 3 mm, it is possible to retrieve screws of 3.5 but even 2.7 mm diameter, made of the same material, which are more advisable because they are less aggressive on the joint

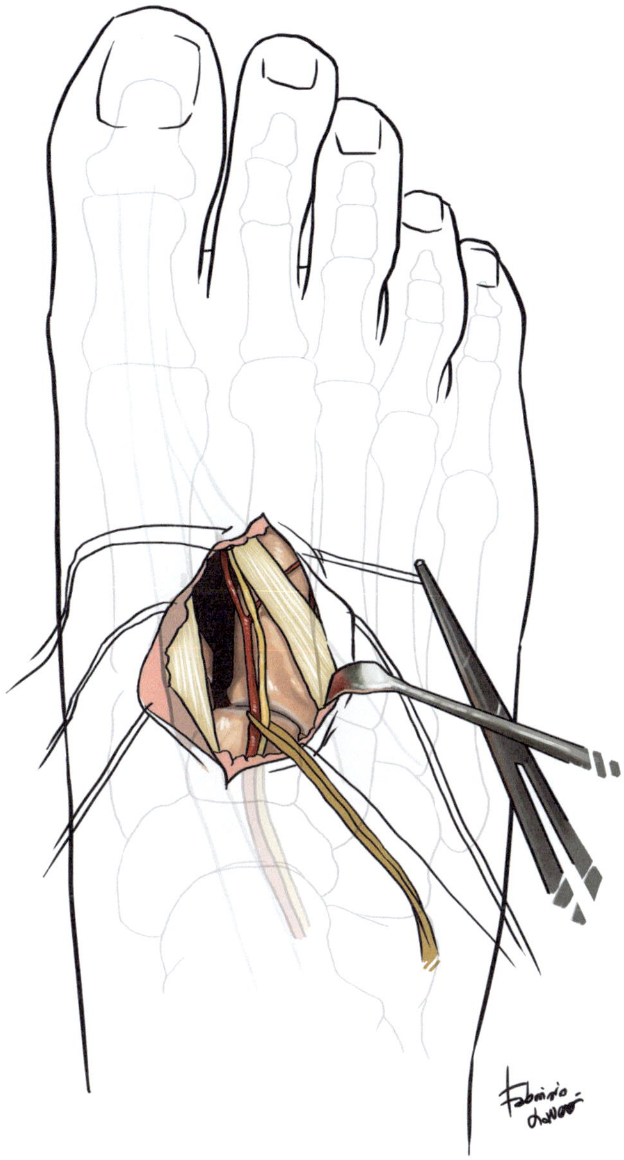

Fig. 6.16 Stabilization of the Lisfranc injuries: after the superficial dissection, it is necessary to isolate and protect the dorsalis pedis neurovascular bundle that flows under the extensor hallucis longus and medial to the extensor hallucis brevis tendon

cartilage. As for the metallic screws, the reduction is well kept because of the compression achieved through the thread of the screw, but, considering the materials they are made of, they are ideal for the stabilization issues of this specific segment (see Fig. 6.19). Indeed these screws lose their mechanic feature in around 5–6 months, an ideal time to obtain a sufficient fibrous healing of the capsular-ligamentous apparatus able to substitute the screw action of maintaining the joint reduction; furthermore, because the PLLA is completely absorbable in a few years' time, the possibility of a rupture of it is not an issue, so that it is absolutely unnecessary to plan a second surgery for the removal [7]. For these reasons, even if the mechanic characteristics are inferior and the surgical technique is more demanding in correlation to the metal hardware [14], because of the threading of the holes before the screw is inserted to avoid any breakage, we usually use these devices every time it is possible in the treatment of the Lisfranc injuries.

In the literature, adverse reactions to some absorbable materials are reported, in particular to polyglycolic acid; such issues are described even for the poly-L-lactic acid but exceptional and sporadic [15], and of these, in more than 10 years of use, we never had a direct experience.

6.3.2.6 Postoperative Care

The stiches are removed after 15 days from surgery; until 40 days from surgery, the affected lower limb must be kept without any weight bearing and with a plaster cast splint in a

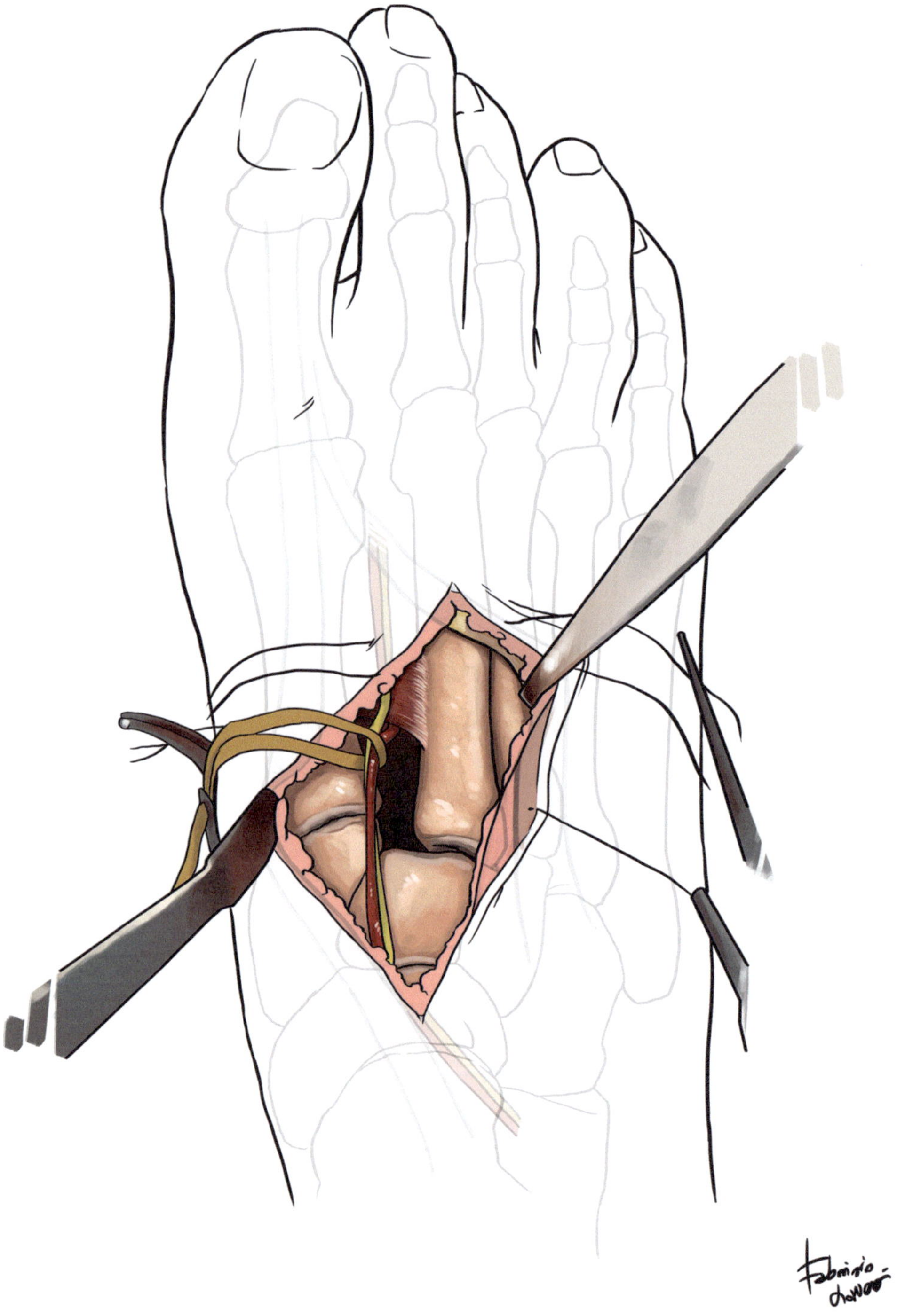

Fig. 6.17 Stabilization of the Lisfranc: after the superficial dissection and protection of the neurovascular dorsal bundle, so to have it free to be moved in any direction, it is followed distally until it deepens into the first intermetatarsal space, arriving to the area in which the base of the second metatarsal bone is, therefore, into the heart of the injury, if a dislocation is present

functional positioning, to avoid any structural equinus contracture; after this period a first X-ray check is done and the removal of percutaneous Kirschner wires if present is done, the active ankle and foot joint mobilization is started, and the recovery of the weight bearing is programmed, usually after 8 weeks from surgery with an insole that will hold up the foot arch and help during the stance. After 3 months, a second X-ray check is done, and the weight bearing is full and free from any support; the patient is invited to start hydrokinetic therapy to quicken the walking reeducation and the functional recovery; the insole is kept in the shoes for at least 6 months after surgery.

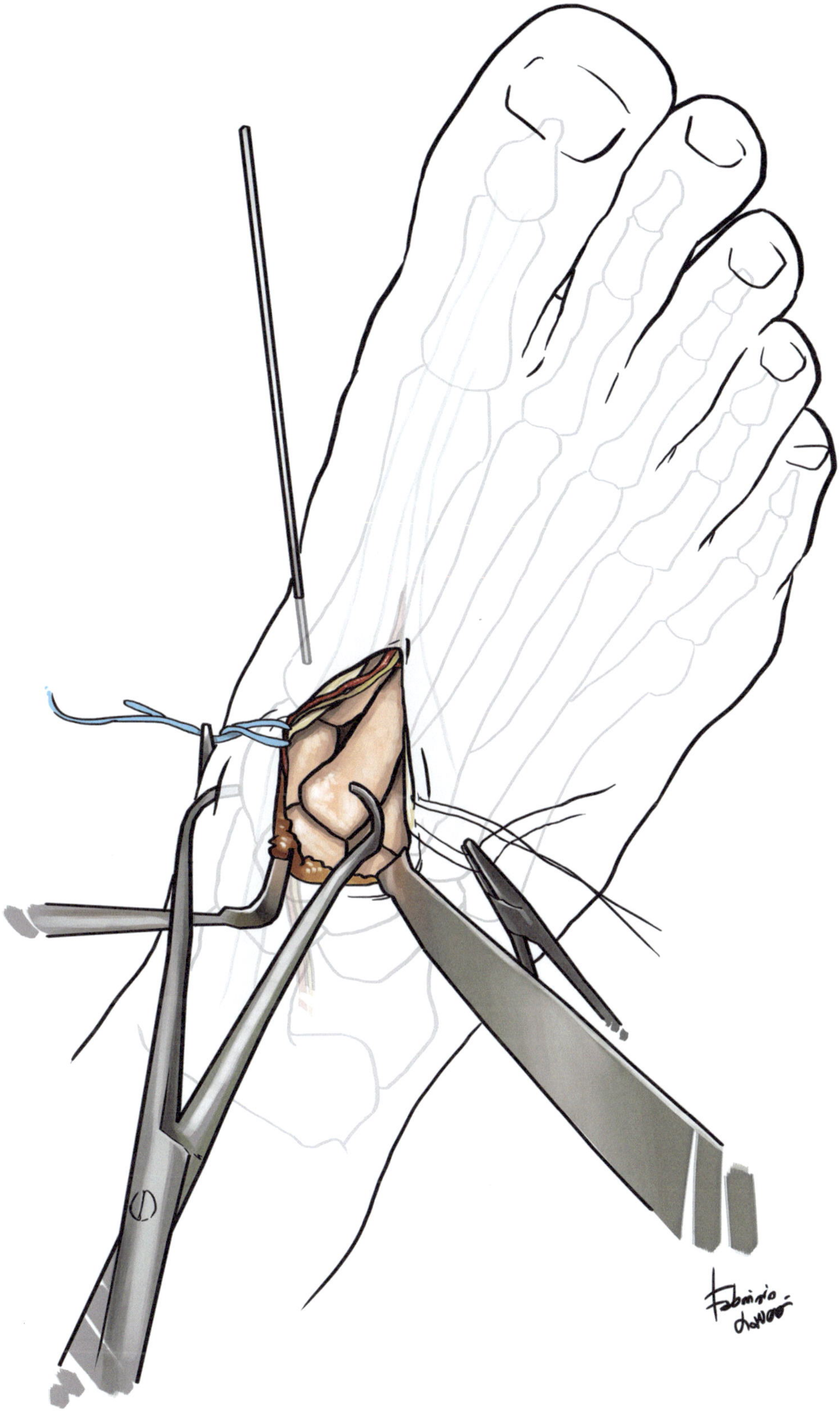

Fig. 6.18 Stabilization of the Lisfranc: the relocation of the second metatarsal base, into the proper slot between the cuneiforms, is the first step to achieve reduction of Lisfranc joint, because it represents the keystone to obtain the normal anatomy of the tarso-metatarsal joints. This manoeuvre can be performed more easily by using some sharp-pointed reduction clamps and finally stabilized through Kirschner wires

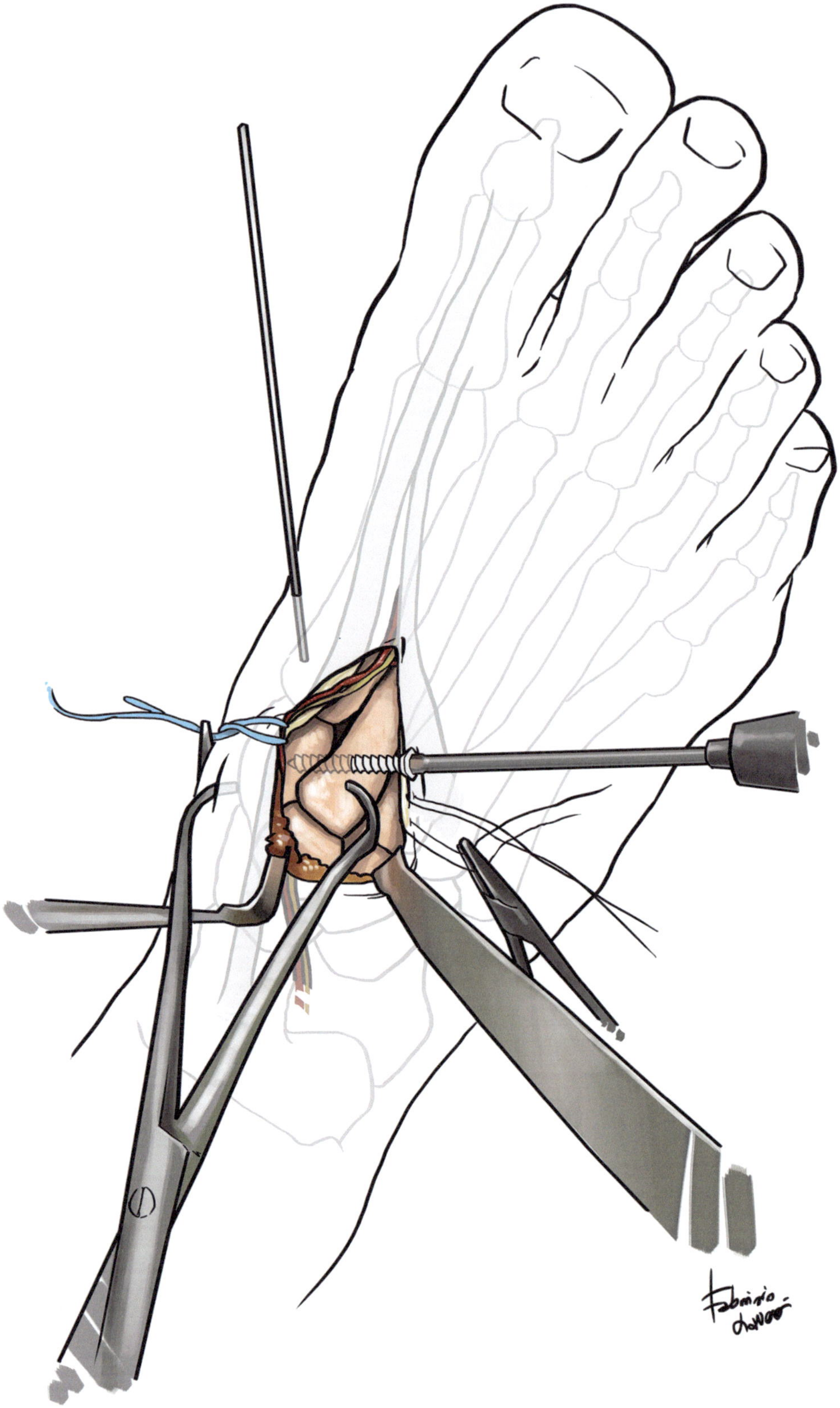

Fig. 6.19 Stabilization of the Lisfranc: the positioning of one or more absorbable screws bridging the joints allows to keep the reduction safer than using only Kirschner wires, and they don't need to be removed

References

1. Court-Brown CM, Zinna S, Ekrol I (2006) Classification and epidemiology of mid-foot fractures. Foot 16:138–141
2. Van Dorp KB, De Vries MR, Van der Elst M et al (2010) Chopart joint injury: a study of outcome and morbidity. J Foot Ankle Surg 49(6):541–545
3. Benirschke SK, Meinberg E, Anderson SA et al (2012) Fractures and dislocations of the midfoot: Lisfranc and Chopart injuries. J Bone Joint Surg Am 94(14):1325–1337
4. Main BJ, Jowett RL (1975) Injuries of the midtarsal joint. J Bone Joint Surg Br 57(1):89–97
5. Bellabarba C, Barei DP, Sanders RW (2007) Dislocation of the foot. In: Coughlin MJ, Mann RA, Saltzman CL (eds) Surgery of the foot and ankle, 8th edn. Mosby Elsevier, Philadelphia, pp 2137–2197
6. Makwana NK, Van Liefland MR (2005) Injuries of the midfoot. Curr Orthop 19:231–242
7. Gogolewski S (2000) Bioresorbable polymers in trauma and bone surgery. Injury 31(Suppl. 4):28–32
8. Sanders RW, Papp S (2007) Fractures of the midfoot and forefoot. In: Coughlin MJ, Mann RA, Saltzman CL (eds) Surgery of the foot and ankle, 8th edn. Mosby Elsevier, Philadelphia, pp 2199–2235
9. Myerson MS, Fisher RT, Burgess AR et al (1986) Fracture dislocations of the tarsometatarsal joints: end results correlated with pathology and treatment. Foot Ankle 6(5):225–242
10. Richter M, Thermann H, Huefner T et al (2004) Chopart joint fracture-dislocation: initial open reduction provides better outcome than closed reduction. Foot Ankle Int 25:340–348
11. Arntz CT, Veith RG, Hansen ST Jr (1988) Fractures and fracture-dislocations of the tarsometatarsal joint. J Bone Joint Surg Am 70(2):173–181
12. Hardcastle PH, Reschauer R, Kutscha-Lissberg E et al (1982) Injuries to the tarsometatarsal joint. Incidence, classification and treatment. J Bone Joint Surg Br 64(3):349–356
13. Ak S, Grose A (2004) Lisfranc injuries. Injury 35(Suppl 2):SB71–SB76
14. Ibrahim AM, Koolen PG, Kim K et al (2015) Absorbable biologically based internal fixation. Clin Podiatr Med Surg 32(1):61–72
15. Rokkanen PU, Böstman O, Hirvensalo E et al (2000) Bioabsorbable fixation in orthopaedic surgery and traumatology. Biomaterials 21(24):2607–2613

7 Surgical Treatment of the Metatarsal and Finger Fractures

Contents

7.1 Fractures of the Metatarsal Bones

The fractures of the metatarsal bones are numerically frequent events, but the surgical treatment indication is generally episodic and sporadic, in consideration of the scarce tendency to develop a secondary displacement, in consequence of their rigid anatomical bond due to the ligamentous components between the single segments [1]. They can be associated with Lisfranc injuries that, if present, they become more important than the metatarsals, in which treatment becomes subordinated to the main injury, while in some cases, they can lead to a disability, because misdiagnosed and consequently healed in a malunion [2–4].

The injuries usually develop in consequence of a direct compression traumatic event when involving the mid-metatarsals and to an indirect torsional trauma for the external metatarsals, first and fifth, with the possibility on the latter to develop avulsion injuries of the base, in consequence of the traction of the peroneus brevis tendon that inserts in this area [5, 6]. A further general possibility of injury mechanism is a fatigue fracture due to a repeated micro-trauma that develops in occasion of reiterated functional overloading (e.g. race walker and marathon runners).

7.1.1 Classification

Aside from the fractures of the base of the fifth metatarsal bone, which are a self-standing topic, the classification usually used for the fractures of this segment is purely descriptive, identifying simply if the injury involves the base, the diaphysis or the distal portion (head or neck) of the metatarsal bone [7], as well as morphologic, discriminating generally if the injuries are simple, where it is possible to recognize one fracture line, usually in consequence of a low-energy stress, or if they are complex, showing the existence of more fracture lines, in consequence of an higher-energy trauma [5].

W. Daghino et al., *Foot and Ankle Trauma Injuries*, https://doi.org/10.1007/978-3-319-69617-1_7

7.1.2 Indications

The surgical treatment indications of these segments are not frequent: they refer to displaced fractures that involve joint segments and to extra-articular displaced fracture that are over the deformity limits of tolerability or with bone exposition [7].

The fractures of the base of the metatarsal bones when the joint is involved fall into the Lisfranc management criteria, while in the other cases, they usually are treated without surgery.

Considering the displacement of the diaphyseal segments, all the injuries of the mid-metatarsal bones that develop a significant dorsal angulation of the distal part are considered worthy of surgical treatment; for the outer metatarsals, the tolerance limits are more strict: the shortenings and the rotation defects of the first [8] and more generally all the injuries in which the displacement provokes an enlargement of the foot [7] are considered unacceptable (see Fig. 7.1).

The fractures of the neck request a surgical reduction if they have a severe displacement or rotation that can lead to an

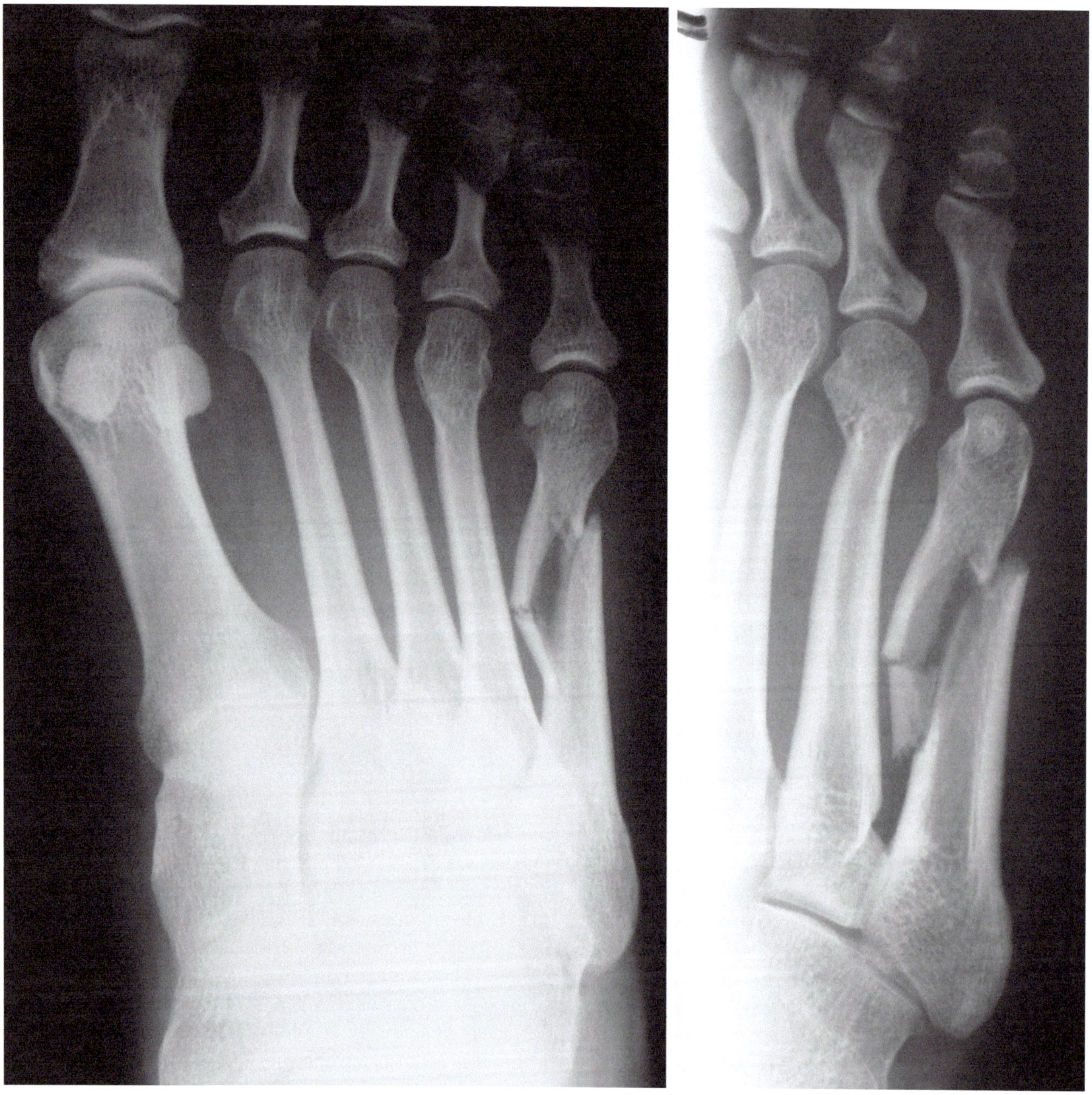

Fig. 7.1 Fracture of the diaphysis of the fifth metatarsal bone: the shortening of the bone segment and the enlargement resulting from the transversal diameter of the foot validate the surgical treatment indication

overloading of the plantar aspects or an exclusion of the weight bearing of the metatarsal head, while if the fracture involves the metatarsal head, the surgical indication if displaced is given if the osteochondral fragments are sufficiently big to be synthetized; otherwise it is necessary to treat them in a conservative way, planning the following treatment of the outcome [7].

In all the cases in which the surgical option is decided, the aim is to achieve a good alignment and to obtain a harmonic metatarsal formula, granting to the patient to have a plantigrade stance and without functional overloads.

7.1.3 Surgical Technique

7.1.3.1 Patient Positioning

The patient is laid on a radiotransparent table, inclined on the healthy side if the injury involved is the fifth metatarsal bone, in all the other cases is supine; the tourniquet is set at the thigh, and a cushion is put under the affected side gluteus to abolish the extrarotation tendency of the lower limb. Mainly if the injury is medial or in the case of a multisegment fracture, it can be useful to elevate the opposite lower limb with the knee flexed on a support, rising or lowering the corresponding portion of the surgical table, to ease the access and reduction manoeuvres of the surgeons; another important advice is to position the affected foot hanging out from the distal part of the bed, allowing to better perform the cranial-caudal and oblique X-ray imaging, which completes the radiological study of the injury (see Fig. 7.2).

After the three X-ray projections have been done, checked that all the surgical table supports do not preclude the imaging to the segments that need to be treated, and saved the X-ray projections for further consultation after the reduction manoeuvres have been performed, it is possible to consider this phase terminated and it is possible to move on to the further steps.

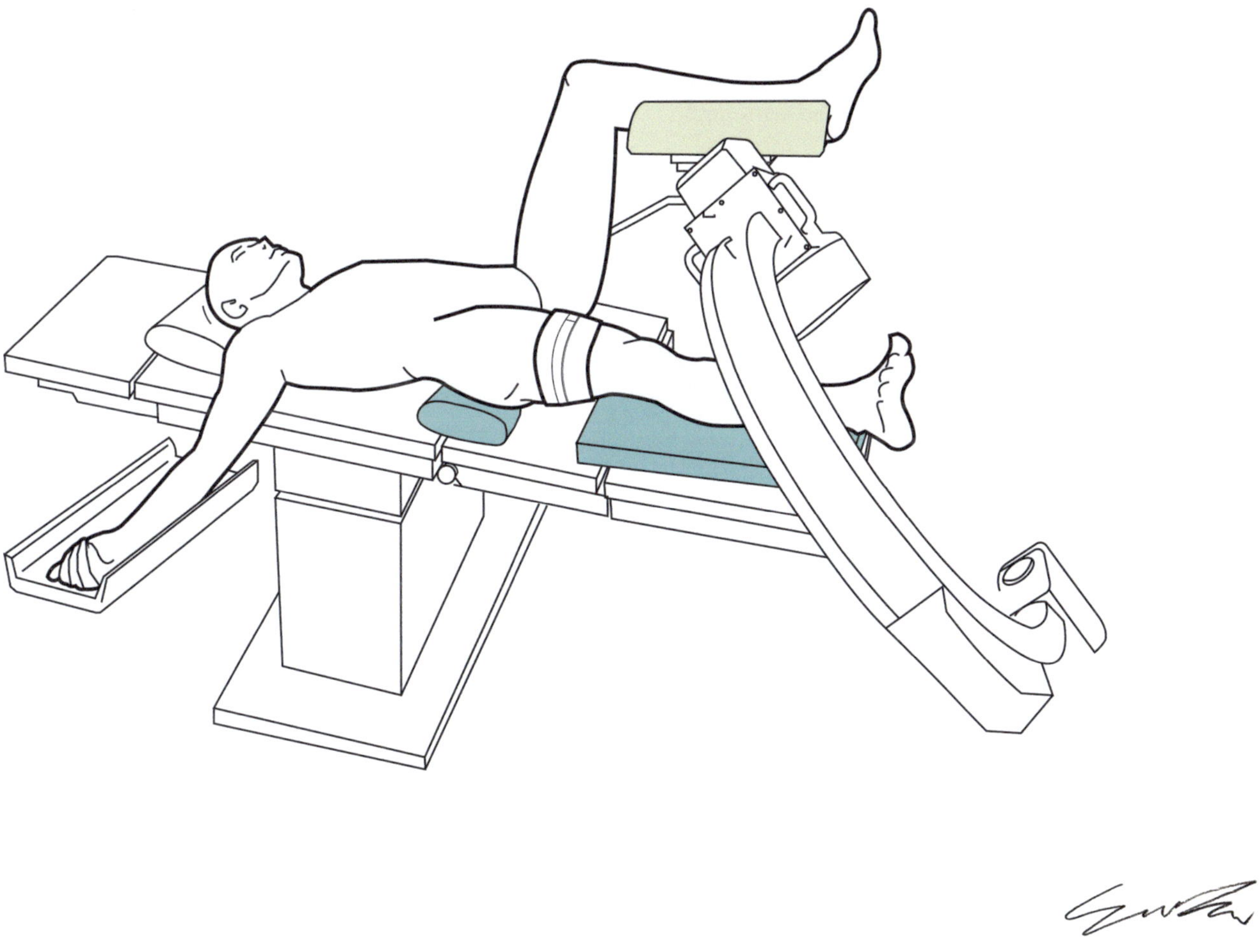

Fig. 7.2 Positioning of the patient for the surgical reduction of the metatarsal fracture: leaving the foot partially hanging out from the table can ease the taking of the fluoroscopic imaging during surgery

7.1.3.2 Surgical Access

The surgical access usually used is dorsal, centred on the fractured segments: for the mid-metatarsals, such approach can be performed on the intermetatarsal space if there are multiple segments involved, allowing to dominate two fragments through one single incision, while for the external metatarsals, usually a dorsal medial incision is done for the first metatarsal bone and a dorsal lateral incision for the fifth metatarsal bone.

As for all the other foot segments, it is important to avoid traction on the skin, retracting the incision through the use of silk wires without using any retractors; when proceeding to the deep dissection, considering that the incision is performed parallel to the terminal branches of the sural and superficial peroneal nerve, usually the neurovascular bundles are out of danger, and to access to the bone surface, it is safe to isolate and retract the extensor tendons, using Hohmann retractors.

7.1.3.3 Reduction Manoeuvres

For all these injuries, it is important to conduct the surgical toilette in the most delicate way possible, being careful to respect any bony asperity, which could be useful to restore the previous anatomy: for this reason, it is advisable to perform the dissection only with the scalpel, avoiding, if possible, the use of periosteum retractors and the use of rongeur to remove the soft tissues, to not ruin any anatomical landmarks, which are very delicate considering the dimensions of the bone segments.

The use of atraumatic anatomical tongs with opposed spiked ends is very useful, because they can be crucial during the reduction manoeuvres, through the application of traction on the distal longitudinal fragments and countertraction on the proximal segments. If the injury is composed of a single fracture line, the reduction must be anatomical, whereas in case of injuries with a higher complexity, it could be necessary to settle for a realignment of the axial orientation and rotation of the segment, which needs to be checked always through fluoroscopy [9].

7.1.3.4 Osteosynthesis/Stabilization

Once the reduction manoeuvres have been completed, it is possible to proceed to the synthesis and/or stabilization, depending on the pattern of the injury.

In the situation in which there is a bony exposition or an important damage of the soft tissues, it is impossible to use an internal fixation; in such cases, as in many other situations where the fragmentation does not allow to achieve the restoration of the bony anatomy, the use of an external fixator, which must have the screws, pins and threaded wires at most of a 3 mm diameter, can be essential for the stabilization. The external fixator types with gliding modules are more useful to restore the axial alignment and allow to manage precisely the length of the bony segment (see Fig. 7.3), which can be essential to restore the correct morphology of the metatarsal formula.

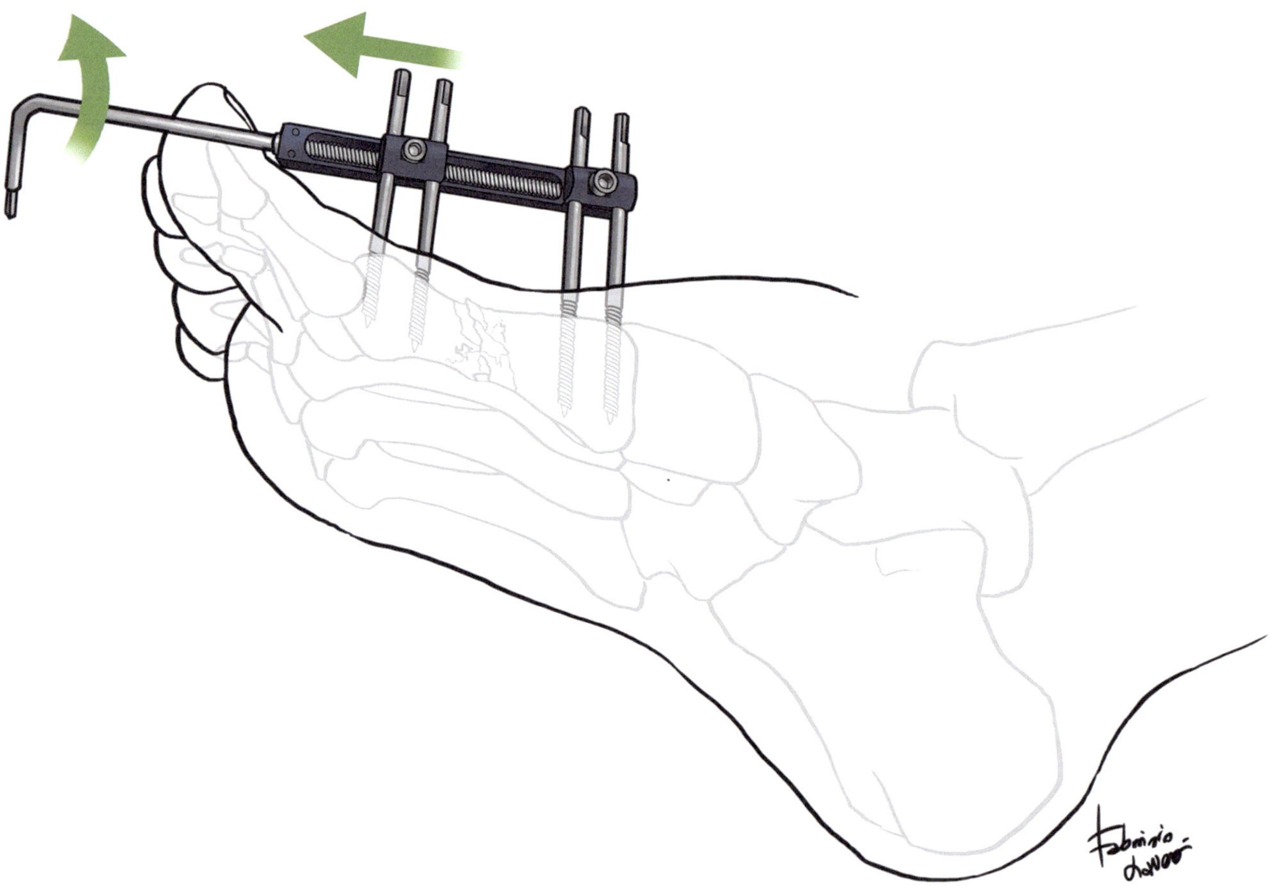

Fig. 7.3 External fixator with sleigh (Orthofix®) positioned for a comminute fracture of the first metatarsal bone diaphysis; the sliding micrometric system allows to dominate more easily the length of the bone even if the fragmentation is important

When an open access to the fracture is possible, in case of extra-articular injuries, involving the diaphysis or the metaphysis, with a transverse or simple fracture line, which do not have a high risk of shortening or losing the reduction through the sliding of the fragments, the best way to achieve a fixation is through the use of Kirschner wires, keeping the stability of the fracture through the three-point fixation achieved with the intramedullary stabilization [8].

The technique foresees the use of at least two wires for segment, with a double point of 1–2 mm diameter, which need to be selected depending on the bone dimensions; generally such wires are introduced into the bone starting from the fracture site, pushing them distally and out under the proximal phalanx of the corresponding finger and afterwards pushing them back from distal to proximal into the medullary canal to the base of the metatarsal bone, after having achieved again the reduction of the fracture (see Fig. 7.4), leaving a distal portion of the Kirschner wire out of the skin, which will allow to remove the wires once the healing is completed.

If the fracture shows any instability such as obliquity or fragmentation, the necessary osteosynthesis will be an internal fixation with free screws if the fracture line is simple or the use of plates and screws if the minimal synthesis is insufficient to grant stability or could lead to mobilization of the fragments due to the complexity of the fracture.

The concept that must be followed is to use the least as possible hardware for the synthesis, which will allow to achieve the necessary stability to neutralize the dislocating forces (see Fig. 7.5): this is because the more the implants used are bulky, the higher is the risk to develop an impingement with the soft tissues and consequently the need of removal. Usually the devices used are mini-osteosynthesis systems with different diameters, between 2 and 2.7 mm, which need to be chosen each time depending on the affected segment and the dimensions of the fragments; using implants that allow to fix the screws onto the plates, it is possible to treat even the fractures with important comminution and more complex, achieving a stability like an internal fixator.

The more recent osteosynthesis systems, such as the one named "compact foot" by Synthes®, usually used in our clinic, use self-threading screws, extremely useful to reduce the inserting time but equally challenging regarding the surgical technique: this is a characteristic common to all the mini-osteosynthesis systems, where the tolerance in the creation of the holes is generally reduced because of the small diameters of the segments; for this reason, even if it could seem contradictory, it is advisable to use (dedicated) motorized instrumentation to perform the drilling and the insertion of the screws, because it is possible to be more precise in the creation of the holes and in the introduction of the screws; only for the last part of the screw insertion, it is necessary to use a screw driver with the hands because it allows to fix the screws dosing the correct strength. If titanium elements are used, this step must be performed with a specific torque limiter inserted into the screw driver, to avoid excessive solicitations during the tightening, which could produce a cold fusion of the elements that could make extremely difficult the eventual removal of the implanted devices. If any osteochondral injuries of the metatarsal head are present and sufficiently big to be synthetized, to reduce the possibility of a mobilization of the devices used for the fixation, which would lead to a painful joint, instead of mini screws or Kirschner wires, commonly used to maintain the reduction, it is possible to use efficiently absorbable poly-L-lactic acid (PLLA) pins for the synthesis.

7.1.3.5 Postoperative Care

Using intramedullary Kirschner wires or external fixators, the fracture healing develops through the formation of bone callus; for this reason, after 6 weeks without weight bearing to protect the devices used for the synthesis, it is usually possible to allow the progressive weight bearing, usually after an X-ray check that shows the correct alignment of the bone segment and the bone healing.

If instead an internal fixation with plates and/or screws has been used, then the healing attended is through direct cortical fusion, longer to be complete; for this reason, the non-weight bearing period is of 2–3 months, allowing the full weight bearing once the biological bone healing is completed.

7.1.4 Fracture of the Fifth Metatarsal Bone Base

Considering the metatarsal bone fractures, a particular case is represented by the fracture of the base of the fifth metatarsal; usually they are caused by adduction forces applied to the forefoot with the ankle plantar flexed, generating injuries due to a rotational and avulsion mechanism [7]. The injuries of this area are more prone to a secondary displacement and/or a difficult healing; for this reason, they are subject to a particular attention, requesting specific therapeutic approaches that are proper only for this metatarsal segment [7].

7.1.4.1 Classification

It is possible to identify in this skeletal segment three categories of injuries (see Fig. 7.6):

1. Fractures of the tuberosity that include the more proximal articular portion of the metatarsal base, which can be fragmented in many pieces, with fracture lines that involve only the joint of the metatarsal base and the cuboid.
2. Fractures of the base that are distal to the tuberosity, which involve the articular portion of the base of the V metatarsal with the base of the IV metatarsal; these are the fractures that can be defined as "Jones fracture", sometimes incorrectly used to describe all the fractures of the base of the fifth metatarsal bone.

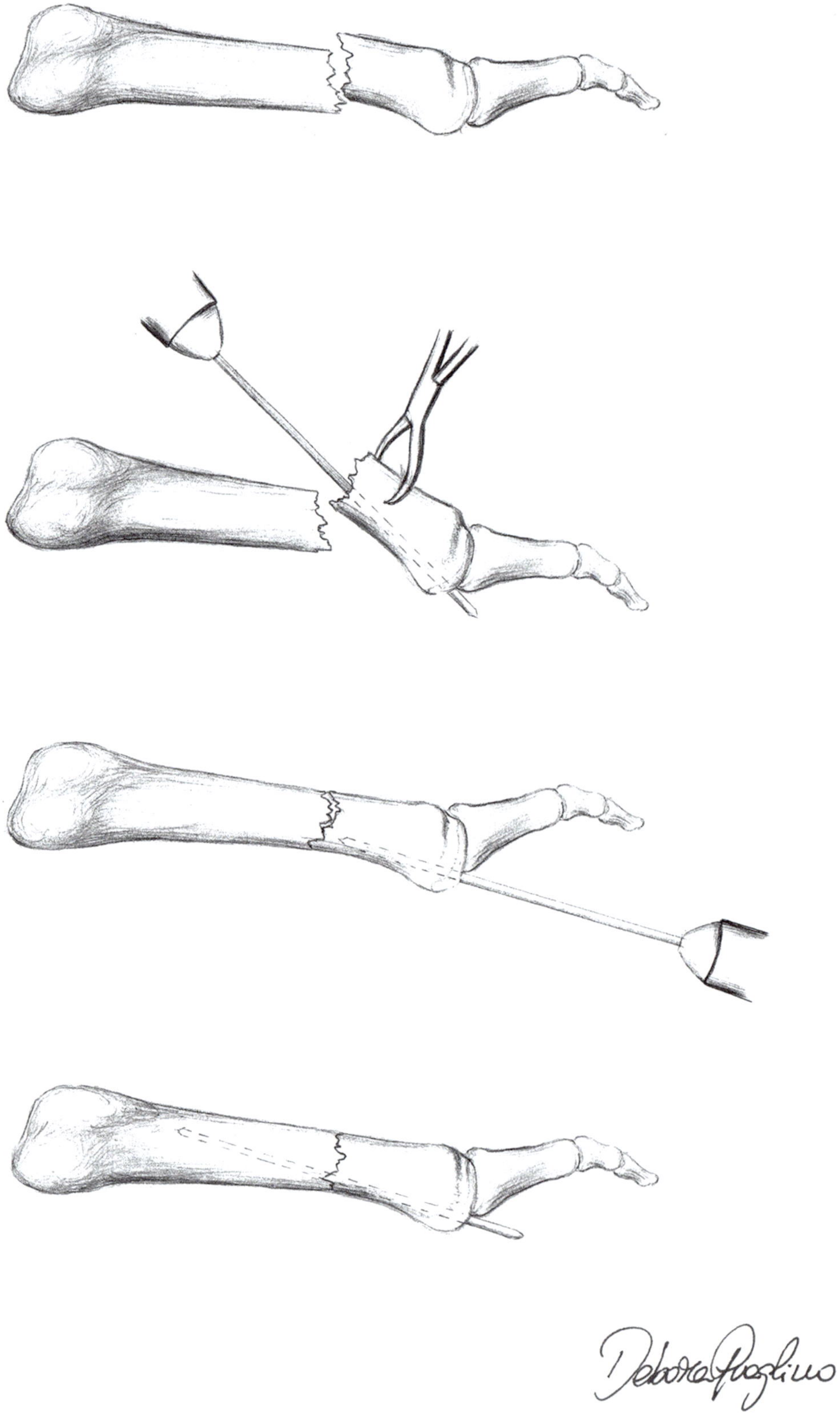

Fig. 7.4 Osteosynthesis sequence with Kirschner wires used as intramedullar devices for the fractures of the metatarsal bone diaphysis: distally the wire is pushed out of the skin under the basal phalanx and from here pushed backwards into the bone, once the reduction is achieved

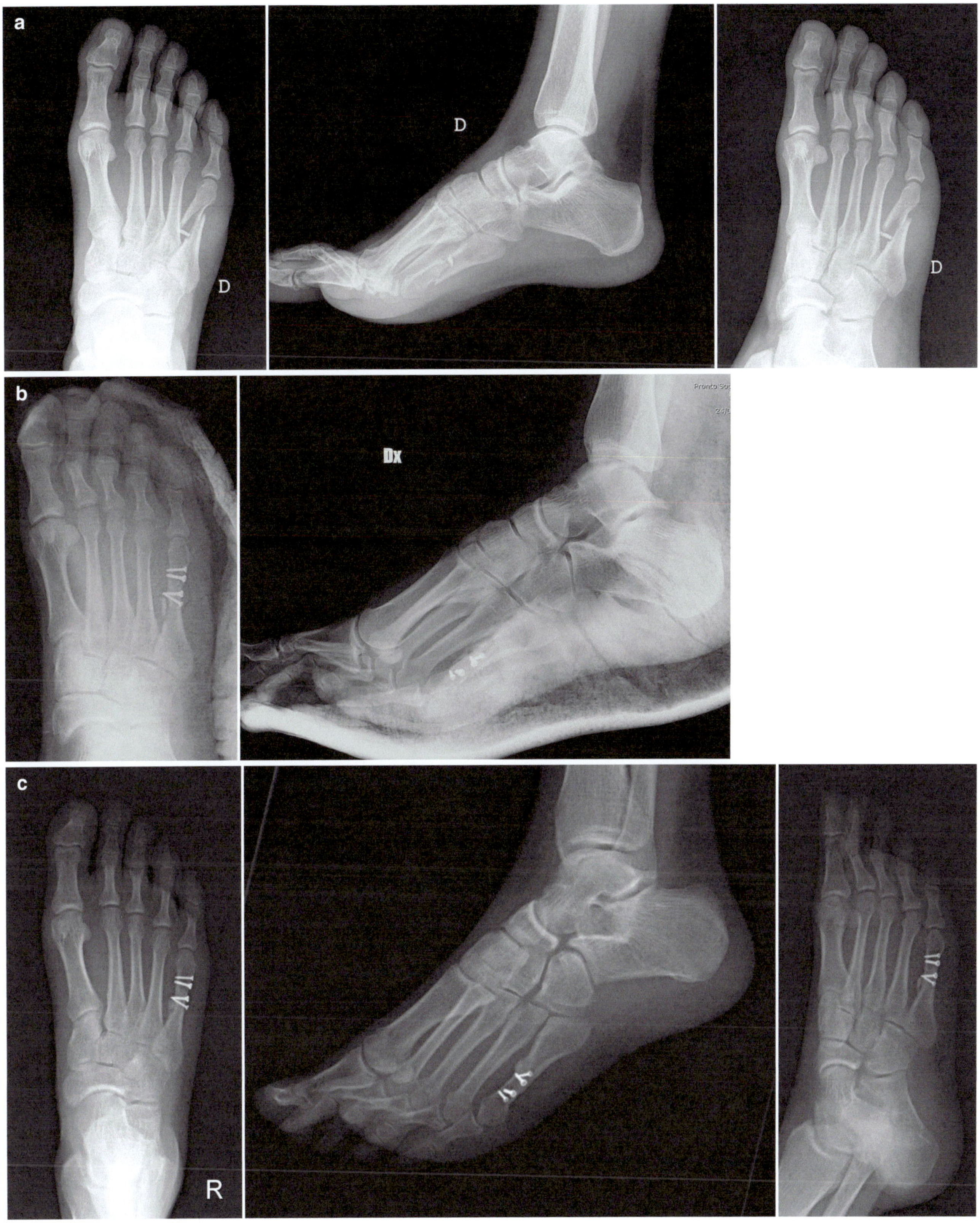

Fig. 7.5 Spiroid fracture of the fifth metatarsal bone diaphysis (**a**); although the presence of a small comminuted fragment, the wide contact surface justified the choice, once the open reduction is completed, of an osteosynthesis with free screws, evidenced in the post-operative imaging (**b**); the follow-up imaging at 4 months (**c**); shows an advanced healing of the bone and the absence of any mobilization of the devices; the hardware removal it is not necessary

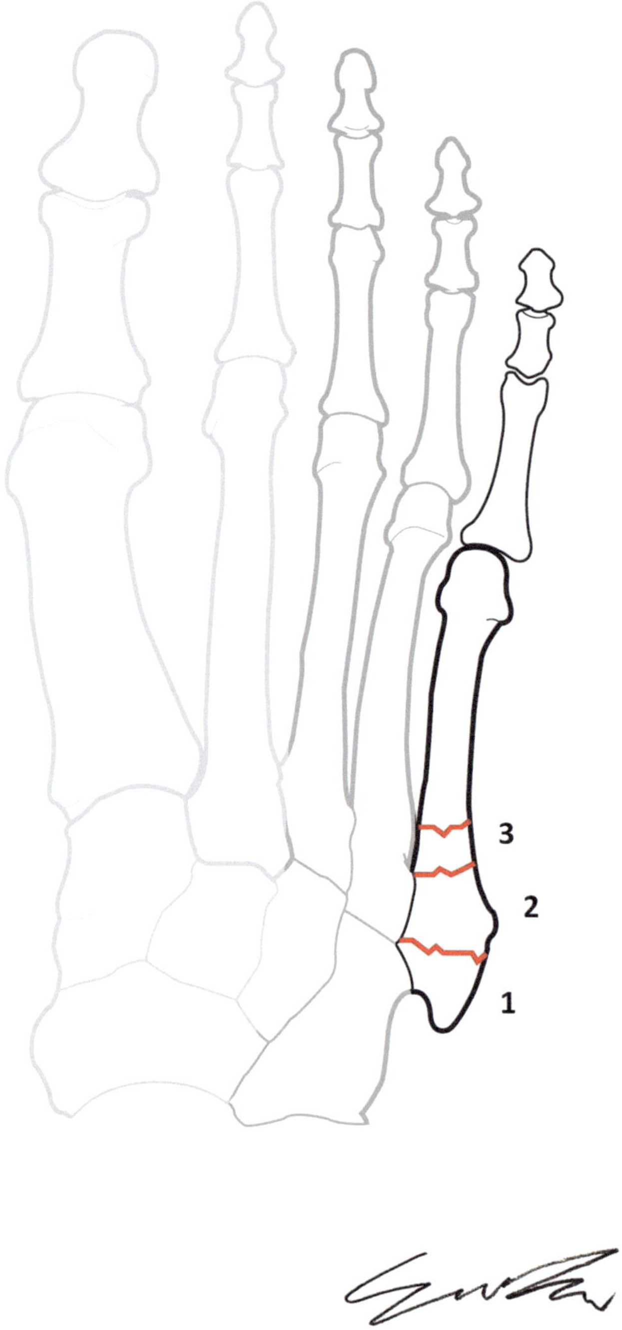

Fig. 7.6 Fracture of the fifth metatarsal bone base: the location of the fracture line distinguishes the fractures of the tuberosity (1), the fractures that involve the joint with the fourth metatarsal bone base, named as "Jones fractures" (2), and the fractures of the proximal diaphysis (3)

3. Fractures of the proximal diaphysis, just distal the zone 2, which develop in consequence of a stress mechanism, and, because they involve an area with a scarce vascularization, as a definition, they have a higher risk of healing problems [10, 11].

7.1.4.2 Surgical Treatment Indications

The fractures of the tuberosity and the Jones fractures are usually treated in a conservative way, except for the conditions where an important dislocation is present or if there is a symptomatic inveterate incomplete consolidation of the fracture; in the case of surgery, the stabilization is achieved through the use of double-threaded screws if there is a single fracture line (see Fig. 7.7) and the use of a tension band or the removal of the fragments and the reinsertion of the tendon if there is a comminuted fracture.

For the stress fractures, considering their chronic condition and the scarce tendency to heal spontaneously, the more

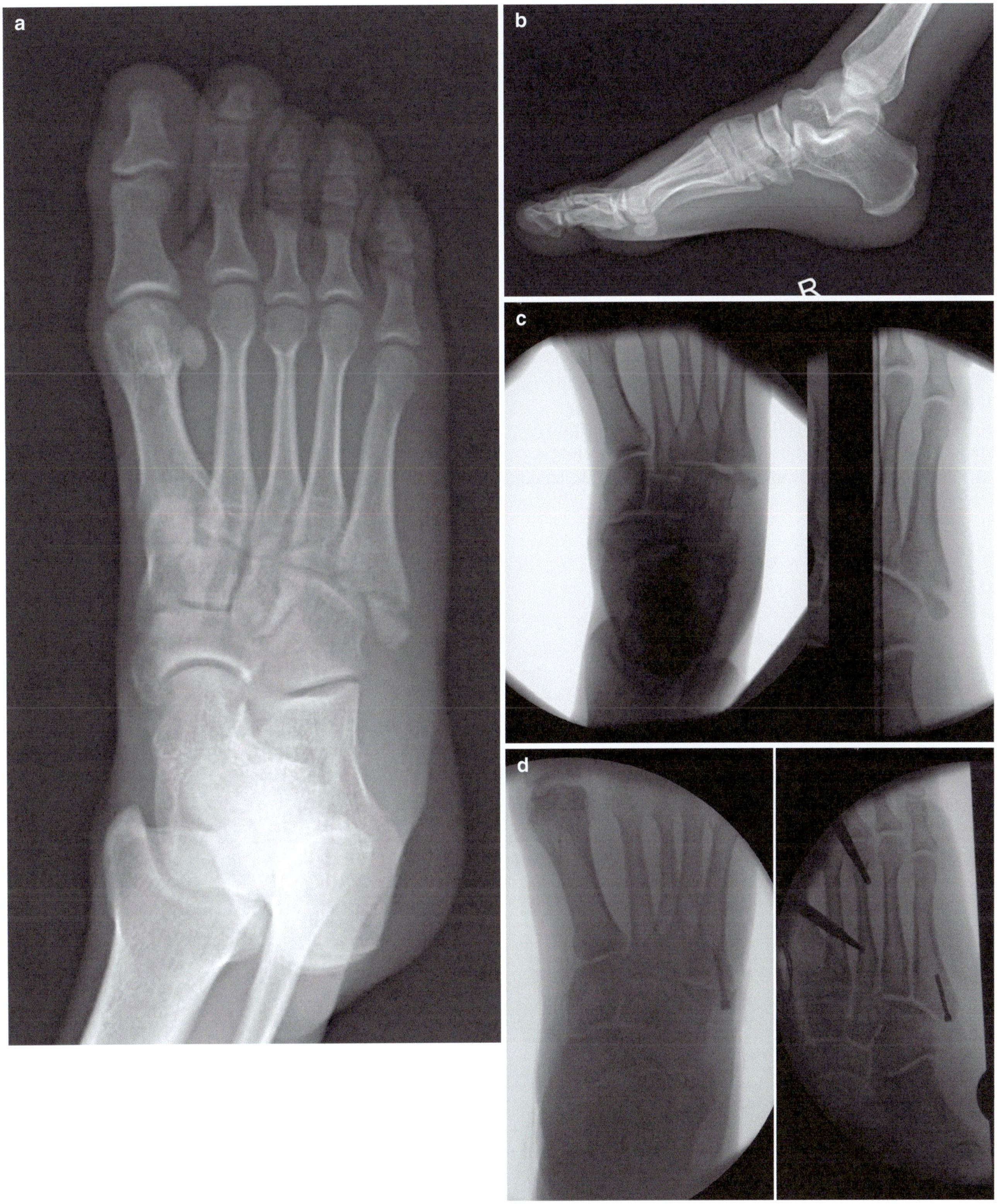

Fig. 7.7 Dislocated tuberosity fractures of the fifth metatarsal bone (**a**, **b**); the fluoroscopy image taken at the beginning of the surgery demonstrates the important size of the dislocated fragment (**c**), for which the indication, once the reduction is achieved, is the osteosynthesis with a cannulated double-threaded screw (**d**)

common indication is the surgical treatment, using a double- or a partially threaded screw, inserted into the medullary canal to achieve compression on the fracture line.

7.1.4.3 Surgical Technique

The patient is laterally laid on the unaffected side, with the tourniquet at the thigh and with the foot that is going to be treated elevated on a cushion to keep a neutral rotation of the hip, checking if it is possible to obtain all the three radiographic projections of the foot (see Fig. 7.8).

A straight incision is performed, over the fractured area; the extremities of the incision are retracted; and a careful dissection of the deep tissues is done until the insertion of the peroneus brevis is exposed, being careful to protect the terminal branches of the sural nerve that eventually could cross the surgical access.

Once the tendon is spotted, in case of an important comminution of the fractured bone segment, it could be necessary to remove the fragments and eventually reinsert the tendon with anchors; if the proximal segment is complete or divided into a few big parts, it is possible to gain access to the bone through the tendon cap and isolate the portions of the fractured bone, acting through cautious and essential surgical dissection, allowing to spot the bone landmarks that will ease the reduction, which must be done with gentle manoeuvres. Once the anatomy is restored, if multiple fragments are present, it is possible to obtain a stabilization through Kirschner wires and a tension band, a technique that has the disadvantage to require the removal of the hardware once the fracture is healed, because of the subcutaneous positioning of the metal components, which could lead to an impingement with the shoes.

When the proximal fragment is single, the more efficient synthesis is achieved through one or two cannulated 3 mm screws, positioned perpendicular to the fracture line (see Fig. 7.9); the double-threaded screws allow to sink completely the screw into the bone head, granting a best tolerability, and always constantly, they are not required to be removed once the injury is healed (see Fig. 7.10). In the more

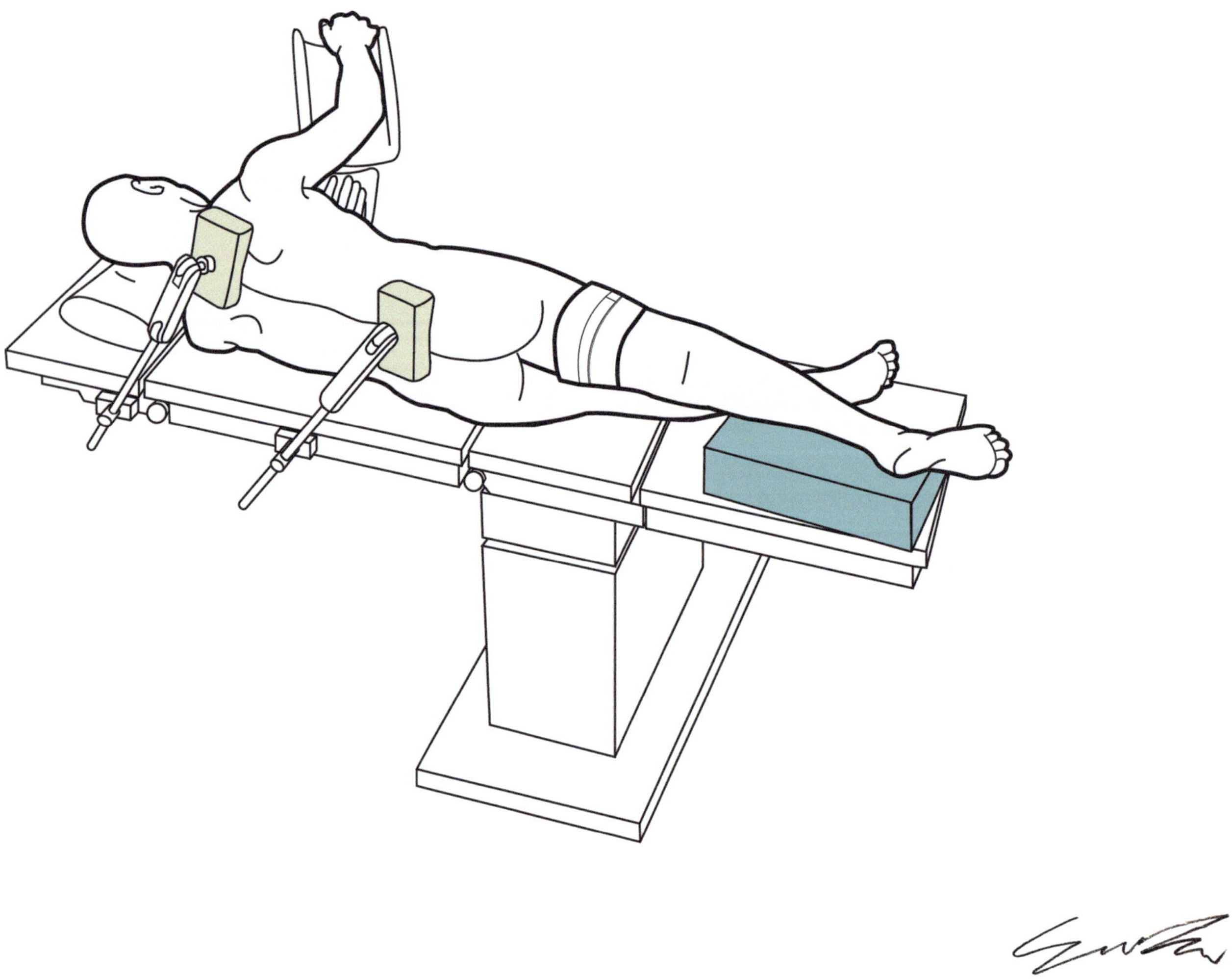

Fig. 7.8 Fracture of the fifth metatarsal bone tuberosity osteosynthesis: patient positioning

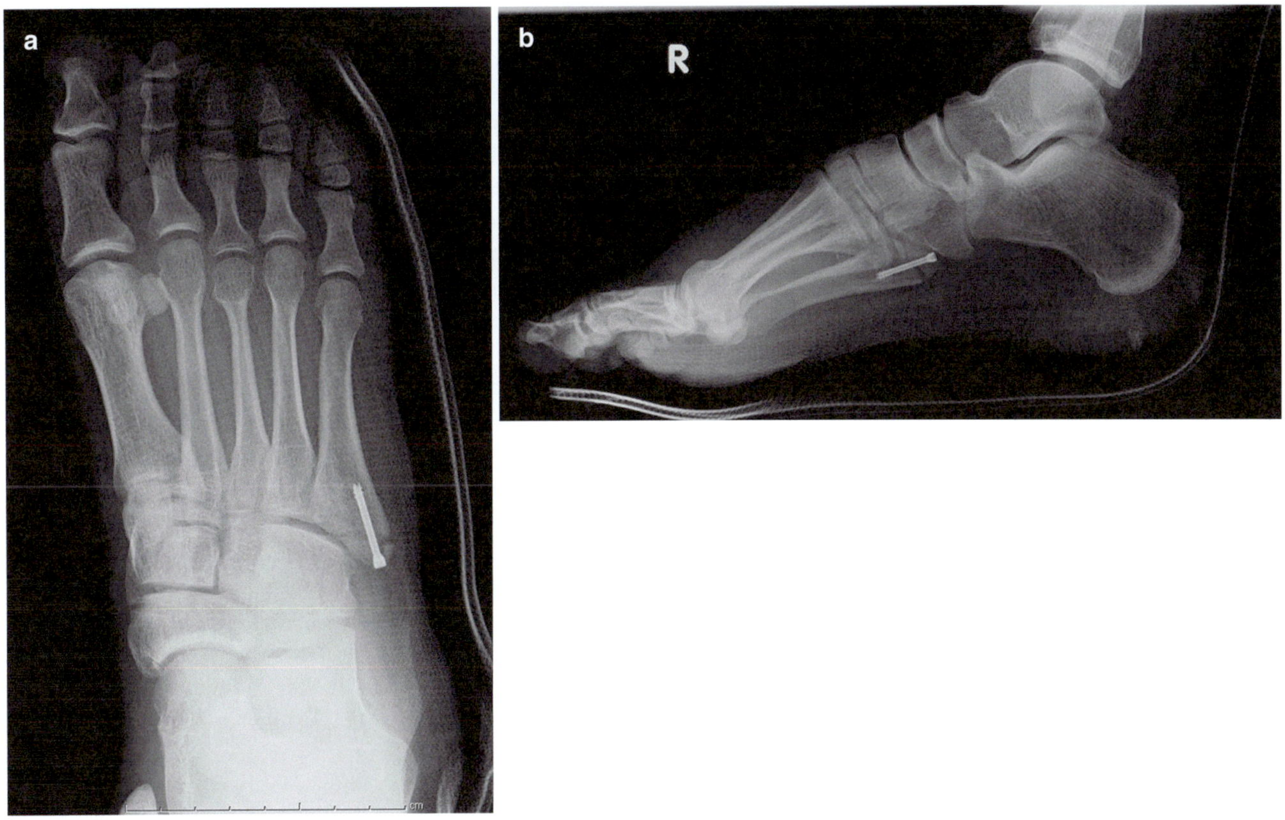

Fig. 7.9 Fracture of the fifth metatarsal bone tuberosity: synthesis with a double-threaded screws; the postoperative check shows the conservation of the reduction in all the projections (**a**, **b**)

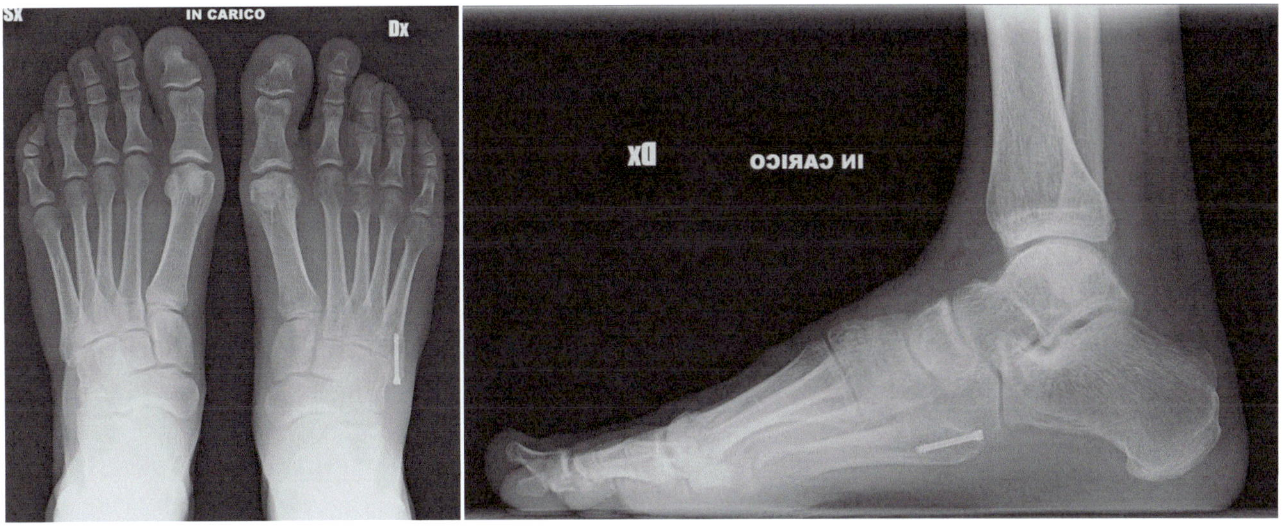

Fig. 7.10 Fracture of the fifth metatarsal bone tuberosity: synthesis with a double-threaded screws; the 6-month follow-up shows the complete healing of the fracture; the screw being sunk into the bone does not create any impingement with shoes and doesn't need to be removed

distal stress fractures, the precarious vascularization and the consequent healing difficulty request the use of screws with a bigger diameter, usually 4.5 mm, inserted into the medullary canal achieving a compression of the fractured site: even in this case, the use of cannulated screws reduces the aggression during the positioning, which is performed only once the pin guide is correctly inserted. Sometimes in the inveterate fractures with the tendency of bone loss, the use of an autologous bone graft to ease the biological component of the surgical treatment can be indicated.

7.1.4.4 Postoperative Care

The plaster cast is kept until the presence of healing is seen through X-rays, usually after 4–6 weeks in the fractures of the tuberosity. In the stress fractures, considering the minimal dislocation and the bigger sturdiness of the performed synthesis, the weight bearing can be allowed precociously, usually after the stich removal at 2 weeks, using a rigid sole shoe or a plastic brace; a protective bracing must be recommended when sport activity has begun [9].

7.2 Fracture of the Fingers

The fractures of the phalangeal bones of the fingers are one of the most frequent in the foot and more generally in the human body, and they represent about 8% of all the fracture [12]; the fractures of the lateral fingers are more common than the fractures of the hallux [13]. Generally they are a consequence of direct trauma, are more frequent to the proximal segments and usually affect the young, usually in consequence of sport injuries.

Even if they present with a high incidence, in consideration of the frequent non-recognizability, the anatomical segment and the low disability generated, the surgical treatment is exceptional [7].

7.2.1 Classification

No specific classifying system is present for the phalangeal fractures of the fingers; for this reason, the only identification is purely descriptive, considering significant for the treatment the level of the bone affected (epiphysis, diaphysis or metaphysis), the grade of dislocation and fragmentation and the articular involvement.

7.2.2 Surgical Treatment Indications

Considering that most of the diaphysis and non-articular injuries can be successfully treated through traction of the finger and the fixation with the adjacent finger through a syndactyly, the indication to a surgical treatment is considered only when an important dislocation of the articular part is present, where the fragment is sufficiently big to be synthetized, and this usually happens only for the hallux fractures. The surgical treatment is more frequently advised in the young, where the simple healing process can lead to non-tolerated limitations that will require a treatment of the outcome, treatment that is considered a good option in the older [14].

7.2.3 Surgical Technique

The patient is supine, with a peripheral anaesthesia and with the tourniquet over the ankle; after starting the fluoroscopic check, which is essential to see if the three-dimensional vision of the bony segment is acquired and nonetheless to acquire in starting images that will be used as a paragon after the reduction manoeuvres have been done, with a gauze set as a tie, the fingers are kept separated from the affected part, and a straight dorsal or medial (for the hallux) incision aimed on the main fractured site that needs to be treated is done, following what has been planned preoperatively.

The skin flaps are retracted with silk wires, avoiding carefully to apply any traction with retractors or hooks on the delicate skin of this area; the dissection through layers is completed and brought directly to the bone, paying attention to respect the neurovascular bundle and to retract laterally or medially the extensor tendon apparatus with retractors (see Fig. 7.11).

Once the main fragments are all exposed, with delicate spatulas and hooks, the reduction is performed, aiming to restore exactly the joint surface, and the osteosynthesis is performed, through free compression screws (see Fig. 7.12) if the bone quality is good; if the fracture is very fragmented or the bone quality is poor not allowing a synthesis with screws, as an alternative, it is possible to fix the achieved reduction with different diameter Kirschner wires on the count of the different fragments (see Figs. 7.13 and 7.14).

7.2.4 Postoperative Care

The treated segment is protected with a metal splint, it is recommended to keep the limb raised, and the weight bearing is proscribed until the stiches are removed, that is, after 2–3 weeks from surgery, with the aim to protect the wound and foot from swelling; afterwards it is possible to begin a partial weight bearing with specific shoes that protect the forefoot from loading. Once the wound is healed, if the osteosynthesis is stable, it is possible to grant an active movement; otherwise if it has been necessary to perform a percutaneous synthesis, the immobilization is recommended for 6 weeks, when the first X-ray is performed, the Kirschner wires are removed, and a progressive weight bearing is allowed.

After 3 months, a weight bearing X-ray of the feet is taken to check the evolution of the healing process and the maintenance of the anatomic axis necessary to grant a good walking dynamics (see Fig. 7.15).

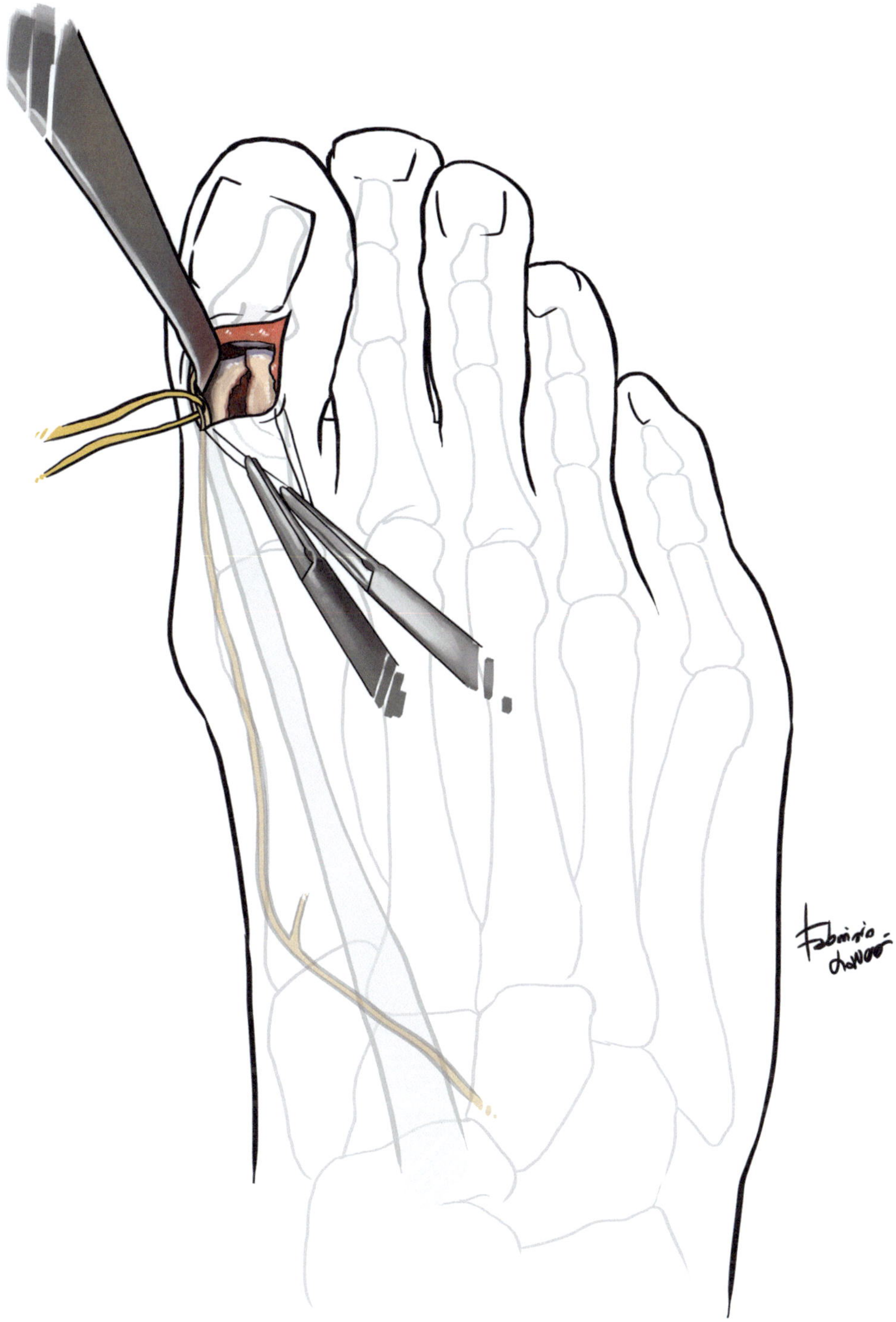

Fig. 7.11 Articular dislocated proximal phalanx fracture of the hallux: dorsal surgical access aimed on the injury, with protection of the dorsomedial neurovascular bundle

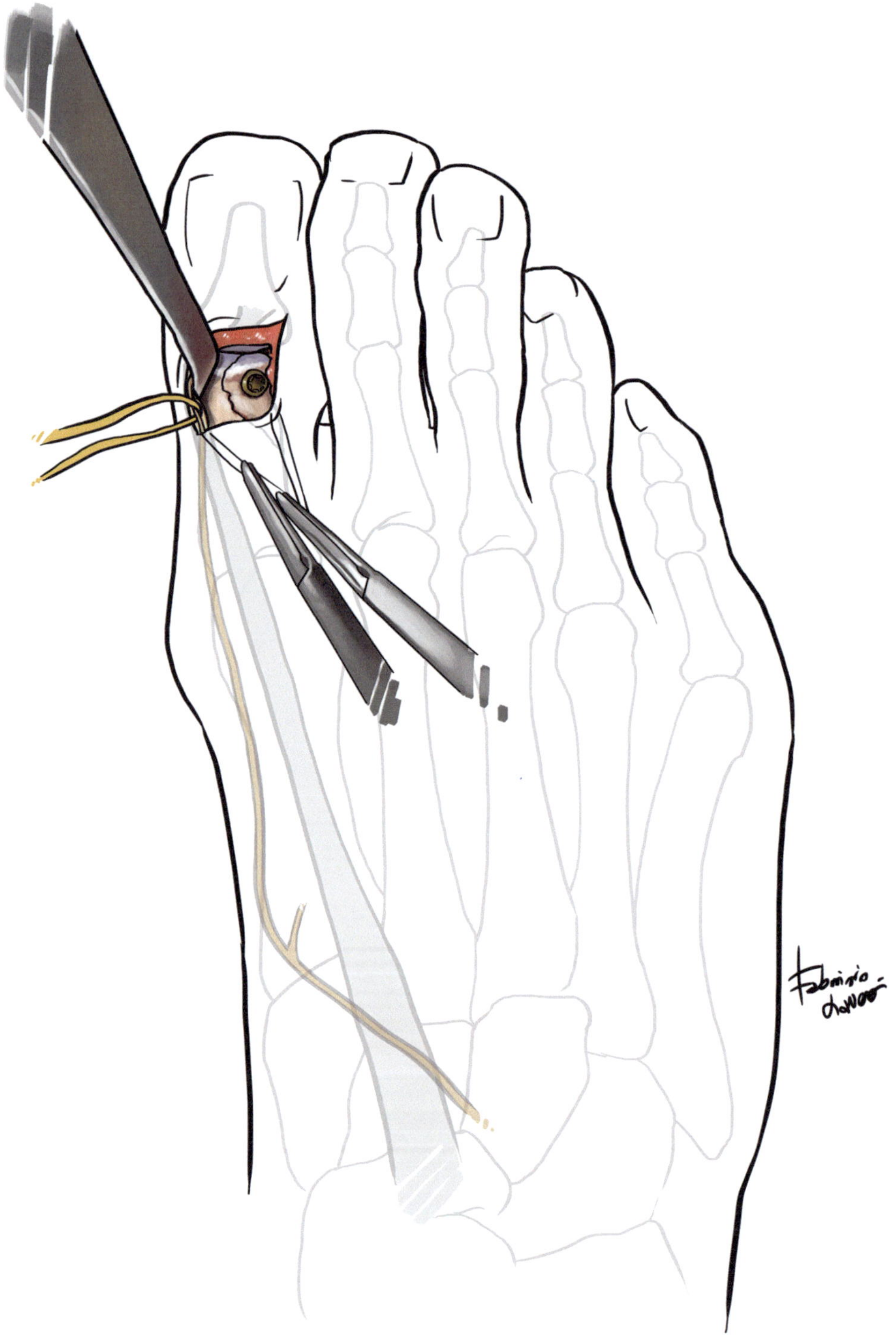

Fig. 7.12 Articular dislocated proximal phalanx fracture of the hallux: after the anatomical reduction of the joint parts, an osteosynthesis with a free compression screw is performed

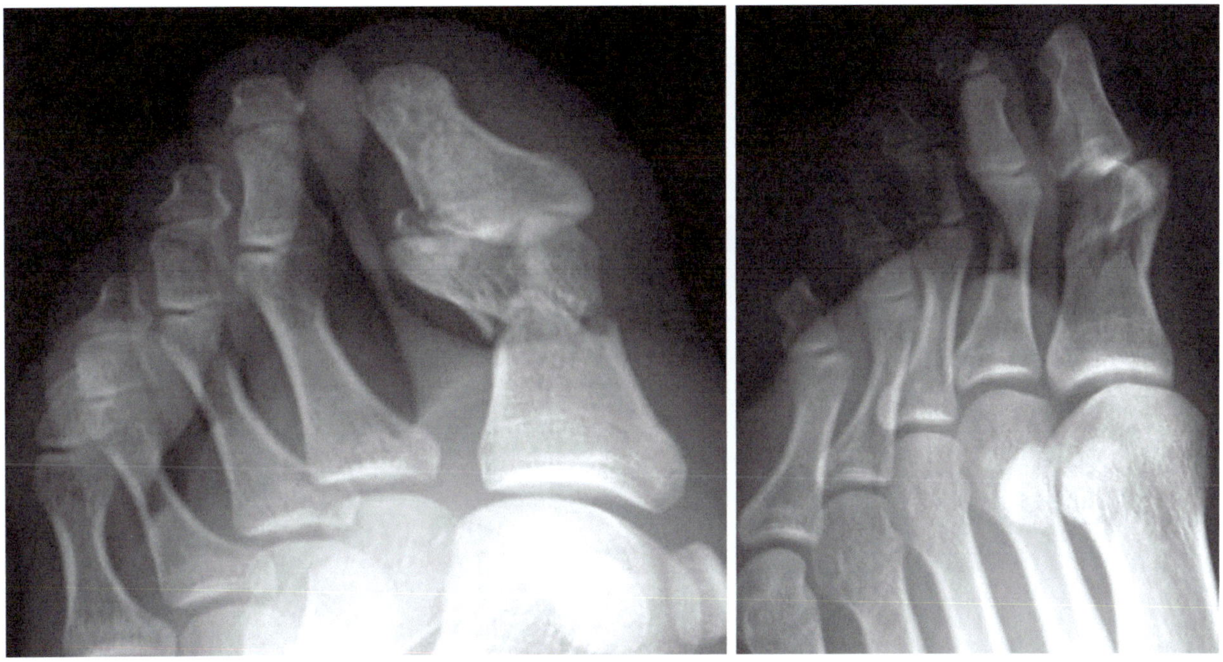

Fig. 7.13 Articular dislocated proximal phalanx fracture of the hallux: in these projections, it is possible to appreciate the comminution of the fragments

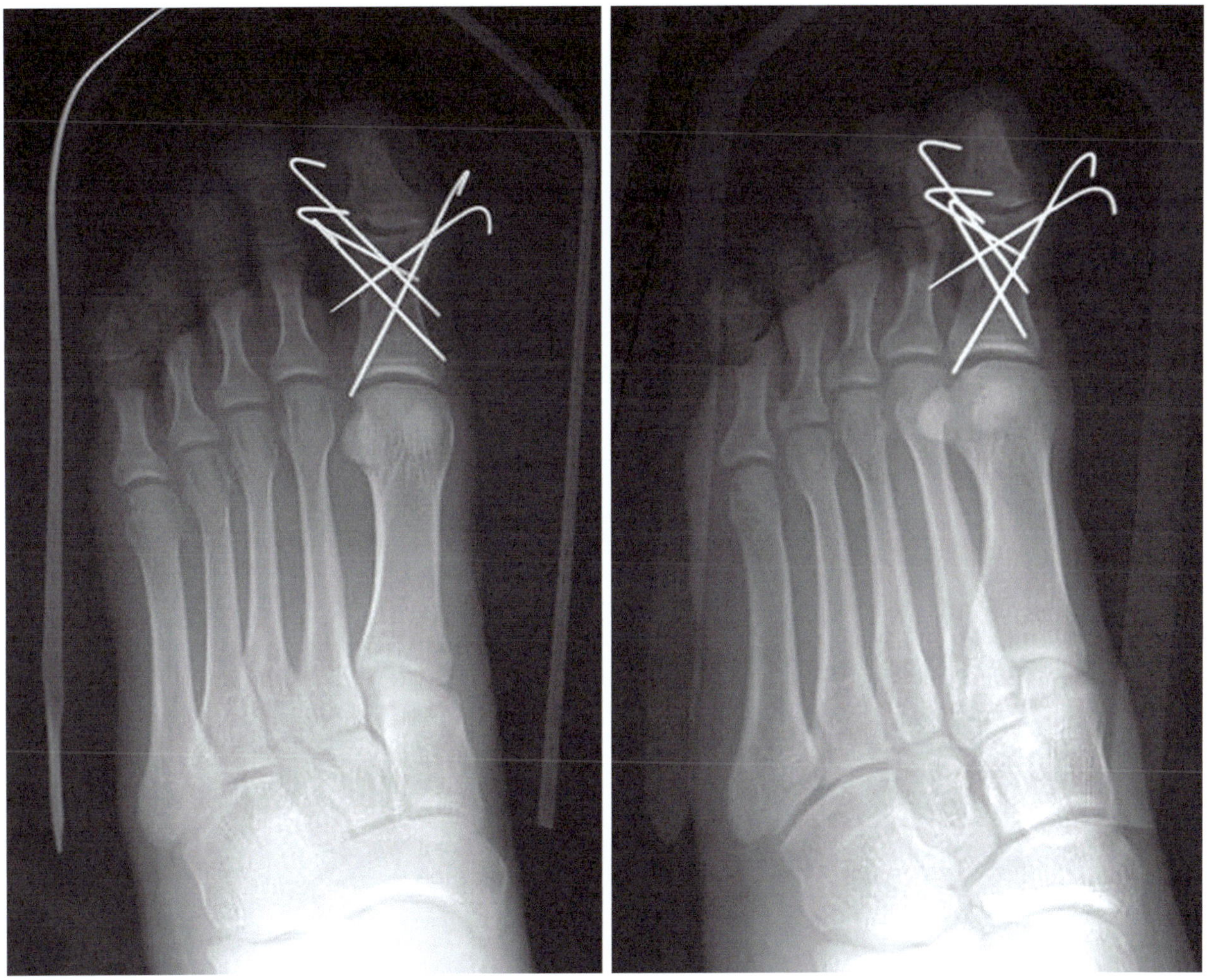

Fig. 7.14 Articular dislocated proximal phalanx fracture of the hallux: after the reduction, considering the comminution of the fragments, a minimal synthesis with Kirschner wires has been chosen

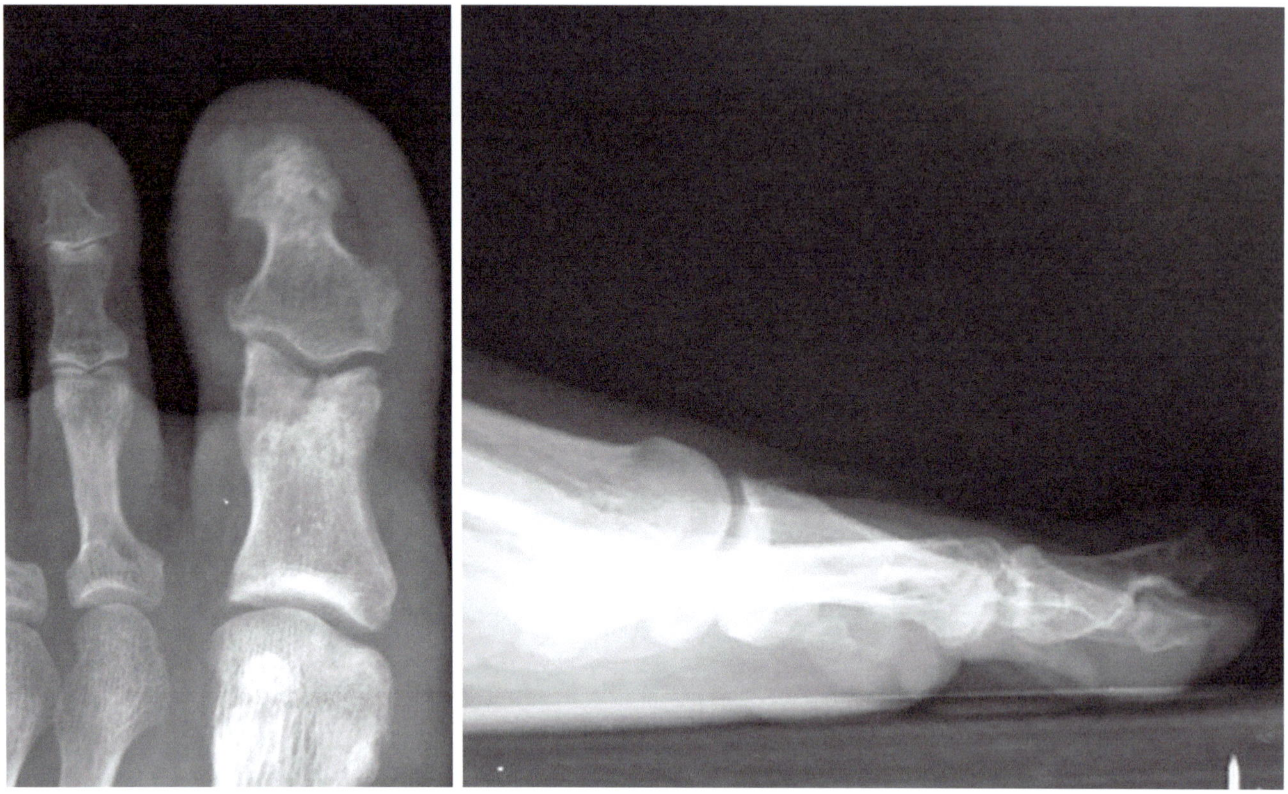

Fig. 7.15 Articular dislocated proximal phalanx fracture of the hallux: the 3-month follow-up shows an advanced healing of the fracture and the conservation of the correct anatomic axis

References

1. Lindholm R (1961) Operative treatment of dislocated simple fracture of the neck of the metatarsal bone. Ann Chir Gynaecol Tenn 50:328–331
2. Key JA, Conwell HE (1946) The management of fractures, dislocations, and sprains. Mosby, St Louis
3. Klenerman L (1976) The foot and its disorders. Blackwell Scientific, Oxford
4. Morrissey EJ (1946) Metatarsal fractures. JBJS 28:594–602
5. Pendarvis JA, Mandracchia VJ, Haverstock BD et al (1999) A new fixation technique for metatarsal fractures. Clin Podiatr Med Surg 16(4):643–657
6. Anderson LD (1977) Injuries of the forefoot. Clin Orthop Relat Res 122:18–27
7. Sanders RW, Papp S (2007) Fractures of the midfoot and forefoot. In: Coughlin MJ, Mann RA, Saltzman CL (eds) Surgery of the foot and ankle, 8th edn. Mosby Elsevier, Philadelphia, pp 2199–2235
8. Heim U, Pfeiffer KM (1987) Internal fixation of small fractures: techniques recommended by the AO group. Springer, Berlin
9. Jackson JB III, Ellington JK, Anderson RB (2014) Fractures of midfoot and forefoot. In: Coughlin MJ, Saltzman CL, Anderson RB (eds) Mann's surgery of the foot and ankle, 9th edn. Saunders, Philadelphia, pp 2154–2186
10. Dameron TB (1975) Fractures and anatomic variations of the proximal portion the fifth metatarsal. JBJS Am 57:788–792
11. Quill GE (1995) Fractures of the proximal fifth metatarsal. Orthop Clin North Am 26:353–361
12. Myerson MS (1991) Injuries to the forefoot and toes. In: Jahss disorders of the foot and ankle: medical and surgical management, 2nd edn. WB Saunders, Philadelphia
13. Bovill EG Jr, Inman VT (1973) Fractures and fracture-dislocations of the foot and ankle. In: DuVries HL, Inman VT (eds) DuVries' surgery of the foot. Mosby, St Louis
14. Jahss MH (1981) Stubbing injuries to the hallux. Foot Ankle 1:327–332

Index

W. Daghino et al., *Foot and Ankle Trauma Injuries*, https://doi.org/10.1007/978-3-319-69617-1

MIX
Papier aus verantwortungsvollen Quellen
Paper from responsible sources
FSC® C105338

If you have any concerns about our products,
you can contact us on
ProductSafety@springernature.com

In case Publisher is established outside the EU,
the EU authorized representative is:
Springer Nature Customer Service Center GmbH
Europaplatz 3, 69115 Heidelberg, Germany

Printed by Libri Plureos GmbH
in Hamburg, Germany